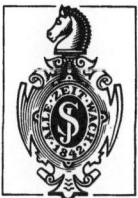

U. Jonas W.F. Thon C.G. Stief (Eds.)

Erectile Dysfunction

With Contributions by
J.H. Abicht, W. Bähren, G.A. Broderick, H. Gall, I. Goldstein
Ph. M. Hanno, U. Hartmann, D. Hauri, M.W. Hengeveld
R.D. Hesch, G. Holzki, U. Jonas, K.-P. Jünemann, F. Kulvelis
R.M. Levin, F.J. Levine, T.F. Lue, W. Scherb, T.H. Schürmeyer
C. Sparwasser, J. Staubesand, W.D. Steers, C.G. Stief
W.F. Thon, K. Van Arsdalen, G. Wagner, A.J. Wein
E. Wespes, U. Wetterauer

With 156 Figures

Springer-Verlag
Berlin Heidelberg New York
London Paris Tokyo
Hong Kong Barcelona
Budapest

Professor Dr. Udo Jonas
Dr. Walter Ferdinand Thon
Dr. Christian Georg Stief

Medizinische Hochschule Hannover
Klinik für Urologie
Konstanty-Gutschow-Straße 8
W-3000 Hannover 61, FRG

ISBN 978-3-662-00988-8   ISBN 978-3-662-00986-4 (eBook)
DOI 10.1007/978-3-662-00986-4

Typesetting: Best-set Typesetter Ltd., Hong Kong
10/3130-543210 – Printed on acid-free paper

Preface

The basic principles of the phenomenon "erection" have been known since the pioneering work of Kölliker, Eckhard and Langley in the nineteenth century. Nonetheless, under the influence of Freud, erectile dysfunction was predominantly attributed to psychogenic factors. A more liberal perception of sexuality since the 1960s, the development of new and refined diagnostic techniques, and the expansion of basic research activity resulted in a new concept of erectile dysfunction, identifying arteriogenic, venogenic, endocrinologic or myopathic (cavernous smooth muscle dysfunction) factors. From this research other considerations such as autonomic innervation, cavernous endothelial intactness or impaired neurotransmitter pool are being introduced into routine clinical assessment. A reevaluation of psychogenic etiology with a consequential new concept of psychogenic impotence is on the rise.

In this book the new concepts of basic knowledge on cavernous smooth muscle function and its supraspinal, spinal, and local control; the new diagnostic approaches in psychogenic and autonomic factors; and the new developments of reconstructive therapeutic options for the patient have been tied together. Outstanding and internationally renowned experts in the field of erectile dysfunction have given detailed insight into the latest basic and clinical developments. Well-established diagnostic and therapeutic techniques are presented by experienced colleagues.

We hope that this book will help the reader to get an overview of the current concepts of erection. Furthermore, we hope that international collaboration in basic and clinical research in the field of erectile dysfunction will render an update necessary in the near future.

Hannover   UDO JONAS
                                             WALTER F. THON
                                             CHRISTIAN G. STIEF

Contents

Therapy

Special Aspects

List of Contributors

Abicht, J.H., Dr., Medizinische Hochschule Hannover,
Klinik für Urologie, Zentrum Chirurgie,
Konstanty-Gutschow-Str. 8, W-3000 Hannover 61, FRG

Bähren, W., Priv.-Doz. Dr., Bundeswehrkrankenhaus Ulm,
Abteilung Radiologie, Oberer Eselsberg 40, W-7900 Ulm, FRG

Broderick, G.A., Assistant Professor of Urology,
Hospital of the University of Pennsylvania, 3400 Spruce Street,
Philadelphia, PA 19104, USA

Gall, H., Dr., Bundeswehrkrankenhaus Ulm, Abteilung III,
Dermatologie, Oberer Eselsberg 40, W-7900 Ulm, FRG

Goldstein, I., M.D., Associate Professor of Urology,
Boston University School of Medicine, Department of Urology,
720 Harrison Avenue, P (606), Boston, MA 02118, USA

Hanno, Ph.M., M.D., Division of Urology, Department of
Surgery, University of Pennsylvania School of Medicine and
the Philadelphia Veterans Administration Medical Center,
Philadelphia, PA 19104, USA

Hartmann, U., Dipl.-Psychologe, Dr., Medizinische Hochschule
Hannover, Arbeitsbereich Klinische Psychologie, Zentrum
Psychologische Medizin, Konstanty-Gutschow-Str. 8,
W-3000 Hannover 61, FRG

Hauri, D., Professor Dr., Universitätsspital Zürich,
Urologische Klinik, Rämistr. 100, 8091 Zürich, Switzerland

Hengeveld, M.W., Dr., Academisch Ziekenhuis Leiden,
Afdeling Psychiatrie, Gebouw 5, Rijnsburgerweg 10,
Postbus 9600, 2300 RC Leiden, The Netherlands

Hesch, R.D., Professor Dr., Medizinische Hochschule Hannover,
Abteilung für Klinische Endokrinologie,
Abteilung Innere Medizin, Konstanty-Gutschow-Str. 8,
W-3000 Hannover 61, FRG

Holzki, G., Dr., Bundeswehrkrankenhaus Ulm, Abteilung III,
  Dermatologie, Oberer Eselsberg 40, W-7900 Ulm, FRG

Jonas, U., Professor Dr., Medizinische Hochschule Hannover,
  Klinik für Urologie, Konstanty-Gutschow-Str. 8,
  W-3000 Hannover 61, FRG

Jünemann, K.-P., Dr., Urologische Klinik, Postfach 10 00 23,
  W-6800 Mannheim 1, FRG

Kulvelis, F., Dr., Staufenburg-Klinik, Burgunderstr. 24,
  W-7601 Durbach, FRG

Levin, R.M., Ph.D., Division of Urology, Department of Surgery,
  University of Pennsylvania School of Medicine
  and the Philadelphia Veterans Administration Medical Center,
  Philadelphia, PA 19104, USA

Levine, F.J., M.D., Boston University School of Medicine,
  Department of Urology, 720 Harrison Avenue, P (606),
  Boston, MA 02118, USA

Lue, T.F., Dr., University of California, Department of Urology,
  U-575, San Francisco, CA 94143-0738, USA

Scherb, W., Dr., Bundeswehrkrankenhaus Ulm, Abteilung VI,
  Neurologie und Psychiatrie, Oberer Eselsberg 40,
  W-7900 Ulm, FRG

Schürmeyer, T.H., Dr., Medizinische Hochschule Hannover,
  Abteilung Klinische Endokrinologie, Abteilung Innere Medizin,
  Konstanty-Gutschow-Str. 8, W-3000 Hannover 61, FRG

Sparwasser, C., Dr., Bundeswehrkrankenhaus Ulm, Urologische
  Abteilung, Oberer Eselsberg 40, W-7900 Ulm, FRG

Staubesand, J., Professor em., Dr., Anatomisches Institut
  der Universität Freiburg, Albertstr. 17, W-7800 Freiburg i. Br.,
  FRG

Steers, W.D., M.D., Assistant Professor of Urology, University
  of Virginia Health Sciences Center, Department of Urology,
  Box 422, Charlottesville, VA 22908, USA

Stief, C.G., Dr., Medizinische Hochschule Hannover,
  Klinik für Urologie, Konstanty-Gutschow-Str. 8,
  W-3000 Hannover 61, FRG

Thon, W.F., Dr., Medizinische Hochschule Hannover,
  Klinik für Urologie Konstanty-Gutschow-Str. 8,
  W-3000 Hannover 61 FRG

Van Arsdalen, K., M.D., Division of Urology,
Department of Surgery, University of Pennsylvania School
of Medicine and the Philadelphia Veterans Administration
Medical Center, Philadelphia, PA 19104, USA

Wagner, G., Dr., University of Copenhagen, The Panum Institute,
Institute of Medical Physiology B, Blegdamsvej 3C, Bygn. 18,
2200 Copenhagen N, Denmark

Wein, A.J., M.D., Division of Urology, Department of Surgery,
University of Pennsylvania School of Medicine
and the Philadelphia Veterans Administration Medical Center,
Philadelphia, PA 19104, USA

Wespes, E., M.D., Ph.D., Cliniques Universitaires de Bruxelles,
Hôpital Erasme, Service d'Urologie, 808, Route de Lennick,
1070 Bruxelles, Belgium

Wetterauer, U., Priv.-Doz. Dr., Klinikum der Universität,
Chirurgische Universitätsklinik, Abteilung Urologie,
Hugstetter Str. 55, W-7800 Freiburg i. Br., FRG

Anatomy, Physiology and Pathophysiology

Anatomy of Male Sexual Function

A.J. Wein, K. Van Arsdalen, Ph.M. Hanno, and R.M. Levin

The physiology of male sexual function in the human involves a complex series of neurologically mediated vascular phenomena which occur within a certain hormonal milieu. Supraspinal psychological and neurological factors are also important, especially in humans, in modifying what are largely reflex phenomena for perpetuation of the species. Masters and Johnson [4] have defined the male sexual response cycle and divided it into four phases for descriptive purposes, although it actually progresses as a continuum (Fig. 1). Each phase involves genital and extra-genital responses that generally occur, whether for procreation or recreation. This chapter will review the pertinent male anatomy and the physiology of erection, emission, ejaculation, and orgasm as defined by experimental work in animals and humans, and by inference from clinical observation. Human data will be emphasized where available, as the human psyche as well as certain anatomic variations make extrapolation of animal data to man very difficult in some cases. Examples of sexual dysfunction will be included only as they help to clarify the normal physiology.

Anatomy

A knowledge of the normal pelvic and genital gross anatomy is helpful in understanding the physiology of male sexual function and the relationship of the organs to the various roles they play. Erection obviously primarily involves the penis, and its neurological and vascular anatomy are therefore important. Seminal emission refers to the deposition of sperm and seminal and prostatic fluid through the ejaculatory and prostatic ducts into the posterior urethra, primarily by contraction of the seminal vesicles and the distal portions of the vas deferens. Ejaculation involves the tonic-clonic contractions of the somatically innervated striated musculature of the pelvic floor and simultaneous closure of the bladder neck, mediated through post-ganglionic sympathetic fibers, normally resulting in antegrade propulsion of the semen through the urethra and out of the penile meatus. The sensation of orgasm is primarily a cerebral phenomenon. Structural aspects important to male sexual function will be emphasized.

U. Jonas et al. (Eds.) Erectile Dysfunction
© Springer-Verlag Berlin Heidelberg 1991

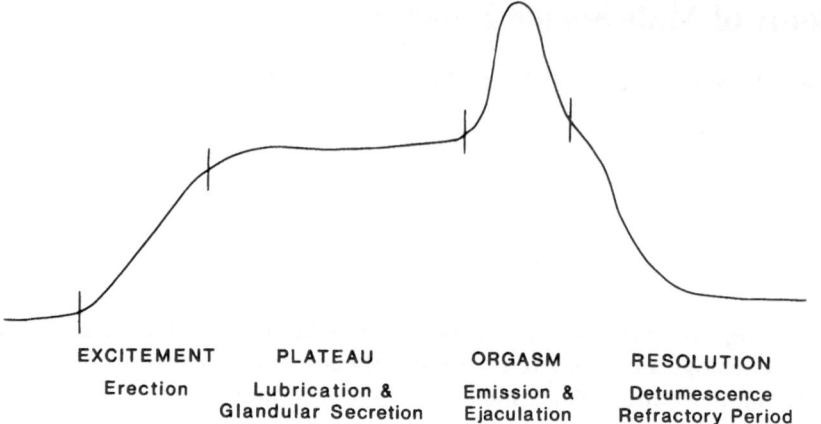

EXCITEMENT   PLATEAU   ORGASM   RESOLUTION

Erection   Lubrication &   Emission &   Detumescence
                  Glandular Secretion   Ejaculation   Refractory Period

Fig. 1. Male sexual response cycle and major genital events occurring at each phase of the cycle. (Adapted from Masters and Johnson [1])

Gross Anatomy of the Penis

The penis is actually composed of an anchored portion and a free or pendulous portion. The bulk of each is composed of three cylindrical masses of

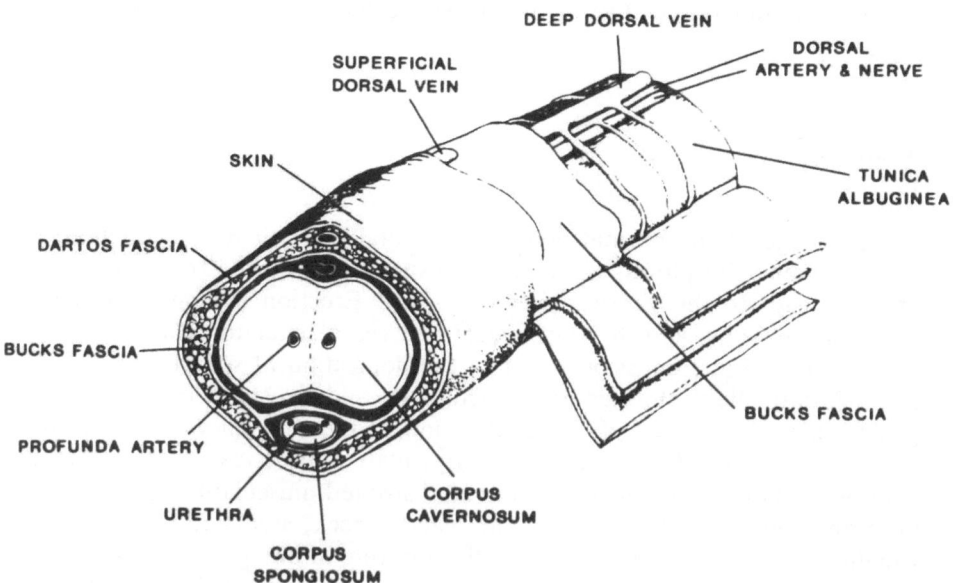

Fig. 2. Anatomy of the pendulous portion of the penis. Note the common perforated septum and the location of the profunda arteries

tissue – two corpora cavernosa and a single ventral corpus spongiosum. Each corporal body is made up of a loose trabecular meshwork of muscular and connective tissues surrounded by a dense fibrous covering called the tunica albuginea (Fig. 2). The corpora cavernosa share a common septum in the pendulous portion of the penis with many perforations that allow free passage of blood from one side to the other, allowing the two to function essentially as a single unit [26]. The corpus spongiosum is unpaired and lies in the ventral groove formed by the two larger cavernosal bodies. The corpus spongiosum contains the urethra and enlarges at its distal end to form the glans penis. The corpora cavernosa indent the proximal part of the glans with their distal ends actually extending into the glans beyond the corona. All of the corporal bodies are surrounded by another dense fascial sheath termed Buck's fascia from which thin fibrous septa extend between the paired corpora cavernosa and the corpus spongiosum [25]. Buck's fascia is an important structure in anchoring the anterior aspect of the penis to the symphysis pubis, as it fuses with the suspensory ligament and joins with Colles' fascia posteriorly at the triangular ligament (Fig. 3). More superficially lies the dartos fascia or Colles'

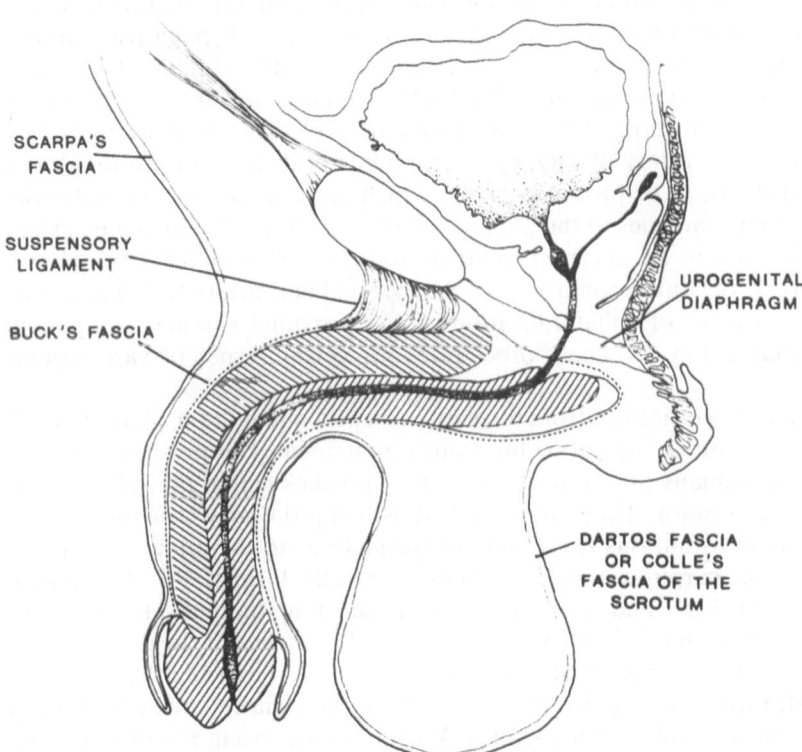

Fig. 3. Fascial relationships of the external genitalia

fascia of the penis, which is just beneath the skin and is continuous with Scarpa's fascia of the abdomen.

The proximal or anchored portions are the crura of the corpora cavernosa. These are firmly attached to the ventral aspects of the ischial rami and therefore diverge and separate from each other at the level of the inferior aspect of the symphysis pubis. Each crus is covered by the ischiocavernosus muscle. Some have felt, in the past, that contraction of this muscle promoted erection by venous compression, but this actually seems to play only a very minor, if any, role in humans [4].

The corpus spongiosum is attached proximally to the ventral aspect of the urogenital diaphragm and covered by the bulbocavernous muscle. This dilated rather bulbous portion is pierced by the urethra after the latter traverses the urogenital diaphragm. The urethra is then surrounded by the corpus spongiosum to the meatus.

Anatomy of the Penile Vasculature

The following description of the vascular supply and venous drainage will include primarily gross anatomic relationships. The hypogastric arteries continue into the deep pelvis and perineum as the internal pudendal arteries via the lesser sciatic foramen and Alcock's canal. Each internal pudendal artery gives off a perineal branch, a bulbar, and a urethral artery before continuing as the artery of the penis. The latter branches to form the dorsal artery and the deep or profunda artery which pierces the crus on each side. The three major arteries to the penis are all paired (Fig. 2). The penile artery may be derived in an aberrant manner from branches of the internal epigastric artery, the obturator artery, or the external iliac artery [17]. These may in turn be sources of collateralization or the proximal vascular component of revascularization or bypass procedures for certain types of vasculogenic impotence.

The dorsal arteries run from the suspensory ligament to the glans beneath Buck's fascia but superficial to the tunica albuginea. The profunda arteries course longitudinally as one to three major branches within the substance of the corpus cavernosa. They are described as being the only structures which are not friable within this tissue, and as lying closer to the midline cribiform septum of the corpus rather than being centrally located [4]. The paired arteries of the bulb and urethra also continue longitudinally to the glans where they anastomose freely with the terminal branches of the dorsal artery [7]. Multiple large anastomotic channels, originally described by Deysach, connect all three major pairs of arteries along their entire course and freely pass through the tunica albuginea [7]. Wagner et al., using plastic corrosion casts, have demonstrated connections which they call "shunt arteries" [27] from the deep arteries to the arteries in the spongiosum and to the dorsal arteries. A potential erectile regulatory function has been ascribed to these, but proof is lacking at this time, and their actual relationship to the previously well demonstrated anastomoses is not clear.

The venous drainage is more complex and potentially much more confusing (Fig. 4). Most reviews and texts use conflicting terms or give little coverage to this part of the anatomy. There is general agreement now that no muscular walled veins occur within the cavernous spaces [17, 26]. One of the clearest and best illustrated discussions of the venous drainage of the penis is contained in the review by Newman and Northup [17]. According to these authors, three major divisions of veins are noted at separate levels – superficial, intermediate, and deep – as well as unnamed emissary, circumflex, and communicating vessels. Together they allow such vast anastomoses that contrast medium, injected under sufficient pressure, will fill all veins and spaces. The superficial level of veins includes the multiple subcutaneous veins that run deep to the dartos fascia but superficial to Buck's fascia; these contribute to the formation of the superficial dorsal vein of the penis in this same plane. This major vessel usually empties into the left saphenous vein. A

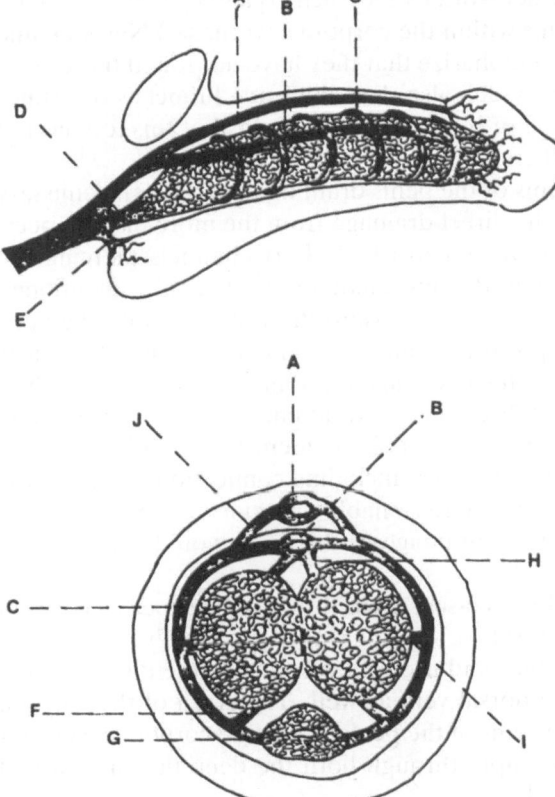

Fig. 4. Veins of the penis. *A*, superficial dorsal vein; *B*, deep (profunda) dorsal vein; *C*, circumflex vein; *D*, deep (profunda) vein of the penis; *E*, bulbar vein; *F*, inferior emissary vein from corpus cavernosum; *G*, superior emissary vein from corpus spongiosum; *H*, superior emissary vein from corpus cavernosum; *I*, lateral emissary vein from corpus cavernosum; *J*, anastomosis between superficial and deep dorsal veins. (From Newman and Northup [17])

similar vessel usually forms posteriorly and empties into the scrotal veins. The intermediate veins lie below Buck's fascia but superficial to the tunica albuginea and include the venae commitantes of the dorsal arteries and the most important vessel at this level, the deep dorsal vein. The major contributions forming the deep dorsal vein are 6–15 short, straight vessels from the glans as well as the emissary and circumflex veins from the corpora cavernosa, to be described. The deep dorsal vein, therefore, drains both the glans and the corpora cavernosa under normal conditions. It passes beneath the arcuate ligament and terminates in the pudendal plexus in the pelvis.

The deep veins of the penis (different from the deep dorsal vein) include the bulbar veins that empty directly into the pudendal vein or pelvic plexus, the anterior and posterior urethral veins, and the deep veins of the corpora cavernosa. The anterior urethral veins join with the posterior emissary veins to produce the circumflex veins that travel around the circumference of the penis superficial to the tunica albuginea and empty into the deep dorsal vein. The posterior urethral veins anastomose with the bulbar veins and empty with the latter as noted above [17].

The deep veins of the corpora cavernosa are often overlooked and consist of four to five large vessels that leave the proximal end of each crus and empty into the pudendal plexus. (Earlier work by Deysach [7] and by Christensen [5] describe deep veins of the penis within the corpora cavernosa.) Newman and Northup [17] and Wagner [26] emphasize that they have not found these veins within the cavernous tissue. Deysach also described side branches or "sluice valves" the allow direct passage of blood into these veins but this too has not been confirmed by other workers.

In addition to the deep veins of the penis draining the crura, the emissary veins provide the majority of the direct drainage from the more distal aspects of the corporal bodies. These veins consist of short channels piercing the tunica albuginea and draining into the intermediate set of veins as mentioned above. Between 9 and 22 anterior emissary veins drain directly into the deep dorsal vein. Similarly, 9–22 posterior emissary veins open into the sulcus between the spongiosum and the cavernosum, join the anterior urethral veins, and thus form the circumflex veins. Lateral emissary veins also empty directly into the circumflex veins. It is readily evident that multiple anastomotic channels and communications exist, including connections between the superficial and deep dorsal veins. A reasonable summary of the important anatomic facts referable to venous drainage of the penis would appear to be as follows:

All tissues superficial to Buck's fascia drain through the superficial dorsal veins into the saphenous, femoral, or scrotal veins. Proximally, the corpus spongiosum drains into the bulbar and urethral veins while the distal portion and glans empty into the deep dorsal vein as well. The crura of the corpora cavernosa empty into the deep veins of the penis, while the corpora cavernosa distal to the arcuate ligament empty through both the deep dorsal vein and the deep veins of the penis [17].

An additional consideration is whether the routes of venous drainage in the penis are the same in the erect state as in the flaccid state. The importance of this becomes evident in considering whether the initiation or maintenance of penile erection involves any active regulation of the venous outflow in addition to the other hemodynamic alterations which seem to occur primarily by alteration of arteriolar flow. Pathologically, the failure to empty the corpora cavernosa through the deep venous system, that is, through the emissary veins to the deep veins of the penis, is seen in priapism. Shunting procedures [23, 30] for this condition bypass the deep venous system of the corpora cavernosa by surgically diverting blood into a portion of the corpus spongiosum or glans. This then allows drainage via the patent dorsal veins into the penis.

Innervation of the Penis

The neural supply of the penis is part of the meshwork which innervates the other pelvic organs concerned with sexual function, as well as the bladder and rectum. Although the pathways are similar, the fibers are obviously not identical [29]. Three types of nerve fibers (sympathetic, parasympathetic, and somatic) from two areas of the spinal cord provide the major innervation. A description of the actual pathways follows and is represented schematically in Fig. 5.

The autonomic nervous system includes motor nerve fibers which originate in the central nervous system and course to the periphery to innervate vessels, viscera and various other structures which are not totally under voluntary control. The basic feature that distinguishes this part of the peripheral nervous system from the strictly voluntary motor portion is that the nerve fibers emanating from the central nervous system do not directly innervate end-organ structures, but rather first synapse in ganglion cells outside the central nervous system. The classic view of the autonomic nervous system distinguishes the sympathetic from the parasympathetic components primarily on the site of origin of the fibers. The sympathetic portion of the autonomic nervous system originates from the thoracolumbar portion of the spinal cord via the ventral roots. The preganglionic fiber then travels to an autonomic ganglion located in the paravertebral sympathetic trunk or somewhat more peripherally. A characteristically long postganglionic fiber then travels to the end-organ. The neurotransmitter at the level of the ganglion is cholinergic (acetylcholine); the neurotransmitter at the end-organ is classically adrenergic (norepinephrine). In contrast, the parasympathetic outflow is via the cranial nerves and the sacral portion of the spinal cord. The preganglionic fiber is characteristically long with the ganglion located very near or in the end-organ. The postganglionic fiber is therefore generally short. All neurotransmission is classically thought to be via cholinergic mechanisms. The dual

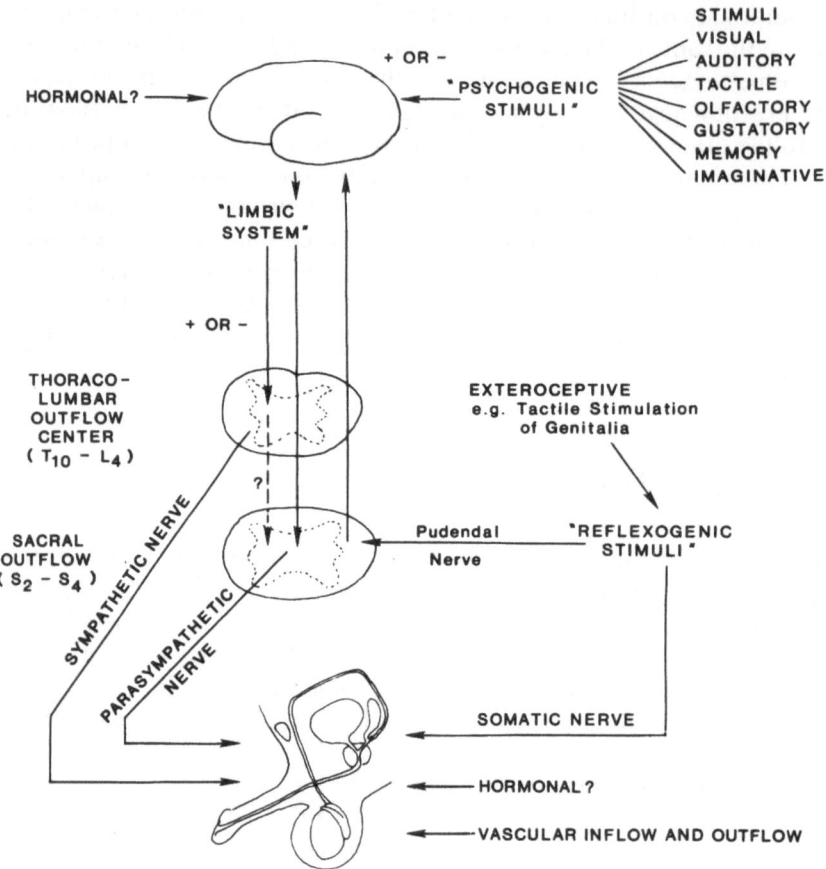

Fig. 5. Schematic representation of the factors involved in erection. (Adapted from Weiss [29])

components of the autonomic nervous system have been felt to be complementary, with one system predominating over the other depending on the circumstance in which the organism finds itself. This relatively simplistic view becomes extremely complex, considering that alternate or additional excitatory and inhibitory neurotransmitters undoubtedly exist at each level of not only the peripheral but central nervous system as well.

The sympathetic outflow involved in male sexual function originates primarily from spinal cord segments T11 to L2, but receives neural contributions from as high as T10 to as low as L4 [19, 22]. These fibers join below the bifurcation of the aorta in the retroperitoneum overlying the lowest lumbar vertebra and the sacral promontory. The size of the collection of fibers here is variable, and hence this grouping has been called either the presacral nerve or the superior hypogastric plexus. This plexus divides into right and left halves that run deep along the side-walls of the pelvis. These distinct collections of nerve fibers are often designated the hypogastric nerves although they are actually neural plexuses [10]. These sympathetic nerves continue to the pelvic or inferior hypogastric plexus where they intermingle with the parasympathetic neural component. These parasympathetic fibers arise primarily as the ventral roots from cord segments S2 to S4 and are designated the pelvic nerves, or the nervi erigentes, after the sacral roots have converged. The inferior hypogastric or pelvic plexus is located lateral to the rectum against the pelvic side-wall and measures approximately 2.5 cm. by 3.5 cm. in size [10]. This mixing and redistribution of nerve fibers gives rise to the vesical plexus, the prostatic plexus, and most distally, the cavernous plexus. Hence, the organs of male sexual function are innervated by anatomically parasympathetic and sympathetic nerves which course through adjacent plexuses and intermingle, and undoubtedly communicate. This great mixture of the autonomic components undoubtedly accounts for the confusion in terminology about what types of neural impulses actually are responsible for the hemodynamic and end-organ changes that result in penile erection. In addition to the difficulty in separating the type of nerve fibers, it also must be realized that the location of all of the ganglia that classically separate pre- from postganglionic fibers is unknown in the human. By the time the level of the pelvic plexus is reached, it is unclear whether one is dealing with pre- or postganglionic, anatomically sympathetic or parasympathetic fibers.

Distinct neural structures along the posterolateral surface of the prostate that appear to conduct the actual impulse responsible for erection have been described in dogs [24], and humans [28]. Direct electrical stimulation of these structures by attached electrodes or by transrectal methods can result in erection. These trunks are undoubtedly derived from the pelvic plexus but whether they can actually be called parasympathetic or sympathetic in the classic sense is doubtful. Walsh [28], Lepor et al [11], Lue [13], and coworkers have clarified the ramifications of these nerves from a precise anatomic standpoint. A prominent neurovascular bundle is located posterolateral to the apex, mid portion and base of the prostate [11]. At the level of the membranous urethra, further neural division occurs into microscopic branches posterolateral and lateral to the membranous urethra. The lateral pelvic fascia fuses with the prostatic capsule anteriorly and anterolaterally, but these are otherwise distinct anatomic structures. The neurovascular bundles are in the leaves of the lateral pelvic fascia outside the prostatic capsule. In general, the nerves are located lateral to the vascular component of the neurovascular bundle (further from the prostatic capsule). Walsh, utilizing his neuroanatomical localizations, has modified the technique of radical retropubic prostatectomy to minimize the risk of injuring the autonomic innervation of the corpora cavernosa and so maximize the potential for erection following this operation [28].

Various studies using light and electron microscopy have attempted to clarify the peripheral neuromorphology and neuropharmacology of the penis.

Benson et al. studied human penile tissue from six transsexual patients after penectomy [2]. Light microscopy after acetylcholinesterase staining for identification of cholinergic neurons showed a scant distribution of these in the corpora cavernosa and an even sparser distribution or a complete absence of these in the corpus spongiosum. These fibers when present often coursed near arterioles and appeared to terminate in the outer tunic of these vessels. Glyoxylic acid fluorescence, indicative of catecholaminergic elements, showed an abundance of such fibers in the corpus cavernosum and fewer in the spongiosum. Interestingly, the fibers appeared not only to end with varicosities on many of the vessels, but also to take a circuitous course through the trabeculae and approach the walls of the cavernous spaces. Whether these are actually innervated or not is not further specified. Baumgarten et al. [1] have shown a dense adrenergic supply to the corpora cavernosa in various animals. Dail and Evan have clearly shown that short adrenergic neurons supply the penis of the rat [6]. Studies by Shirai et al. conflict with the above, however. They utilized techniques similar to those of Benson and associates in their evaluation of penile tissue removed for cancer; however, they demonstrated an abundance of cholinergic fibers in the corpora cavernosa and relatively few adrenergic fibers [21].

The ultrastructural examination of the neural components within the corporal tissue by Benson et al. serves both to help clarify and further complicate the picture of microscopic neuroanatomy [2]. Electron microscopy reveals the presence of mostly unmyelinated bundles of two to six fibers. Vesicles of various descriptions were found within the nerve varicosities. Small, highly electron-dense vesicles thought to contain norepinephrine were observed. Typical small clear vesicles, usually associated with cholinergic neurotransmitters, were not evident. Other vesicles of different sizes and densities were observed and were felt to be compatible with those described for peptidergic or purinergic nerve fibers. These findings would appear to indicate a predominant adrenergic innervation, a scant cholinergic innervation, and also the existence of other neurotransmitter mechanisms in this area.

Other studies support these ideas. Melman et al. have demonstrated an abundance of norepinephrine in the cavernous tissue as well as the absence of the enzyme choline acetyltransferase, responsible for the conversion of acetyl-CoA plus choline to acetylcholine [15, 16]. Polak et al [20] and Gu et al. [9] have shown that the nerves innervating the erectile tissue of the penis contain several regulatory peptides, most predominantly vaso active intestinal polypeptide (VIP). These VIP containing nerves were found intimately connected with the arteries and arterioles of the erectile tissue, whereas the other peptide containing nerves were not. It is obvious that even the autonomic neuromorphology of the penis has been far from completely elucidated at this time, and even the possibilities are by no means universally agreed upon. It is not yet known whether it is proper to call the nerves identified beyond the pelvic plexus as sympathetic or parasympathetic, from the classic anatomic standpoint.

The relevant somatic innervation also emanates from the second through the fourth sacral segments as the pudendal nerve, which leaves the pelvis with the internal pudendal artery and innervates structures of the perineum and external genitalia with motor and sensory branches. Perineal branches innervate the bulbocavernous and ischiocavernous muscles, the urogenital diaphragm and the skin of the genitalia. The somatic innervation of the urogenital diaphragm may not be as simple as previously believed, particularly regarding the striated muscle component within and adjacent to the wall of the urethra. Only type 1 (slow twitch) muscle fibers were found by Gosling et al. [8] in the external urethral sphincter, with a mixture of type I and type II (fast twitch) muscle fibers found in the periurethral levator ani muscle. Functionally this is compatible with prolonged periods of tone by the external sphincter – needed in the active maintenance of urinary continence – without fatigue. The fast twitch fibers of the periurethral levator ani muscle enable rapid forceful contraction and closure of the urethra. Of interest from the standpoint of neurological control however, is the absence of muscle spindles from the external urethral sphincter itself but their presence in the levator ani [8]. These structures are useful in reflex and voluntary control of tone in typical striated muscle and their absence in the external sphincter indicates a potentially different mechanism and pathway for the control of this muscle, perhaps through the pelvic nerve. This is compatible with clinical observations that pudendal neurectomy does not always relieve the functional outlet obstruction caused by what is termed striated sphincter dyssnergia. The penile skin is supplied primarily by branches of the dorsal nerves of the penis. These nerves are the distal continuations of the pudendal nerves that travel from the pelvis adjacent to the inferior pubic ramus and superior to the crus and come to lie on the dorsal aspect of the penis, parallel and lateral to the dorsal penile arteries [26]. The major role at this level appears to be sensory.

Anatomy of Other Relevant Pelvic Organs

The periurethral glands (of Littré) and the bulbourethral glands lubricate the anterior urethra, especially during the plateau phase of the sexual response cycle. The bulbourethral glands or Cowper's glands lie within the substance of the deep transverse perineus muscle of the urogenital diaphragm [10]. Their ducts travel in the corpus spongiosum and terminate in the bulbous urethra. Clear fluid from these glands is expressed by contraction of the surrounding extrinsic muscle. Blood supply is from the artery of the bulb and innervation is from the inferior hypogastric plexus [12]. The structures which ultimately provide the seminal fluid associated with emission and ejaculation include the prostate and the seminal vesicles. The anatomic relationships of these structures are described elsewhere [12]. An important point to emphasise in considering male sexual function is that each of these glandular, muscular structures are capable both of secretion and active expression of secretions under neurological stimulation. The ejaculatory duct results from fusion of the ampulla of the vas deferens and the ipsilateral duct of the seminal vesicle. This duct, along with the multiple prostatic ducts, opens into the posterior urethra. The blood supply to these organs is from branches of the inferior vesical arteries. A vast plexus of veins drains these areas and receives the penile veins as previously noted. Innervation is by the adjacent subsidiary plexuses of the inferior hypogastric plexus. The contributions from the testes, epididymides and vasa will not be considered further.

References

1. Baumgarten HC, Falek B, Lange W (1969) Adrenergic nerves in the corpora cavern-ous penis of some mammals. Z Zellforsch 95:58
2. Benson GS, McConnell J, Lipshultz LI, Corriere JN Jr, Wood J (1980) Neuromor-phology and neuropharmacology of the human penis. J Clin Invest 65:506
3. Benson GS, McConnell JA, Schmidt, WA (1981) Penile polsters: Functional structures or atherosclerotic changes? J Urol 125:800
4. Benson GS, Lipshultz LI, McConnell J (1981) Mechanism of human erection, emis-sion and ejaculation: current clinical concepts. In: von Eschenbach AC, Rodriguez DB (eds) Sexual rehabilitation of the urologic cancer patient. GK Hall Medical Publishers, Boston, Chap 5
5. Christensen GC (1954) Angioarchitecture of the canine penis and the process of erec-tion. Am J Anat 95:227
6. Dail WG, Evan AP Jr (1974) Experimental evidence indicating that the penis of the rat is innervated by short adrenergic neurons. Am J Anat 141:203
7. Deysach LJ (1939) The comparative morphology of the erectile tissue of the penis with especial emphasis on the probable mechanism of erection. Am J Anat 64:111
8. Gosling JA, Dixon JS, Critchley HOD, Thompson SA (1981) A comparative study of the human external sphincter and periurethral levator ani muscles. Br J Urol 53:35
9. Gu J, Polak JM, Probert L, Islam KN, Marangos PJ, Mina S, Adrian TE, McGregor GP, O'Shaughnessy DJ, Bloom, SR (1981) Peptidergic innervation of the human male genital tract. J Urol 130:386
10. Hollingshead WH (1967) Textbook of anatomy. Harper and Row, New York, Chap 21, pp 714–717
11. Lepor H, Gregerman M, Crosby R, Mostofi FK, Walsh PC (1985) Precise localization of the autonomic nerves from the pelvic plexus to the corpora cavernosa: a detailed anatomical study of the adult male pelvis. J Urol 133:207
12. Lich R Jr, Howerton LW, Amin M (1979) Anatomy and surgical approach to the urogenital tract in the male. In: Harrison JH, Gittes RF, Perlmutter AD, Stamey TA, Walsh PC (eds) Campbell's urology. Saunders, Philadelphia, Chap 1
13. Lue TF, Zeinch SJ, Schmidt RA, Tanagho, EA (1984) Neuroanatomy of penile erec-tion: its relevance to iatrogenic impotence. J Urol 131:273
14. Masters WH, Johnson, VE (1966) Human sexual response. Little, Brown & Co, Boston
15. Melman A, Henry, D (1979) The possible role of the catecholamines of the corpora in penile erection. J Urol 121:419
16. Melman A, Henry DP, Felten DL, O'Connor BL (1980) Alteration of the penile cor-pora in patients with erectile impotence. Invest Urol 17:474
17. Newman HF, Northup JD (1981) Mechanism of human penile erection: an overview. Urology 17:399
18. Newman HF, Reiss H (1982) Method for exposure of cavernous artery. Urology 19:61

19. Newman HF, Reiss H, Northup JD (1982) Physical basis of emission, ejaculation and orgasm in the male. Urology 19:341
20. Polak JM, Gu J, Mina S, Bloom SR (1981) VIPergic nerves in the penis. Lancet 2:217
21. Shirai M, Saski K, Rikimaru A (1972) Histochemical investigation on the distribution of adrenergic and cholinergic nerves in the human penis. Tohoku J Exp Med 107:403
22. Siroky MB, Krane RJ (1979) Physiology of male sexual function. In: Krane RJ, Siroky MB (eds) Clinical neuro-urology. Little, Brown & Co, Boston, Chap 3
23. Steinn JJ, Martin DC (1974) Priapism. Urology 3:8
24. Tanagho E, Lue T, Takamura T, Schmidt R (1982) Mechanism of penile erection. Presented at the XIX International Congress of the Société Internationale d'Urologie, September 8
25. Thomas AJ Jr, Pierce JM Jr (1979) Sexual function. In: Harrison JH, Gittes RF, Perlmutter AD, Stamey TA, Walsh PC (eds) Campbell's Urology. Saunders, Philadelphia, Chap 61
26. Wagner G (1981) Erection, Anatomy. In: Wagner G, Green R (eds) Impotence. Plenum Press, New York, Chap 1
27. Wagner G, Bro-Rasmussen F, Willis EA, Nielsen MH (1982) New theory on the mechanism of erection involving hitherto undescribed vessels. Lancet 1:416
28. Walsh PC, Donker PJ (1982) Impotence following radical prostatectomy: insight into etiology and prevention. J Urol 128:492
29. Weiss HD (1972) The physiology of human penile erection. Ann Int Med 76:793
30. Winter CC (1976) Cure of idiopathic priapism: new procedure for creating fistula between glans penis and corpora cavernosa. Urology 8:389

Innervation of the Cavernous Tissue*

W.D. Steers

Penile erection is a vascular event under the control of the autonomic nervous system which regulates both vasodilator and vasoconstrictor responses [40]. Unlike other visceral structures, neural input to the sex organs is essential for proper function. Any interruption of neural pathways or disorders affecting the neuroeffector junction can produce impotence.

An understanding of the organization and of transmitters within neural pathways to the penis provides insight into the mechanisms responsible for penile erection and those processes leading to impotence. This knowledge may also lead to the development of improved pharmacological therapies for sexual dysfunction.

Parasympathetic Innervation

The parasympathetic nervous system provides the major excitatory input to the penis, responsible for vasodilation of the penile vasculature and erection [40]. Parasympathetic preganglionic input to the human penis originates within the second through fourth segments of the sacral spinal cord [6, 31] (Fig. 1). These preganglionic neurons are situated in the intermediolateral cell column and send dendritic projections to laminae V, VII, IX and X of the spinal cord [41, 44, 48–50] (Fig. 2). The distribution of axonal processes suggests that sacral preganglionic neurons receive afferent (sensory) information from visceral and somatic structures (Fig. 2). Dendrites also project to regions containing descending axons from supraspinal centers that integrate and coordinate the autonomic nervous system, such as the hypothalamus, reticular formation, and midbrain (for reviews see [20, 76]). Lue et al. [41] have suggested that the preganglionic neurons innervating the penis are located somewhat laterally in the sacral parasympathetic nucleus.

As the sacral roots (S2 − S4) exit the spinal canal through the sacral foramen they divide into autonomic and somatic branches (Fig. 1). Afferent and efferent components of parasympathetic outflow travel more ventrally to form the pelvic nerves and project to a group of peripheral ganglion cells within the pelvic plexus [27].

*This work was supported by NIH Grants 5K11 DK 01732-2 and 1R29 NS28566-01.

U. Jonas et al. (Eds.) Erectile Dysfunction

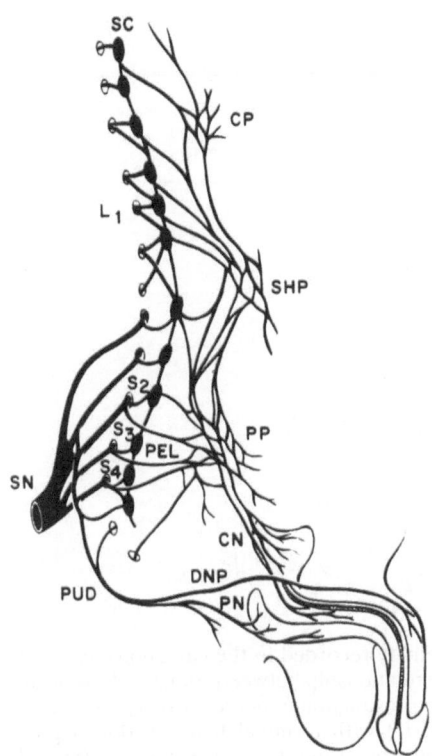

Fig. 1. Innervation to the penis. Thoracolumbar sympathetic outflow arises from the T9–L2 spinal cord segments and travels by either lumbar splanchnic nerves to the prevertebral ganglia (celiac plexus, *CP*; superior hypogastric plexus, *SHP*) and eventually to the hypogastric nerve or by the vertebral sympathetic chain ganglia (SC) and via the pelvic nerve (*PEL*) to the pelvic plexus (*PP*). Parasympathetic input to the cavernous tissues arises from the sacral (S2 to S4) spinal cord segments and travels in the PEL to the PP. The cavernous nerves represent the final common pathway for autonomic innervation to the penis. Somatic motoneurons also originate in the S2 to S4 cord segments and are conveyed by the pudendal nerve (*PUD*) whose terminal branches are the dorsal nerve of the penis (*DNP*) and perineal nerve (*PN*). *SN*, sciatic nerve

It is uncertain whether visceral afferents conveyed by the pelvic nerve participate in physiological events associated with erectile function. In other autonomic pathways visceral afferents are postulated to relay sensory information essential for reflexogenic processes. They also modulate the immune system, and function as motor neurons by influencing events such as vascular permeability, efferent neuronal function, and smooth muscle contraction [16, 42].

The pelvic plexus is a 4–5 cm long curvilinear network of neurons oriented in a sagittal plane and lying in the pelvic fascia on either side of the prostate and rectum in humans [38, 47, 54] (Fig. 1). Connective, vascular, and lymphatic tissues obscure this network of nerves in vivo. However topographical analysis in fetuses reveals that this network does not share a common fascial layer with vascular structures [6, 15]. Loose bundles of fibers from the pelvic plexus cross the midline in three ways: (1) decussate posterior to the rectum, (2) between the rectum and bladder, and (3) anterior to the bladder [6].

In rodents, the pelvic plexus is topographically organized with the ganglion cells supplying the penis located primarily at the origin of the cavernous

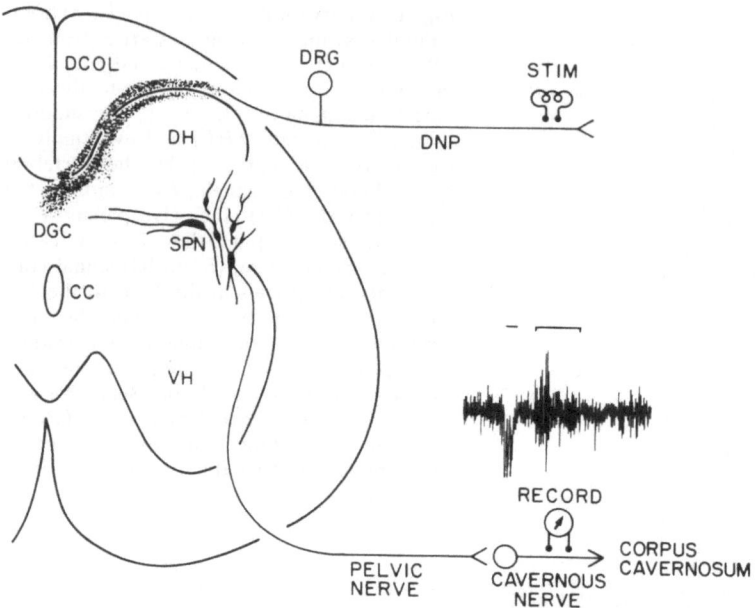

Fig. 2. Axonal tracing data and evoked reflex activity recorded in the cavernous nerve of the rat. Horseradish peroxidase data demonstrate relationship between somatic afferents in dorsal nerve of the penis (*DNP*) and sacral preganglionic nerves (*SPN*). Afferent projections to medial portion of dorsal horn (*DH*) with terminal fields in dorsal grey commissure (*DGC*) and lamine II–IV. SPN sends dendrites to ventral horn (*VH*) and vicinity of afferent terminals in DH and DGC. Electrical stimulation (*STIM*) of DNP elicited 80–120 ms discharge recorded on cavernous nerve which was abolished by pelvic nerve lesioning but remained following thoracic (T6) spinal cord transection. Stimulus 20 V, 0.7 Hz. *Bar* over stimulus artifact; *bracket* over response. (Axonal tracing data from Booth et al. [3]; Nunez et al. [52]; electrophysiology data from Steers et al. [78]

nerves [10–13, 28, 73]; Fig. 3A. In humans, individual plexuses for different pelvic organs cannot be distinguished [23]. Furthermore, the morphology of postganglionic neurons varies between species. For example, in the cat and monkey postganglionic neurons in the pelvic plexus have numerous dendrites, while ganglion cells in the rat lack such processes [81]; Fig. 3B. Morphological studies of other autonomic ganglion cells suggest that as one moves up the phylogenic tree, these neurons acquire a more complex geometry [59, 60]. This geometry is correlated with an increasing capacity for integration and communication between adjacent neurons. Indeed, the pelvic plexus functions as an integration and relay center for sacral and thoracolumbar preganglionic axons which synapse on postganglionic neurons supplying the penis. In addition to communication between neurons contact between neurons and their target tissue (corpora cavernosa) probably influences transmitter expression and morphology [37].

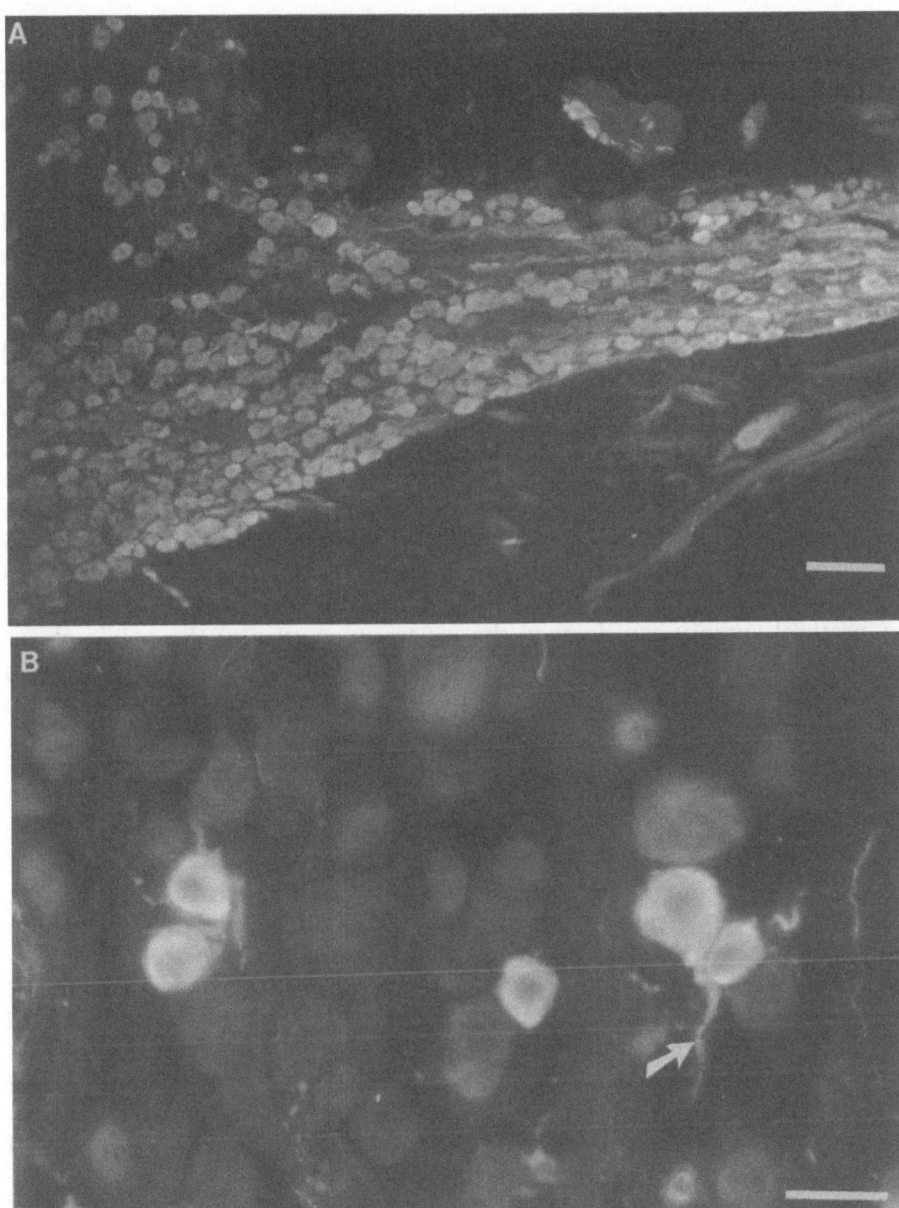

Fig. 3A,B. Immunocytochemical staining for vasoactive intestinal polypeptide (*VIP*) neurons in the cavernous nerve and adjacent pelvic ganglion. **A** VIP immunoreactive (IR) neurons in the cavernous nerve (*right*) and proximal pelvic ganglion (*left*) of the rat. ×10. **B** Higher magnification ×40) of neurons in cavernous nerves that are IR for VIP. Note single axonal process (*arrow*). VIP antibody from Peninsula (1/250 dilution) with colchicine pretreatment of tissue. *Calibration bar* represents 100 µm in **A** and 25 µm in **B**. (From Keast [28])

Not all axons conveyed by hypogastric or pelvic nerves synapse in the pelvic plexus [32, 43, 53, 57, 78]. Afferent and sympathetic postganglionic neurons pass through this plexus en route to the penis [3, 8, 13, 78]. However, some investigators have suggested that axon collaterals from afferent neurons may influence the neural function of ganglion cells in this plexus [53, 57].

The cavernous nerves can be visualized during pelvic surgery or cadaveric dissection [38, 82] and have been shown to travel in the pelvic fascia external to the prostatic capsule. More recently, Higgins and Gosling [23] described a series of ganglia lying in a similar position along the prostate. The cavernous nerves project along the posterolateral aspect of the prostate and at the prostatic apex they lie only millimeters from the urethral lumen. Fritsch [15] has shown that the cavernous nerves exit the pelvis by two routes. One group of fibers lies between the fascia of the levator ani and urethra en route to the penis while other branches appear to enter the striated urethral sphincter. At the level of the membranous urethra, the cavernous nerves are situated at the 3 and 9 o'clock positions, while distal to this point, some fibers penetrate the tunica albuginea of the corpus spongiosum. Other branches lying at the 1 and 11 o'clock positions enter the corpora cavernosa with the pudendal artery and cavernous veins. Thus, it is easy to envision how venous ligation, pelvic or urethral surgery can damage the cavernous nerves or the pelvic plexus producing neurogenic impotence [47, 82]. Recently investigators have been able to use nerve grafts in rats to restore erectile function following cavernous nerve ablation [61].

Sympathetic Pathways

The sympathetic nervous system is capable of mediating both penile erection and detumescence [14, 19, 75]. Sympathetic innervation to the corpora cavernosa in humans originates from preganglionic neurons in the intermediolateral gray matter at the levels of the ninth thoracic to second lumbar spinal cord [36]. Axonal tracing and degeneration studies in animals have revealed that preganglionic sympathetic neurons are located in the intermediolateral nuclei and the dorsal commissure [55, 66]. Dendrites from thoracolumbar preganglionic neurons are distributed mediolaterally toward the central canal and ventrally. This arrangement of dendritic projections allows preganglionic neurons to receive input from descending supraspinal centers. In addition, the proximity of the dendrites to afferent projections in lamina V raises the possibility of viscerovisceral convergence. One potential role for viscerovisceral convergence may be in coordinating concurrent visceral functions responsible for a variety of physiological events such as cardiovascular responses, seminal emission and bladder neck closure during sexual activity. Although coordination of visceral function may involve supraspinal centers, these data raise the possibility that spinal mechanisms may also play a role.

Thoracolumbar preganglionic axons travel by two routes to the penis [3, 8, 13, 34, 63, 71]. Fibers leaving the ventral roots enter the white rami and project to postganglionic neurons in the paravertebral chain ganglia (Fig. 1). These neurons give rise to axons which travel in gray rami on their way to lumbosacral chain ganglia which supply the corpora cavernosa. After leaving the thoracolumbar foramen, sympathetic preganglionic fibers may also pass through the chain ganglia to form the lumbar splanchnic nerves. The lumbar splanchnic nerves then project to prevertebral ganglia including the hypogastric plexus. Although sympathetic postganglionic neurons to the pelvic viscera have been thought to arise primarily from the hypogastric plexus, axonal tracing studies in animals suggest that many ganglion cells reside in the pelvic plexus, the cavernous nerve or in ganglia near the pelvic target organ [3, 8, 13, 29]. Sympathetic pathways entering the pelvic plexus are capable of modulating the function of parasympathetic neurons [17].

Somatic Pathways

Somatic afferents from the penis travel in a branch of the pudendal nerve known as the dorsal nerve of the penis (DNP) (Fig. 1). Afferent input conveyed by the DNP is essential for eliciting reflexogenic erections [4, 19]. Recent electrophysiological experiments in rodents have also shown that the cavernous nerves contain somatic afferents [78]. These afferents appear to arise from the perineum and possibly the urethra. In humans, cadaveric dissection and surgery for venogenic impotence also confirm connections between the DNP and the cavernous nerves [38].

Somatic motoneurons in the second, third, and fourth segments of the sacral spinal cord may also be important for sexual function since efferent activity conveyed by the pudendal nerve facilitates rigidity during penile erection [35]. Motoneurons originating in a region termed Onuf's nucleus in humans travel in the pudendal nerve to the bulbocavernous and ischiocavernous muscles as well as to other striated muscles of the pelvis and perineum [81]. Motoneurons within Onuf's nucleus in the rat [46, 69], cat [39] and dog [33] are topographically organized, according to whether they project to the urethra, penis, or striated pelvic floor muscles. In the primate, Onuf's nucleus gives rise to rostrocaudal projections as well as to axons which travel dorsomedially to the central canal or dorsolaterally to the intermediolateral gray matter [64]. Projections to these two regions imply that pudendal motoneurons receive input from supraspinal centers and may influence activity of preganglionic neurons (Fig. 2). Synaptic connections between somatic and visceral neurons could facilitate coordination between autonomic (penile erection) and somatic (ejaculation) events associated with sexual behavior.

Cadaveric dissections have been used to trace the course of the pudendal nerve [27]. These studies reveal that the sacral nerve roots divide into anterior and posterior bundles. The pudendal nerve is formed from the more posterior branch of the second through fourth sacral nerve roots. This nerve travels superior to the sacrospinal ligament on the coccygeal muscle and lateral to the coccygeal bone. More caudally, the pudendal nerve traverses the medial portion of the ischiorectal fossa in a fascial sheath known as Alcock's canal.

The first branch of the pudendal nerve is the DNP which separates from the main nerve trunk near the point where the pudendal artery and vein join the pudendal nerve. The DNP projects above the obturator internus muscle and beneath the levator ani muscle. It then enters the urogenital diaphragm before passing through the suspensory ligament to enter the dorsum of the penis.

Histochemistry and Immunocytochemistry

Histochemical studies have confirmed that sacral preganglionic neurons contain the neurotransmitter acetylcholine. Preganglionic neurons are also immunoreactive for neuropeptides such as leucine-enkephalin (L-ENK), calcitonin gene-related peptide (CGRP), and vasoactive intestinal polypeptide (VIP) (for reviews see [21, 42]). These neurons may also use purines as transmitters or neuromodulators [72]. In the vicinity of sacral preganglionic neurons are axonal processes which arise from afferent neurons, interneurons, and cells located in supraspinal centers (for review see [76]). These axons contain serotonin, norepinephrine, cholecystokinin, somatostatin, bombesin, neurotensin, neuropeptide Y (NPY), enkephalins, dynorphin, substance P, VIP, and oxytocin.

Afferent nerves in parasympathetic pathways originate from the sacral dorsal root ganglia and send axonal projections to the dorsal horn of the spinal cord. These pelvic afferents are immunoreactive for numerous neuropeptides including VIP, somatostatin, cholecystokinin, substance P and CGRP (for reviews see [21, 42]). Dorsal root transection combined with immunocytochemical staining has been used to distinguish those substances which arise from dorsal ganglion cells (afferents) from those intrinsic to the spinal cord.

Histochemical examination of human penile tissue, obtained at the time of prosthetic surgery for impotence or penectomy during gender reassignment, has been used to provide insight into possible transmitters within nerves supplying the vascular smooth muscle of the cavernous tissues. These include: acetylcholine, norepinephrine, VIP, NPY, somatostatin, CGRP, substance P, and ATP. In addition to heterogeneity based on size or immunoreactivity, regional differences in the density of innervation have been found. Using neuron-specific enolase, Gu et al. [22] have shown that the outer erectile tissue of the corpus cavernosum is more densely innervated than the inner portion. These investigators also demonstrated that the proximal portion of erectile tissue contains more nerve fibers than the distal segment. This finding correlates with morphological studies showing greater amounts of vascular smooth muscle in the proximal penis.

Traditionally, the action of postganglionic parasympathetic neurons is thought to be mediated through the release of acetylcholine based on histochemical and pharmacological data. Histochemical identification of cholinergic neurons in the peripheral nervous system has relied on staining for the enzyme acetylcholinesterase (AChE). Using this method of detection, AChE-positive ganglion cells in the pelvic plexus have been identified [10, 12, 14, 23, 53]. However, AChE-positive fibers appear in limited numbers in the corpora cavernosa and corpus spongiosum [1, 45, 74]; Fig. 4A. AChE-positive fibers are distributed in small bundles near the arterioles, or as individual fibers. Biochemical studies document synthesis and release of acetylcholine by nerves within human cavernous tissues [2]. In addition, bilateral cavernous nerve ablation in rodents is associated with loss of erectile function and depletion of acetylcholine-synthesizing enzymes within the penis [9]. Thus, anatomical, biochemical, and physiological evidence exists for cholinergic innervation to the penis. However pharmacological data suggest that acetylcholine is not the sole transmitter responsible for penile erection [19, 76].

Postganglionic cholinergic neurons are often associated with parasympathetic pathways. However, combined immunocytochemical and axonal tracing studies as well as electrophysiological analysis, lesioning and pharmacological experiments suggest that cholinergic mechanisms may also participate in vasodilation of penile vasculature mediated by sympathetic pathways [12, 75].

Sympathetic activity is usually linked with adrenergic mechanisms. Therefore it is not surprising that adrenergic fibers have been identified within the penis using histofluorescent techniques [1, 45, 67, 74]. Catecholamine fluorescent varicosities have been found within cavernous tissues (Fig. 4B). Furthermore, these adrenergic varicosities outnumber AChE-positive fibers in the penis [1]. Similar to cholinergic nerves, adrenergic varicosities are found between smooth muscle trabeculae and surrounding blood vessels. The endogenous synthesis and release of norepinephrine in cavernous tissues has been documented [67]. Thus, sympathetic activity in the cavernous tissues probably relies on both adrenergic and cholinergic mechanisms.

Based on retrograde tracing studies in the cat and rat, adrenergic and cholinergic input to the penis is thought to originate from ganglion cells located (1) along the cavernous nerves, (2) in the pelvic plexus, and (3) in the lumbosacral sympathetic chain [3, 8, 13]. It is of interest that combined retrograde labeling and cytochemical staining show that no neurons projecting to the penis from the pelvic ganglion of the rat contain tyrosine hydroxylase (TH), an enzyme marker for adrenergic neurons. However, numerous AChE-positive cells supplied by the hypogastric nerve can be identified in this ganglion [12, 28]; (Fig. 5). This finding suggests that most adrenergic input to the

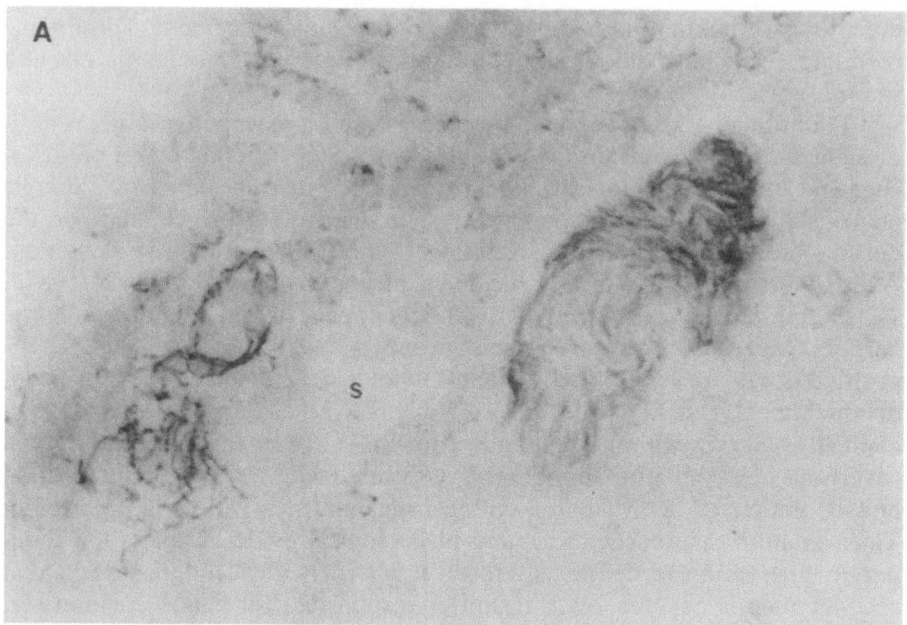

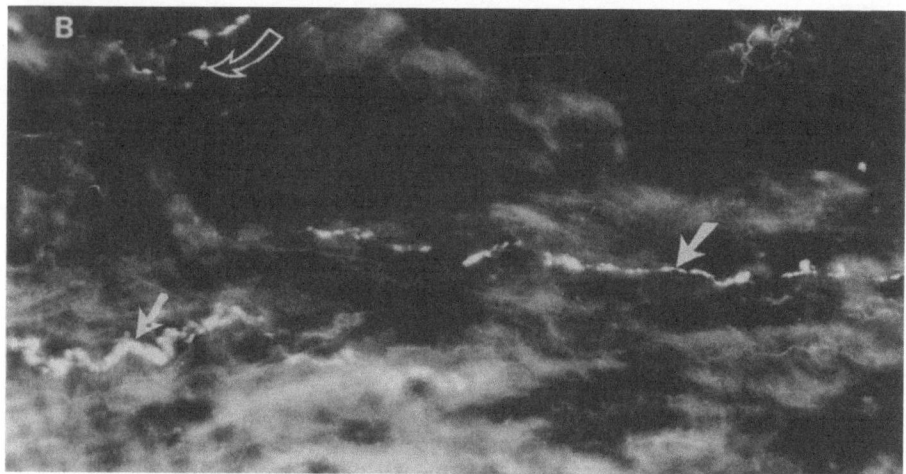

Fig. 4A,B. Histochemical staining for acetylcholinesterase and catecholamines in human corpus cavernosum. **A** Acetylcholinesterase staining around an arteriole (*left*) and within nerve bundle (*right*) on frozen section (×20). **B** Glyoxylic acid-processed frozen section showing catecholamine fluorescent varicosities (*filled arrows*) between trabecular smooth muscle and around blood vessel (*open arrow*; ×36). (From Benson et al. [1])

penis probably arises outside the pelvic plexus, possibly from the sympathetic chain ganglia. In addition, penile neurons in the pelvic plexus are surrounded by fibers or basket-like configurations immunoreactive for substances known to be present in some sacral preganglionic neurons (Fig. 5). Overall the

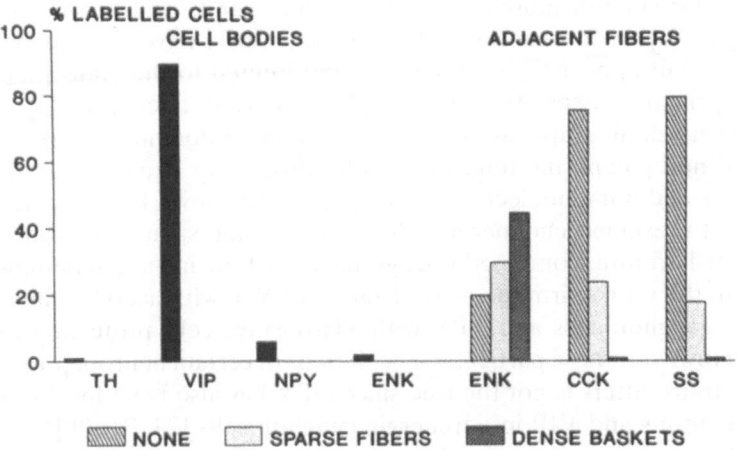

Fig. 5. Summary of immunocytochemical characterization of retrogradely labeled penile neurons in rat. Majority of neurons are immunoreactive (*IR*) for VIP. No penile neurons were positive for TH in the pelvic ganglia. NPY colocalized with some VIP-positive cells in presumed cholinergic neurons. Few enkephalin (*ENK*) staining cells were observed. Surrounding retrogradely labeled penile neurons were fibers positive for ENK, cholecystokinin (*CCK*) and somatostatin (*SS*) which probably represent preganglionic fibers. (Modified from Keast and de Groat [28])

histochemical characteristics of penile neurons in the pelvic ganglion of the rat appear to be quite distinct from those supplying the bladder and colon.

Autonomic nerves have been found to synthesize and release substances other than acetylcholine and norepinephrine which may function as transmitters or neuromodulators. Since neuropeptides are recognized as mediators of noncholinergic and nonadrenergic transmission at various sites in the peripheral and central nervous systems, their identification within the penis has suggested a physiological role in penile erection or detumescence. Immunocytochemistry and radioimmunoassay techniques have demonstrated VIP, NPY, substance P, somatostatin, enkephalins and CGRP within the penis [7, 22, 26, 56, 77, 80, 83, 84].

The distributions of VIP, NPY, and somatostatin immunoreactive fibers within penile tissues are similar to cholinergic and adrenergic varicosities. VIP immunoreactive fibers are found within the trabecular smooth muscle and along arterioles and venules in human corpora cavernosa [56, 77, 84]. In addition to varicosities, neuronal cell bodies staining for VIP have been identified within the penis [22]. NPY-staining fibers are mostly concentrated in the inner adventitia of arterioles and venules within the penis as well as between trabecular smooth muscle [7, 83]. Keast and de Groat [28] have reported that 7% of retrogradely labeled neurons from the penis in the pelvic ganglion of the rat are immunoreactive for NPY (Fig. 5). Likewise, somatostatin immunoreactive varicosities are found along penile blood vessels and between trabecular smooth muscle and surrounding penile neurons in the pelvic plexus [22, 28]. A few substance P-containing fibers have been identified in the penis but appear to be superficial and limited to the glans [22]. Substance P is primarily associated with peripheral sensory fibers [16, 42].

VIP and acetylcholine appear to coexist in many autonomic neurons, while NPY and norepinephrine tend to be colocalized. For example, ultrastructural studies and immunoelectron microscopy have shown the presence of both VIP and presumed cholinergic vesicles within the same varicosities [77] (Fig. 6). Furthermore, combined retrograde axonal tracing and immunocytochemistry in the rat confirm the colocalization of VIP with acetylcholinesterase-positive ganglion cells and NPY with TH-positive cells projecting to the penis [12]. However, these particular associations of certain neuropeptides and traditional transmitters is not the rule since NPY has also been localized in cholinergic neurons and VIP in adrenergic ganglion cells [24, 25, 28].

Acetylcholine, norepinephrine, and neuropeptides directly effect corporal smooth muscle contractility, neural transmission and the release of transmitters from nerve terminals within cavernous tissues (for review see [16]). Furthermore these substances may influence a variety of cavernous tissue-derived compounds such as arachidonic acid metabolites, endothelium-derived relaxing factors (EDRF), or endothelial contracting factors such as endothelin [2, 67, 68]. Thus, the peripheral neural regulation and pharmacology of corporal tissue is quite complex with potential interactions between multiple transmitters, local factors and smooth muscle. The multiplicity of transmitters and efferent mechanisms may explain in part why penile erection

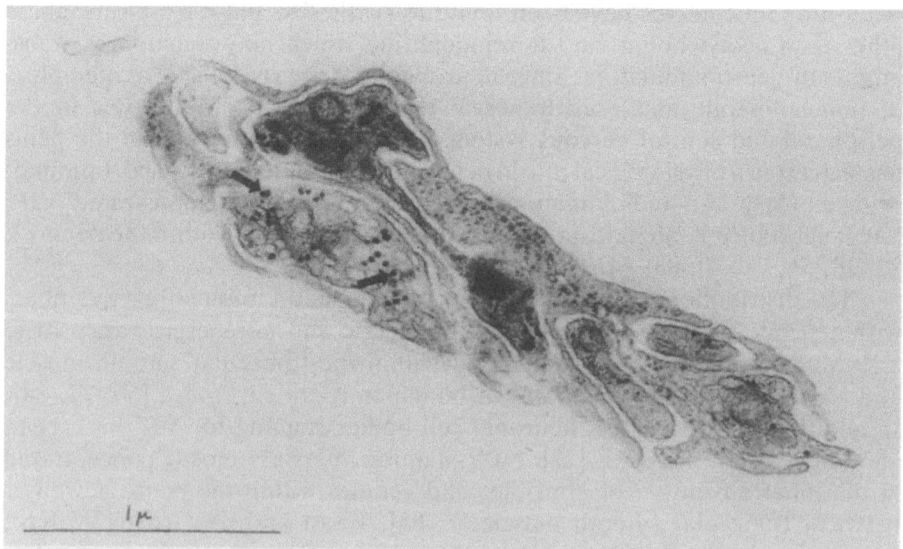

Fig. 6. Election micrograph of VIP immunoreactive vesicles (*arrows*) in varicosity from human corpus cavernosum. (From McConnell [45]) ×20 000

and detumescence is sensitive to drugs and a wide variety of pathological states including neurological diseases and metabolic disorders.

Neurophysiology

Pelvic nerve or sacral spinal root stimulation in man produces penile erection [5] while destruction of these nerves causes loss of reflexogenic erections [4]. Likewise, stimulation of the cavernous nerves produces vasodilation of blood vessels supplying the corpora cavernosa of primates [40], dogs [79] and rats [62, 78]. Therefore, sacral parasympathetic input conveyed by the pelvic and cavernous nerves is considered the primary vasodilator pathway to the penis.

Stimulation of the hypogastric nerve in some species such as the rabbit produces both erectile and detumescence responses [75]. On the other hand lumbar sympathetic chain stimulation elicits detumescence or inhibits the ability to obtain electrically evoked penile erection [34]. More recently Dail et al. [14] have suggested that following injury of parasympathetic pathways to the penis, stimulation of hypogastric nerves, which prior to injury did not produce penile erection, elicits erectile responses. This result is similar to the neural plasticity that occurs in autonomic pathways to the bladder following lower motoneuron injury [18].

Stimulation of the hypogastric nerves in man has no obvious effect on penile erection [5]. Furthermore, extensive sympathectomies in humans do not abolish erections or produce priapism [30, 65]. Yet patients with sacral spinal cord lesions or conus medullaris injury often maintain psychogenic erections through hypogastric pathways which suggests a vasodilator role for sympathetic pathways to the penis [4, 19]. The recent animal studies by Dail et al. [14] may, in this latter situation, indicate a de novo role for preganglionic sympathetic neurons which re-innervate postganglionic parasympathetic neurons deprived of neural input.

Electrophysiological techniques have been used to examine the axonal composition and reflex activity in the cavernous nerves of the rat [58, 78]. Stimulation of the pelvic nerve, hypogastric nerve or sympathetic chain elicits synaptic and axonal volleys in the cavernous nerve (Fig. 7A–F). Cholinergic synaptic transmission in peripheral ganglia is confirmed using nicotinic ganglionic blockade (Fig. 7B,D). Furthermore, stimulation of the DNP evokes central reflex (50–150 ms latency) activity in the cavernous nerve (Fig. 2). These DNP evoked reflexes are eliminated by pelvic and occasionally hypogastric nerve lesioning but not by thoracic spinal cord transection, indicating that DNP reflexes originate in the lumbosacral spinal cord. Furthermore, electrophysiological experiments support the notion of significant somato-visceral convergence as corroborated by anatomical data showing the close proximity of preganglionic dendritic projections to somatic afferents from the penis (Fig. 2), [3, 52]. Finally, it is tempting to speculate that the DNP to

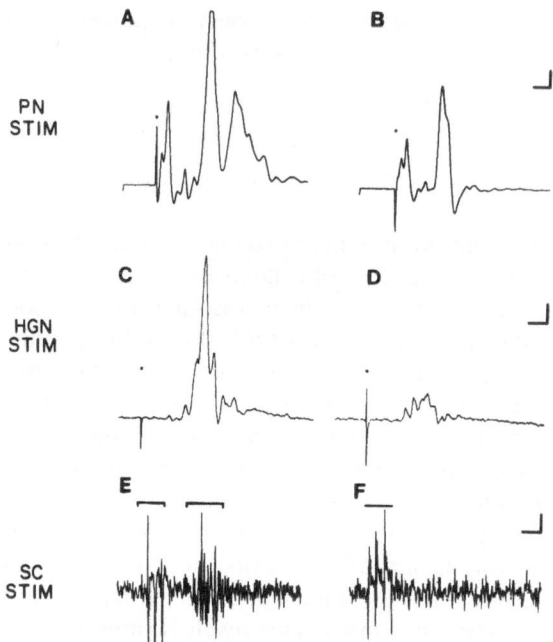

Fig. 7A–F. Short latency electrophysiological responses recorded from cavernous nerves following electrical stimulation of pelvic nerve (**A**, **B**), hypogastric nerve (**C**, **D**), and sympathetic chain (**E**, **F**). **A** Evoked responses in cavernous nerve before ganglionic blockade (GB) in response to pelvic nerve (*PN*) stimulation (6 V, 3Hz). **B** After GB, change in discharge represents loss of cholinergic synaptic responses with continued PN stimulation (5 V, 3 Hz). Remaining discharge represents either afferent or nonsynaptic postganglionic volleys. **C** Discharge recorded on cavernous nerve following hypogastric (*HGN*) stimulation (10 V, 3Hz). **D** After GB, loss of responses with HGN stimulation indicates significant cholinergic synaptic transmission. **E** Sympathetic chain (*SC*)-evoked response in cavernous nerves (4 V, 30 Hz, three trains). **F** Loss of SC-evoked response after pelvic nerve transection indicating SC input to penis in pelvic nerve pathways. *Dots* in **A–D**, *first bracket* in **E**, and *line* in **F** correspond to stimulus artifacts. *Second bracket* in **E** represents response. *Vertical calibration* 100 mV, *horizontal* 5 ms in **A**, **B**; 50 uV, 10 ms in **C**, **D**; and 5 uV, 20 ms in **E**, **F**. (From Steers et al. [78])

cavernous nerve reflex represents the electrophysiological correlate to tactile-induced erections.

Electrophysiological data also support the concept of viscerovisceral convergence within the sacral spinal cord. Stimulation of afferents within the pelvic nerve has been shown to elicit central reflex activity in the cavernous nerve [78]. Since afferents within the pelvic nerve originate from several pelvic viscera including the bladder and colon, these afferents may activate or inhibit preganglionic neurons projecting to the cavernous nerve. This hypothesis of viscerovisceral convergence within the sacral spinal cord may explain the mechanism by which vascular responses in the cavernous tissues can be influenced by neural input from other pelvic organs. Examples of viscerovisceral convergence may include the ability of colonic or bladder distension to effect erectile function or the coordination of such functions as voiding, defecation and penile erection at the level of the spinal cord.

Summary

Anatomical and electrophysiological data have led to a refinement in our understanding of the neural regulation of penile erection and coordination of sexual function with other autonomic and somatic events. Since neurogenic impotence is often a diagnosis of exclusion, a more complete understanding of the peripheral and central neural pathways to the cavernous tissues may lead to improved clinical testing. Furthermore, identification of transmitters within these pathways may facilitate the development of drugs which block vasoconstrictor pathways or augment vasodilator pathways to the penis, allowing advances in pharmacological therapy for organic and psychogenic impotence.

Acknowledgement. The author would like to acknowledge the work of Bobra Slaughter in preparing and proof-reading this manuscript.

References

1. Benson GS, McConnell J, Lipschultz LI, Corriere JN (1980) Neuromorphology and neuropharmacology of the human penis. J Clin Invest 65:506–513
2. Blanco R, Saenz de Tejada I, Goldstein I, Krane RT, Wotiz HH, Cohen RA (1988) Cholinergic neurotransmission in human corpus cavernosum II. Acetylcholine synthesis. Am J Physiol 254:H468–H472
3. Booth AM, Roppolo JA, de Groat WC (1986) Distribution of cells and fibers projecting to the penis of the cat. Abst Soc Neurosci 12:1056
4. Bors E, Comarr AE (1960) Neurological disturbances in sexual function with special reference to 529 patients with spinal cord injury. Urol Surv 10:191–222
5. Brindley GS (1986) Sacral root and hypogastric plexus stimulators and what these models tell us about autonomic actions on the bladder and urethra. Clin Sci (Suppl 14) 70:41s–44s
6. Calabrisi P (1956) The nerve supply of the erectile cavernous tissue of the genitalia in the human embryo and fetus. Anat Rec 125:713–723
7. Carrillo Y, Fernandez E, Dail WG et al. (1989) Neuropeptide Y innervation of penile erectile tissue. Abst Soc Neurosci 15:631
8. Chung SK, McKenna KE (1987) The autonomic innervation of the penis and clitoris of the rat. Abst Soc Neurosci 13:272
9. Dail WG, Hamill RW (1989) Parasympathetic nerves in penile erectile tissue of the rat containing choline acetyltransferase. Brain Res 487:165–170
10. Dail WG, Moll MA, Weber K (1983) Localization of vasoactive intestinal polypeptide in penile erectile tissue and in the major pelvic ganglion of the rat. Neurosci 10: 1379–1386

11. Dail WG, Manzanares K, Moll MA, Minorsky N (1985) The hypogastric nerve inner-vates a population of penile neurons in the pelvic plexus. Neurosci 16:1041–1046
12. Dail WG, Minorsky N, Moll MA (1986) The hypogastric nerve pathway to penile erectile tissue: histochemical evidence supporting a vasodilator role. J Auton Nerv Syst 15:341–349
13. Dail WG, Trujillo D, Walton G, Rosas D de la (1987) Autonomic composition of reproductive organs of the rat. Abstr Soc Neurosci 13:272
14. Dail WG, Walton G, Olmsted MP (1989) Penile erection on the rat: Stimulation of the hypogastric nerve elicits increases in penile pressure after chronic interruption of the sacral parasympathetic outflow. J Auton Nerv Sys 28:251–258
15. Fritsch H (1989) Topography of the pelvic autonomic nerves in human fetuses be-tween 21–29 weeks of gestation. Anat Embryol 180:57–64
16. de Groat WC (1987) Neuropeptides in pelvic afferent pathways. Experimentia 43: 801–813
17. de Groat WC, Booth AM (1980) Inhibition and facilitation in parasympathetic ganglia. Fed Proc 39:2990–2996
18. de Groat WC, Kawatani M (1989) Reorganization of sympathetic preganglionic con-nections in cat bladder ganglia following parasympathetic denervation. J Physiol (London) 409:431–449
19. de Groat WC, Steers WD (1988) Neuroanatomy and neurophysiology of penile erection. In: Tanagho EA, Lue TF, McClure RD (eds) Contemporary management of impotence and infertility. Williams and Wilkins, Baltimore, pp 3–27
20. de Groat WC, Steers WC (1990) Autonomic regulation of the urinary bladder and sexual organs. In: Spyer RM, Loewy A (eds) Central regulation of autonomic func-tions. Oxford Univ Press, Oxford
21. de Groat WC, Kawatani M, Hisamitsu T, Lowe I, Morgan C, Roppolo J, Booth AM, Nadelhaft I, Kuo D, Thor K (1983) The role of neuropeptides in the sacral autonomic reflex pathway of the cat. J Auton Nerv Syst 7:339–350
22. Gu J, Polak JM, Probert L, Islam KN, Marangos PJ, Mina S, Adrian TE, McGregor GP, OShaughnessy DJ, Bloom SR (1983) Peptidergic innervation of human male genital tract. J Urol 130:386–391
23. Higgins JRA, Gosling JA (1989) Studies on the structure and intrinsic innervation of the normal human prostate. Prostate (Suppl) 2:5–16
24. Hill EL, Elde RC (1989) Vasoactive intestinal peptide distribution and colocalization with dopamine beta hydroxylase in sympathetic chain ganglia of pig. J Auton Nerve Sys 27:229–239
25. Jarvi R, Helen M, Huikko P, Hervonen M (1986) Neuropeptide Y (NPY)-like immunoreactivity in rat sympathetic neurons and small granule-containing cells. Neurosci Lett 67:233–237
26. Juenemann KP, Lue TF, Luo JA, Jadallah SA, Nunes LL, Tanagho EA (1987) The role of vasoactive intestinal polypeptide as a neurotransmitter within canine penile erection. A combined in vivo and immunohistochemical study. J Urol 138:871–877
27. Juenemann KP, Lue TF, Schmidt RA, Tanagho EA (1988) Clinical significance of sacral and pudendal nerve anatomy. J Urol 139:74–80
28. Keast JF, de Groat WC (1989) Immunocytochemical characterization of pelvic neurons which project to the bladder, colon or penis in rats. J Comp Neurol 288:307–394
29. Keast JF, Booth AM, de Groat WC (1989) Distribution of neurons in the major pelvic ganglion of the rat which supply bladder, colon or penis. Cell Tiss Res 156:105–112
30. Kedia KR, Markland C, Fraley EE (1975) Sexual function following high retroperi-toneal lymphadenectomy. J Urol 114:237–239
31. Kimmel DL (1958) The development of the pelvic plexus and the distribution of the pelvic splanchnic nerves in the human embryo and fetus. J Comp Neurol 110:271–298
32. Kuo DC, Hisamitsu T, de Groat WC (1984) A sympathetic projection from sacral para-vertebral ganglia to pelvic nerve and postganglionic nerves on the surface of the urinary bladder and large intestine of the cat. J Comp Neurol 226:77–86
33. Kuzukara S, Kanazawa I, Nakanishi T (1980) Topographical localization of the Onuf's nuclear neurons innervating the rectal and vesical striated sphincter muscles: a

retrograde fluorescent double labelling study in cat and dog. Neurosci Lett 16:125–130

34. Langley JN, Anderson HR (1895) The innervation of the pelvic and adjoining viscera. J Physiol (London) 19:71–130

35. Lavoisier P, Proulx J, Courtois F, Carufel F de, Durand L-G (1988) Relationship between perineal muscle contractions, penile tumescence and penile rigidity during nocturnal erections. J Urol 139:176–179

36. Learmonth JR (1931) A contribution to the neurophysiology of the urinary bladder in man. Brain 54:147–176

37. Leblanc G, Landis S (1986) Development of choline acetyl-transferase (CAT) in the sympathetic innervation of the rat sweat glands. J Neurosci 6:260–265

38. Lepor H, Gregerman M, Crosby R, Mostofi FR, Walsh PC (1985) Precise localization of the autonomic nerves from the pelvic plexus to the corpora cavernosa: a detailed anatomical study of the adult male pelvis. J Urol 133:207–212

39. Li Q, Leedy G, Beattie MS, Bresnahan JC (1988) Cat motoneurons innervating urethral and anal sphincters have different dendritic arbors. Abstr Soc Neurosci 14:337

40. Lue TF, Takamura T, Schmidt AR et al (1983) Hemodynamics of erection in the monkey. J Urol 130:1237–1241

41. Lue TF, Zeineh SJ, Schmidt RA, Tanagho EA (1984) Neuroanatomy of penile erection: its relevance to iatrogenic impotence. J Urol 131:273–280

42. Maggi CA, Meli A (1986) The role of neuropeptides in the regulation of the micturition reflex. J Auton Pharmacol 6:133–162

43. Mallory B, Steers WD, de Groat WC (1989) Electrophysiological study of micturition reflexes in the rat. Am J Physiol 257:R410–R421

44. Mawe G, Breshnahan JC, Beattie MS (1986) A light and electron microscopic analysis of the sacral parasympathetic nucleus after labelling primary afferent and efferent elements with HRP. J Comp Neurol 250:33–57

45. McConnell J, Benson GS, Wood JG (1982) Autonomic innervation of the urogenital system: adrenergic and cholinergic elements. Brain Res Bull 9:679–694

46. McKenna KE, Nadelhaft I (1986) The organization of the pudendal nerve in the male and female rat. J Comp Neurol 248:532–549

47. Mundy AR (1982) An anatomical explanation for bladder dysfunction following rectal and uterine surgery. Br J Urol 54:501–504

48. Nadelhaft I, de Groat WC, Morgan C (1980) Location and morphology of parasympathetic pregnanglionic neurons in the sacral spinal cord of the cat revealed by retrograde axonal transport of horseradish peroxidase. J Comp Neurol 193:265–291

49. Nadelhaft I, Roppolo JR, Morgan C, de Groat WC (1983) Parasympathetic preganglionic neurons and visceral primary afferents in monkey sacral spinal cord revealed following application of horseradish peroxidase to pelvic nerve. J Comp Neurol 216:36–52

50. Nadelhaft I, Booth AM (1984) The location and morphology of preganglionic neurons and the distribution of visceral afferents from the rat pelvic nerve: a horseradish peroxidase study. J Comp Neurol 226:238–245

51. Neuhuber W (1982) The central projections of visceral primary afferent neurons of the inferior mesenteric plexus and hypogastric nerve and location of the related sensory and preganglionic sympathetic cell bodies in the rat. Anat Embryol 164:413–425

52. Nunez R, Gross GH, Sachs BD (1986) Origin and central projections of rat dorsal penile nerve: possible direct projections to autonomic and somatic neurons by primary afferents of nonmuscle origin. J Comp Neurol 247:417–429

53. Papka RE, Traurig HH (1988) Interactions between chemically identified nerve fibers and neurons in female rat paracervical ganglia. Abstr Soc Neurosci 14:354

54. Pearson AA, Sauter RW (1970) Nerve contributions to the pelvic plexus and umbilical cord. Am J Anat 128:485–498

55. Petras JM, Cummings JF (1978) Sympathetic and parasympathetic innervation of the urinary bladder and urethra. Brain Res 153:363–369

56. Polak JM, Gu J, Mina S, Bloom SR (1981) Vipergic nerves in the penis. Lancet 2:217–219

57. Purinton PT, Fletcher TF, Bradley WE (1971) Sensory perikarya in autonomic ganglia. Nature 231:63–64
58. Purinton PT, Fletcher TF, Bradley WE (1976) Innervation of pelvic viscera in the rat. Evoked potentials in nerves to bladder and penis. Invest Urol 14:28–32
59. Purves D, Hume RI (1981) The relation of postsynaptic geometry to the number of presynaptic axons that innervate autonomic ganglion cells. J Neurosci 5:441–452
60. Purves D, Snider WD, Voyvodic JT (1988) Trophic regulation of nerve cell morphology and innervation in the autonomic nervous system. Nature 336:123–128
61. Quinlan DM, Nelson RJ, Walsh PC (1989a) Cavernous nerve grafts to restore erectile function in the rat. J Urol 141:186A
62. Quinlan DM, Nelson RJ, Partin AW, Mostwin JL, Walsh PC (1989b) The rat as a model for the study of penile erection. J Urol 141:656–661
63. Root S, Bard P (1947) The mediation of feline erection through sympathetic pathways with some remarks on sexual behavior after deafferentation of the genitalia. Am J Physiol 151:80–90
64. Roppolo JR, Nadelhaft I, de Groat WC (1985) The organization of pudendal motoneurons and primary afferent projections in the spinal cord of the rhesus monkey revealed by horseradish peroxidase. J Comp Neurol 234:475–488
65. Rose SJ (1953) An investigation into sterility after lumbar ganglionectomy. Br Med J 1:247–250
66. Rubin E, Purves D (1980) Segmental organization of sympathetic preganglionic neurons in the mammalian spinal cord. J Comp Neurol 192:163–174
67. Saenz de Tejada I, Kim N, Lagan I, Krane RJ, Goldstein I (1989a) Regulation of adrenergic activity in penile corpus cavernosum. J Urol 142:1117–1121
68. Saenz de Tejada I, Goldstein I, Azadoi K, Krane RJ, Cohen RA (1989b) Impaired neurogenic and endothelium mediated relaxation of penile smooth muscle from diabetic men with impotence. N Engl J Med 320:1025–1030
69. Schroder HD (1980) Organization of the motoneurons innervating the pelvic muscles of the male rat. J Comp Neurol 192:567–587
70. Schroder HD (1981) Onuf's nucleus X: a morphological study of a human spinal nucleus. Anat Embryol 162:443–953
71. Semans JH, Langworthy OR (1938) Observations on the neurophysiology of sexual function in the male cat. J Urol 40:836–846
72. Senba E, Daddona PE, Nagy JI (1987) A subpopulation of preganglionic parasympathetic neurons in the rat contain adenosine deaminase. Neurosci 20:487–502
73. Shimizu T, Egan-Konopha LM, Ohta Y, Sun NY (1982) Localization of postganglionic neurons to the male genital organs in the major pelvic ganglion of the rat. Tohoku J Exp Med 136:351–352
74. Shirai M, Sasaki K, Rikimaru A (1972) Histochemical investigation on the distribution of adrenergic and cholinergic nerves in human penis. Tohoku J Exp Med 107:403–404
75. Sjostrand NO, Klinge E (1979) Principal mechanisms controlling penile retraction and protrusion in rabbits. Acta Physiol Scand 106:199–214
76. Steers WD (1990) Neural regulation of penile erection. Semin Urol 8:66–79
77. Steers WD, McConnell J, Benson GS (1984) Anatomical localization and some pharmacological effects of vasoactive intestinal polypeptide in human and monkey corpus cavernosum. J Urol 132:1048–1053
78. Steers WD, Mallory B, de Groat WC (1988) Electrophysiological study of neural activity in penile nerve of the rat. Am J Physiol 254:R989–R1000
79. Stief C, Benard F, Bosch R, Aboseif S, Nunes L, Lue TF, Tanagho EA (1989) Acetylcholine as a possible neurotransmitter in penile erection. J Urol 141:1444–1448
80. Stief CG, Bernard F, Bosch R, Aboseif SR, Lue TF, Tanagho EA (1990) A possible role for calcitonin gene-related peptide in the regulation of the smooth muscle tone of the bladder and penis. J Urol 143:392–397
81. Tabatabai M, Booth AM, de Groat WC (1986) Morphological and electrophysiological properties of pelvic ganglion cells in the rat. Brain Res 382:61–70
82. Walsh PC, Donker P (1982) Impotence following radical prostatectomy: insight into etiology and prevention. J Urol 128:492–497

83. Wespes E, Schiffman S, Vanderhaeghen JJ, Schulman CC (1988) Light and electron microscopic demonstration of neuropeptide Y in the human penis with some pharmacologic aspects. Proc 3rd Biennial World Meeting on Impotence, Boston, p 44
84. Willis E, Ottesen B, Wagner G, Sundler F, Fahrenkrug J (1983) Vasoactive intestinal polypeptide as a putative transmitter in penile erection. Life Sci 33:383–491

Ultrastructural Findings in Patients with Erectile Dysfunction

J. Staubesand, U. Wetterauer, and F. Kulvelis

The increasingly efficient diagnosis of erectile dysfunction (ED) during recent years has established that pathological organic changes are to be found in more than half of these patients. In addition to the extensive older literature, a large amount of recent histological – but little ultrastructural – research is available [1, 2, 14]. We therefore decided it would be rewarding to compare the ultrastructure of the corpora cavernosa penis (CCP) in patients with and without ED, in the hope that a pathomorphological basis for the condition might be revealed.

Surgical biopsies a few millimeters in width and depth were obtained from 32 patients and immediately fixed by immersion. Specimens from patients ($n = 6$) with normal erections, but observable penile deviation corrected by the Nesbit procedure served as controls. One or more of the following conditions were confirmed preoperatively in 26 of the patients with ED: venous leakage, arteriosclerosis, diabetes mellitus, primary ED, and fibrosis.

Since the tunica albuginea is not without significance for erection and rigidity of the CCP [2, 4, 7], we paid particular attention to the collagen fibrils within it, and in our earlier research on the ultrastructure of these fibrils in various diseases of connective tissue and blood vessels we were always able to confirm changes in the form of intra- and extrafibrillar collagen dysplasia [15]. Contrary to our expectations, however, the collagen fibrils of the tunica albuginea in patients with ED show disturbances neither in their texture nor in their fine structure. Even in the presence of organic disease, their oblique criss-cross arrangement remains unchanged.

On the other hand, the vessels of the CCP are markedly altered in the group of patients with ED (Fig. 1). Depending upon the type of basic disease and its severity, an increased number of vacuolated cells in the endothelium, for instance, and osmiophilic shrinkage necroses in the smooth muscle cells of the media are, amongst other signs of degeneration such as medial fibrosis (Fig. 1a), to be observed. In some isolated cases no lumen at all can be detected, particularly in the smaller vessels (Figs. 1b, c). Slight pathological changes can even be reconized in young patients (Fig. 1b). The findings in the blood vessels support the clinical diagnosis and explain the poor prospect of preoperative corpus cavernosum autoinjection therapy (CAT) in cases of long-standing diabetes mellitus or severe arteriosclerosis. In seven patients,

U. Jonas et al. (Eds.) Erectile Dysfunction
© Springer-Verlag Berlin Heidelberg 1991

four of whom had shown no clinical signs of manifest arterial disease, calcium microspheres were seen in the interstitial tissue of the trabeculae, in the basal membrane of the endothelium or in the subendothelium (Fig. 2b), and also singly in the tunica albuginea (Fig. 2a).

Collections of thrombocytes – occasionally already at the stage of viscous metamorphosis – were found not infrequently within the blood sinuses of the erectile tissue and also singly in the subalbugineal venous plexus.

Normally fibrin is precipitated during the coagulation of shed blood [18], but we only observed platelet thromboses in two out of eight patients. This morphological finding may suggest that increased fibrinolytic activity occurs in the CCP [13]; this has, admittedly, not yet been confirmed. The biological sense of an endogenous fibrinolysis in the CCP is suggested in view of the minimal blood-flow in the sinuses during erection.

The smooth muscle in the interstitial tissue of the CCP has proved itself to be of great physiological and pathological significance for the process of erection [11, 12]. Very often – that is to say, in 75% of the patients we examined – degenerative signs appear such as the deposition of lipid drops in the cytoplasm (Fig. 3a), or even complete cell death in the form of shrinkage necrosis (Fig. 3b). These changes are often associated with an intensification in the arrangement of the smooth muscle cells into bundles. The frequency of this finding leads one to suspect that it is of considerable pathophysiological significance.

Neurogenic causes of ED were assumed in about 10% of all cases, and we have reason to believe that this percentage – at least in a contributory sense – should really be substantially higher. In every second patient, we encountered the pathological occurrence of paraneuritic fibrous long-spacing collagen [3, 9] among the intracavernous nerves close to the Schwann cells (Fig. 4a, b). We consider it possible that a neural disturbance of metabolism (probably arising sui generis) underlies ED much more frequently than is reported in the literature, and that this is bound up with the pathomorphological substrate fibrous long-spacing collagen.

During our work on the intracavernous nerves, we observed other pathological changes in the perineurium and Schwann cells. We also found, in patients, a greater amount of collagen within the peripheral nerves than in the control group, as well as damage to axons. Should these neuropathological findings be confirmed, this would explain the disturbance of the erectile mechanism [5–8, 10]. This complex of findings will have to be borne in mind by those planning systems of drug therapy in the future.

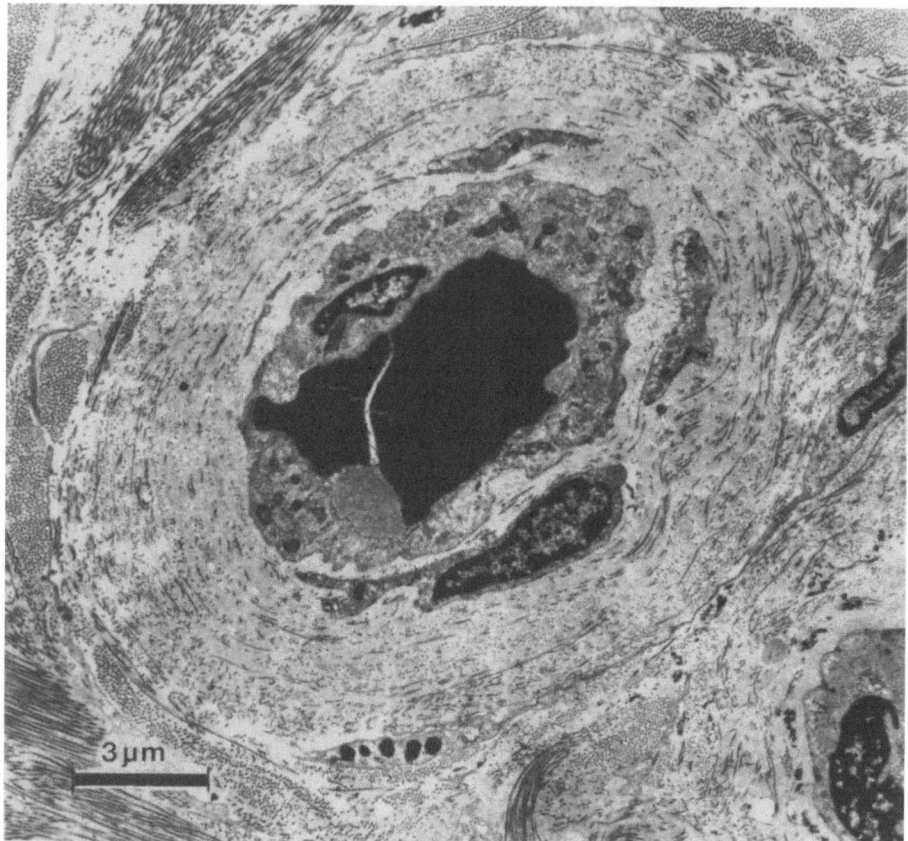

Fig. 1a

Fig. 1a–c. Immersion fixation performed in three patients to investigate the blood vessels

Fig. 1a. Patient W.E. aged 48 years and with ED, diabetes mellitus Type I, raised blood-lipid level, nicotine abuse, and venous leakage. A small blood vessel from the tunica albuginea with marked medial fibrosis. Only a few smooth muscle cells still present. Sectioned erythrocytes can be seen in the reduced lumen. Primary magnification × 2900; for final enlargement see scale

Fig. 1b. Patient N.G. aged 19 years and with ED and venous leakage. The lumen of the intracavernous vessel is barely still recognizable. Here and there vacuoles are present in the endothelial and muscle cells. Primary magnification × 1400; for final enlargement see scale

Fig. 1c. Patient A.A. aged 38 years and with ED, arteriosclerosis, and diabetes mellitus Type I. Small blood vessel from the CCP; lumen no longer present. Endothelial cells cannot be unequivocally identified. Most of the medial myocytes have bizarre shapes. Primary magnification × 650; for final enlargement see scale

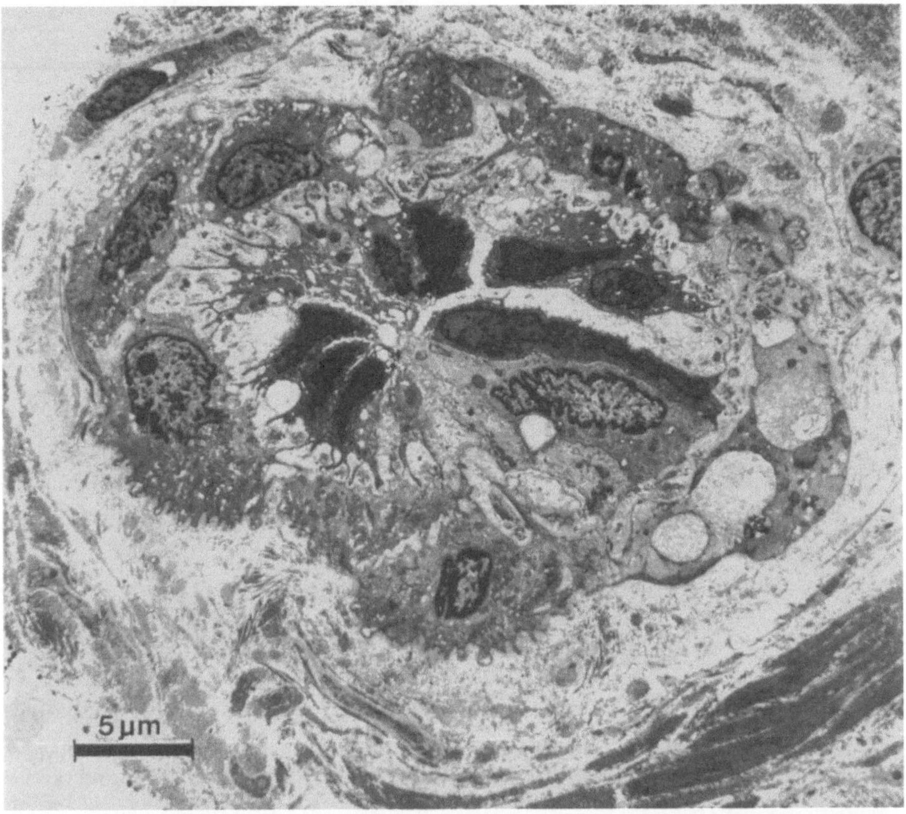

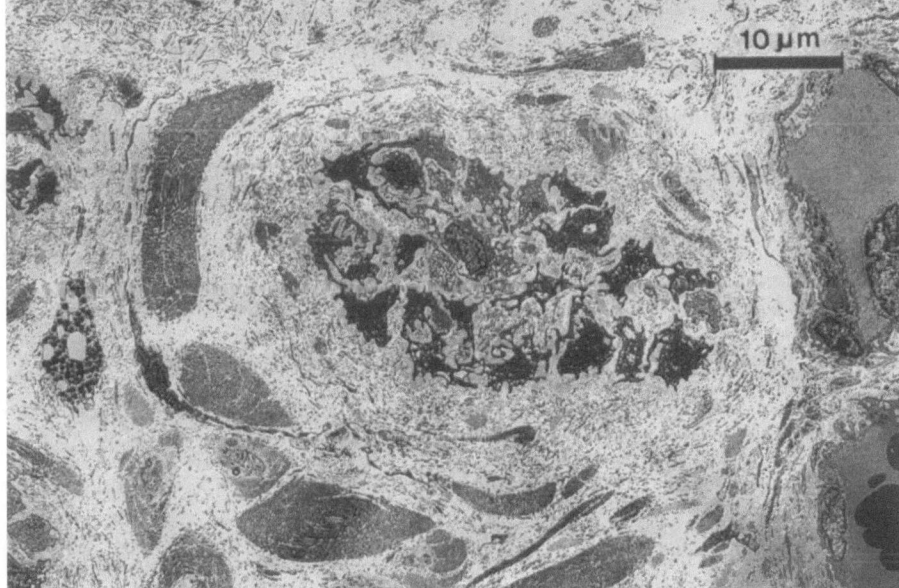

Fig. 1b

Fig. 1c

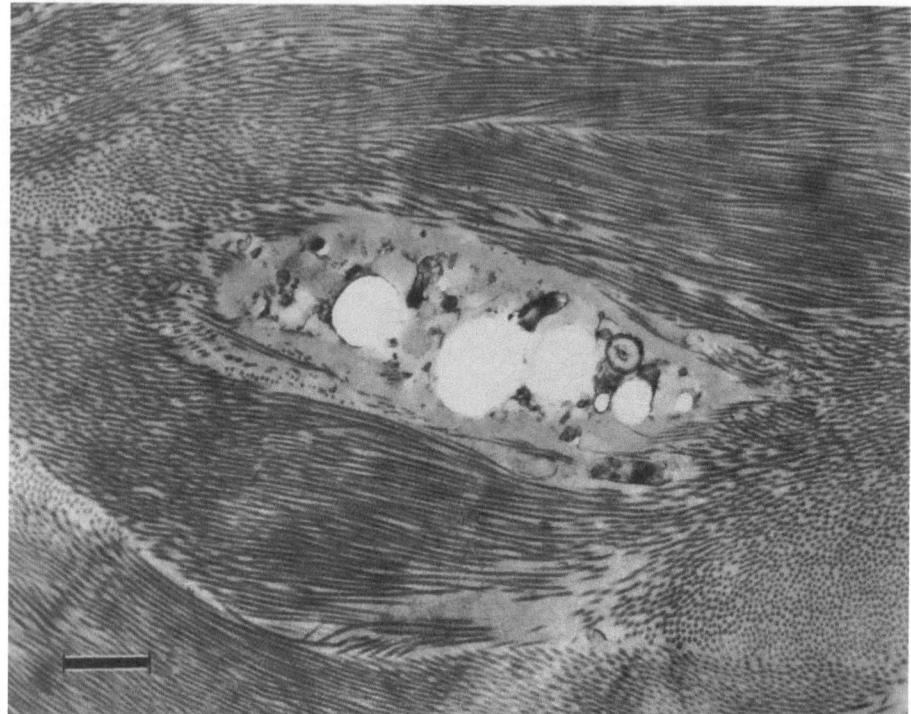

Fig. 2a, b. Immersion fixation showing calcium microspheres in patient W.E. aged 48 years and with ED, diabetes mellitus Type I, raised blood-lipid level, nicotine abuse, and venous leakage

Fig. 2a. Cord of connective tissue from the middle of CCP. A group of calcium concretions (microspheres) is lying between unaltered bundles of collagen fibrils. Primary magnification × 2900; for final enlargement see scale

References

1. Benson GS, McConnell J, Lipshultz LI, et al. (1980) Neuromorphology and neuropharmacology of the human penis. J Clin Invest 65:506–1513
2. Bossart MI, Spjut HJ, Scott FB (1980) Ultrastructural analysis of human penile corpus cavernosum. Urology 15:448–456
3. Bruns RR (1984) Beaded filaments and long-spacing fibrils: relation to the type VI collegen. J Ultrastr Res 89:136–145
4. Gelbard M (1982) The disposition and function of elastic and collagenous fibers in the tunic of the corpus cavernosum. J Urol 128:850–851
5. Goldstein AMB, Meehan JP, Zakhary R, et al. (1982) New observations on microarchitecture of corpora cavernosa in man and possible relationship to the mechanism of erection. Urology 20:259–266
6. Goldstein AMB, Morrow JW, Meehan JP, et al. (1984) Special microanatomical features surrounding the intracorpora cavernosa nerves and their probable function during erection. J Urol 132:44–46

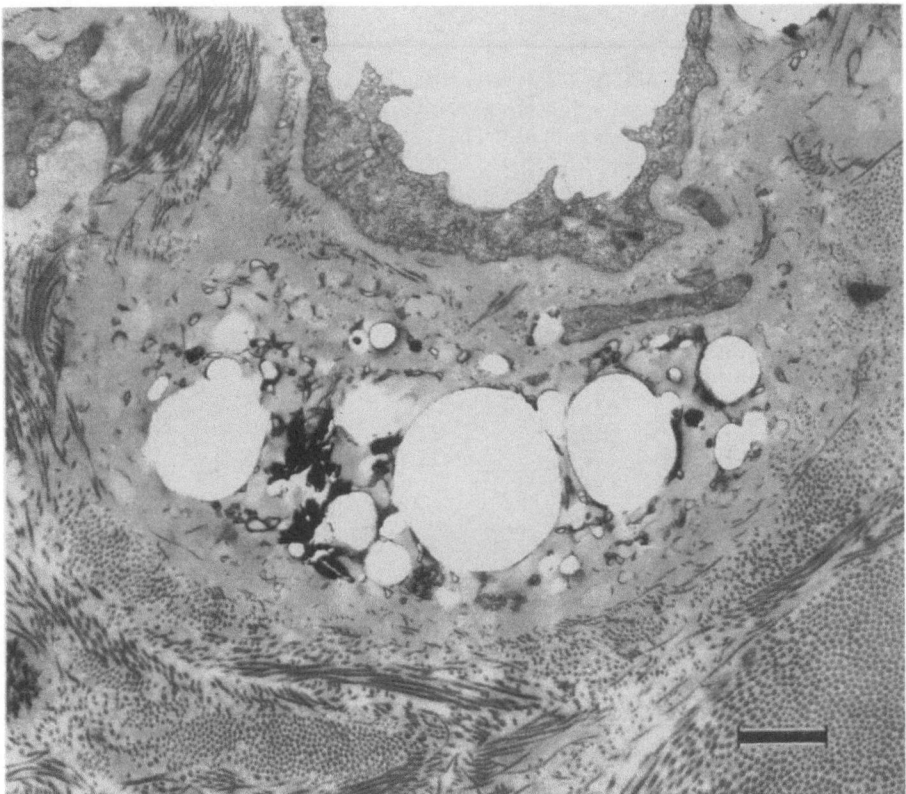

Fig. 2b. Blood lacuna from the middle of CCP. Below the endothelium at the top of the picture: a larger collection of calcium concretions (calcium microspheres – the calcium has mostly been washed out during the preparation). Primary magnification × 5100; for final enlargement see scale

7. Jeremy JY, Mikhailidis DP, Dandona P (1986) Muscarinic stimulation of prostacyclin synthesis by the rat penis. Eur J Pharmacol 123:67–71
8. Lue TF, Takamura T, Schmidt RA, et al. (1983) Hemodynamics of erection in the monkey. J Urol 130:1237
9. Luse SA (1960) Electron microscopic studies of brain tumors. Neurology 10:881–905
10. Ottesen B, Wagner G, Virag R, Fahrenkrug J (1984) Penile erection: possible role for VIP as a neurotransmitter. Br Med J 288:9
11. Saenz de Tejada I, Goldstein I, Blanco R (1985) Smooth muscle of the corpora cavernosa: role in penile erection. Surg Forum 36:623
12. Saenz de Tejada I, Goldstein I, Azadzoi K, et al. (1989) Impaired neurogenic and endoethelium-mediated relaxation of penile smooth muscle from diabetic men with impotence. New Engl J Med 320:1025–1030
13. Speiser, W (1987) Das antithrombotische Potential des Gefäßendothels. Hämostaseologie 7:63–72
14. Spycher MA, Hauri D (1986) The ultrastructure of the erectile tissue in priapism. J Urol 135:142–147
15. Staubesand J, Fischer N (1980) The ultrastructural characteristics of abnormal collagen fibrils in various organs. Connect Tissue Res 7:213–217

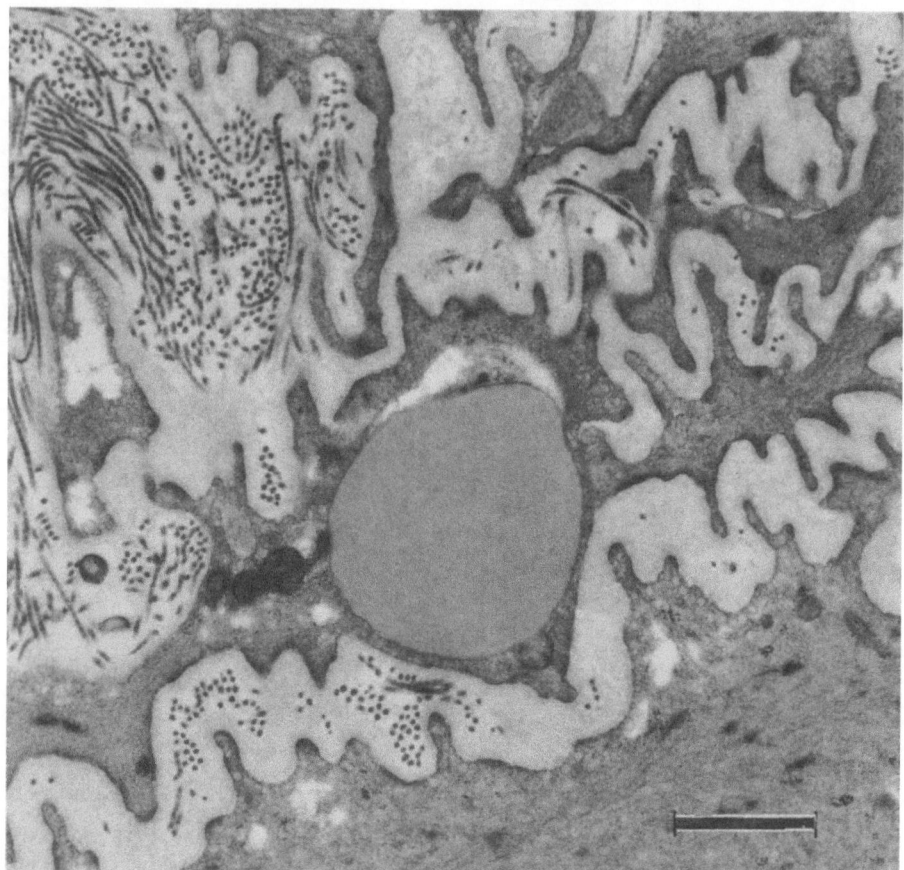

Fig. 3a, b. Immersion fixation showing interstitial smooth muscle cells in patient J.B. aged 65 years and with ED, congenital penile deviation, previous prostatectomy for carcinoma, and cholesterol 308 mg/100 ml

Fig. 3a. Smooth muscle cells from the interstitial tissue of the CCP interdigitating with each other by means of fine processes. A lipid vacuole in one of the cells. Primary magnification ×7100; for final enlargement see scale

16. Staubesand J, Kulvelis F, Wetterauer U (1988) Das Corpus cavernosum penis bei Patienten mit Erektionsstörungen – eine ultrastrukturelle Studie. Verh Anat Ges 83 (Anat Anz Suppl 166):427–428
17. Tudoriu T, Bourmer H (1983) The hemodynamics of erection at the level of the penis and its local deterioration. J Urol 129:741–745
18. Weisel JW (1986) The electron microscope band pattern of human fibrin: various stains, lateral order, and carbohydrate localization. J Ultrastr Mol Res 96:176–188

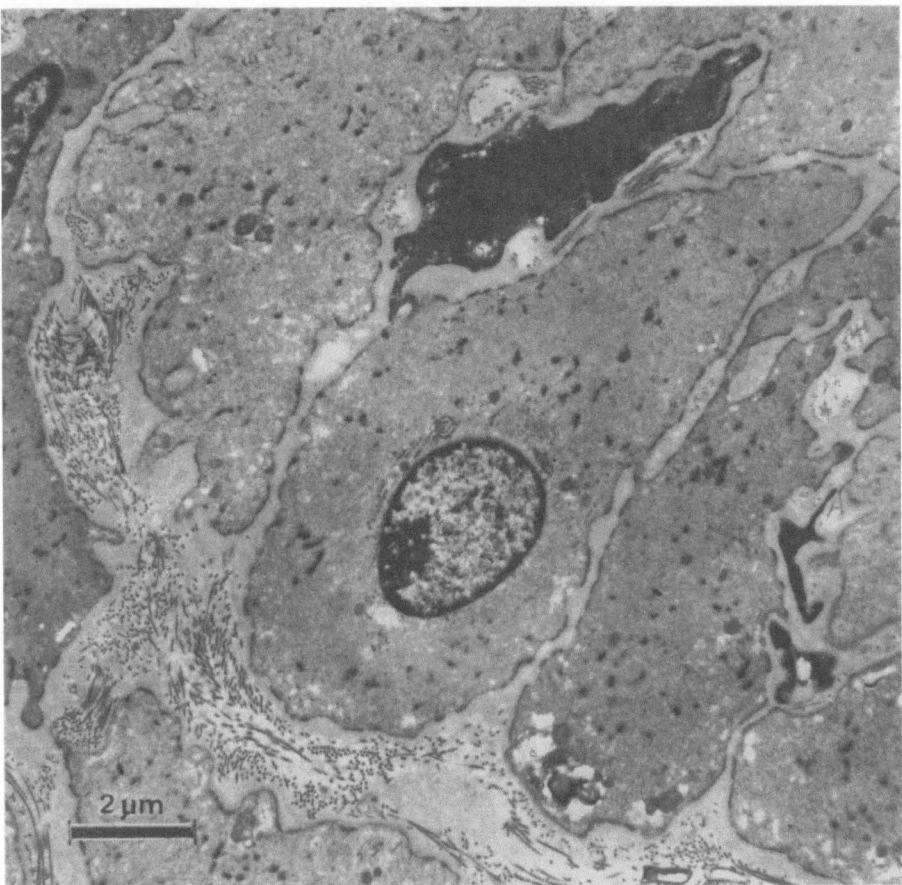

Fig. 3b. Interstitial smooth muscle cells from CCP. A dying cell at the upper border of the figure (osmiophilic shrinkage necrosis). Primary magnification × 2900; for final enlargement see scale

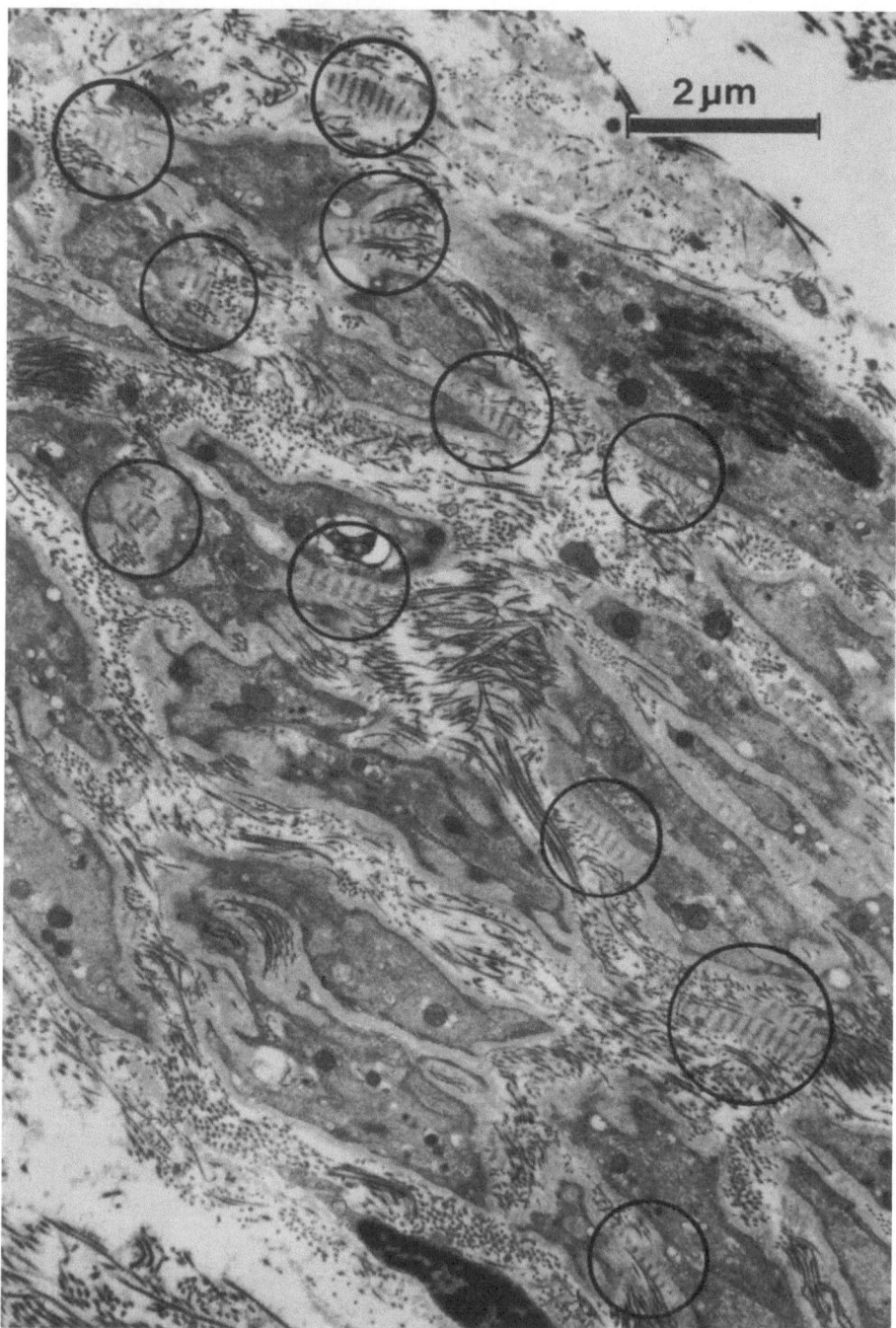

Fig. 4a, b. Immersion fixation performed in two patients showing neural tissue. **a** Patient W.A. aged 41 years and with ED since puberty, smoker (10 cigarettes per day), and venous leakage. Paraneural tissue from the boundary zone between cavernous tissue and the tunica albuginea. Fibrous long-spacing collagen is marked with *circles*. Primary magnification × 3700; for final enlargement see scale

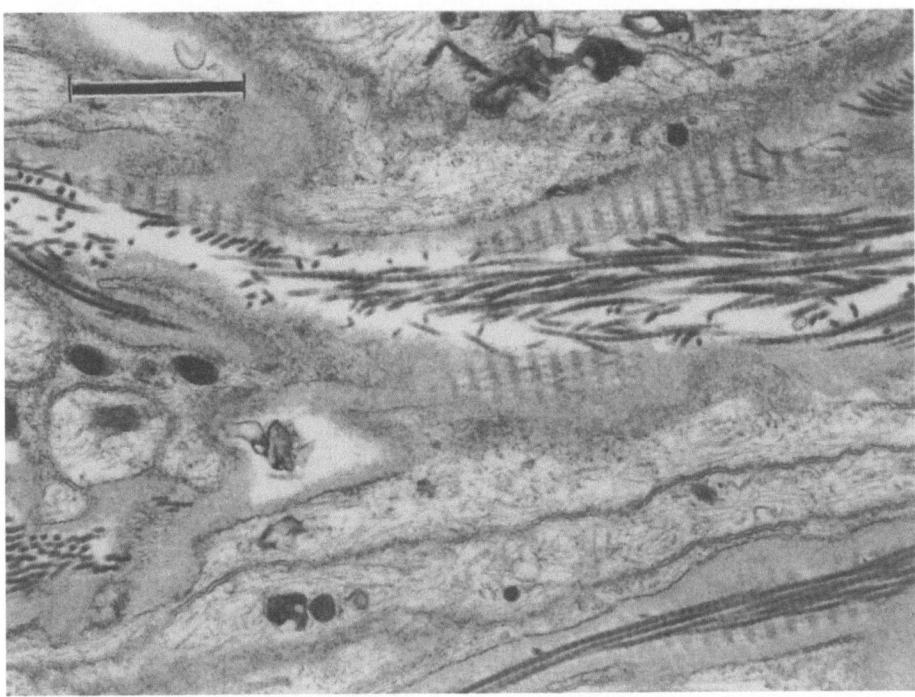

Fig. 4b. Patient A.L. aged 59 years and with ED, diabetes mellitus, and venous leakage. Intracavernous nerve in longitudinal section. Unmyelinated nerve fibers with Schwann cells. In four places (mostly in the immediate neighborhood of the thickened basal membrane), long-spacing collagen can be recognized among the typical collagen fibrils. Its periodicity is approximately twice that of normal collagen; i.e., about 125 nm. Primary magnification × 13 100; for final enlargement see scale (1 μm)

Physiology of Penile Erection

T.F. Lue

Introduction

Better understanding of the physiology of penile erection has been made possible by innovative laboratory and clinical research in the past decade. Penile erection involves psychological, neurological, hormonal, arterial, venous, and sinusoidal factors. Advances in the understanding of these factors have markedly improved the diagnosis and treatment of impotence and the care of tens of thousands of patients with impotence. This chapter will discuss the basic physiology involved in the erectile process.

Vascular Anatomy and Physiology of the Penis

Vascular Anatomy

The penis is composed of three spongy cylinders encased in a fascia sheath (Buck's fascia). The extremely loose penile skin and the subcutaneous connective tissues permit considerable elongation and expansion of the corpora within the coverings. The three cylinders are the paired corpora cavernosa and a single corpus spongiosum. The corpus cavernosum consists of a thick fibro-elastic sheath (tunica albuginea) and spongy erectile tissue. The crura (roots) of the corpora cavernosa arise from the inferior pubic rami and join at the hilum of the penis to form the pendulous portion. A fibrous fascial sheet (suspensory ligament) attaches the hilar portion of the corpora cavernosa to the periosteum of the pubic bone to provide support of the penis. The urethra-containing corpus spongiosum lies in the ventral groove formed by the paired corpora cavernosa. Its expanded proximal portion, the bulb, is attached to the inferior layer of the genitourinary diaphragm. Distally, the corpus spongiosum expands to form a conical mass (the glans penis). The tunica albuginea of the corpus spongiosum is much thinner than that of the corpora cavernosa. At the glans penis, the tunica albuginea is practically absent. The three corpora and the glans penis are composed of multiple blood-filled cavernous spaces (sinusoids) separated by trabeculae of supporting

U. Jonas et al. (Eds.) Erectile Dysfunction
© Springer-Verlag Berlin Heidelberg 1991

connective tissues containing smooth muscles cells, arterioles, venules, and terminal nerve endings. The sinusoids are lined with endothelial cells with possible secretory function, which may be important in the erectile process.

The paired internal pudendal artery, a branch of the hypogastric artery, is usually the main blood supply to the penis. After giving off the perineal artery, the penile artery branches to form the bulbourethral, the dorsal, and the cavernous arteries. The bulbourethral branch supplies the bulb, corpus spongiosum, and the glans to some extent. The paired cavernous artery is primarily responsible for tumescence of the corpora cavernosa and the dorsal artery for engorgement of the glans penis during erection [45]. Accessory pudendal arteries from the external iliac, obturator, or inferior vesical arteries supplying part of the penis are not uncommon. Occasionally, the accessory pudendal artery may be the only blood supply to the corpora cavernosa [5].

The venous drainage from the three corpora originates in tiny venules leading from the peripheral sinusoidal spaces under the tunica albuginea. These venules travel in the trabeculae between the tunica and the peripheral sinusoids for some distance to form the subtunical venular plexus before exiting as the emissary veins [5]. In the mid- and distal shaft, these emissary veins course obliquely through the tunica albuginea. The majority of these veins exit dorsally to join the deep dorsal vein or laterally to the circumflex veins. Some of the emissary veins exit ventrally to join the periurethral veins. In the proximal corpora cavernosa and the crura, these emissary veins empty into the cavernous vein and the crural veins. These veins in turn join the urethral veins to form the internal pudendal vein. Because of the lack of tunica, the sinusoids of the glans penis empty directly into many large and small veins, which form a retrocoronal plexus, the origin of the deep dorsal vein. Along its course, the deep dorsal vein receives several circumflex veins and eventually turns upward behind the pubic bone to become the periprostatic plexus. The superficial dorsal veins are small venous channels in the subcutaneous layer draining the skin and subcutaneous tissue of the penis. The superficial dorsal vein usually empties into the saphenous vein.

Vascular Physiology

Hemodynamics of Penile Erection

The hemodynamics of penile erection have been a controversial subject for a long time. In the nineteenth century, venous occlusion was thought to be the main factor in achieving and maintaining erection [51]. More recent investigators [11, 8, 31, 12] have stressed increased arterial blood flow during erection. Studies of radioactive xenon washout and cavernosography during visual sexual stimulation in volunteers have yielded conflicting results. Shirai et al. concluded that the venous flow is increased, whereas Wagner et al. concluded that the venous flow is decreased during erection. Recent studies in simian and canine models during electrical stimulation of the erection nerves

SIX PHASES OF PENILE ERECTION

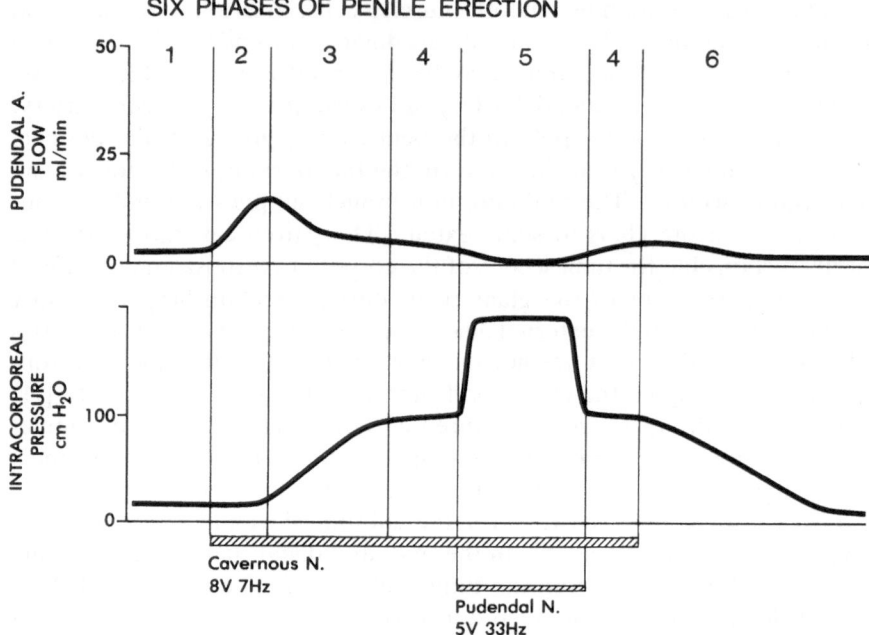

Fig. 1. Six phases of penile erection. (From [28])

and in humans following intracavernous injection of pharmacological agents have clarified some of the controversial issues on the different phases of erection and the blood flow changes. The hemodynamic event can be divided into six phases (Fig. 1) [28]:

1. The flaccid phase. Only a small amount of inflow enters the three corpora and the glans penis due to the high resistance of the penile arterioles and the cavernous smooth muscles.
2. The latent phase. Upon stimulation of the cavernous nerves, there is an immediate increase in flow through the penile artery during both the systolic and diastolic phases. The pressure in the corpora cavernosa remains the same for a period of about 10 s. This is the time of isotonic filling of the cavernous spaces without change of pressure. Some elongation of the penis can be seen in monkeys during this phase, but the penis remains soft.
3. The tumescence phase. The intracavernous pressure begins to increase after the sinusoidal spaces are filled to some degree. The inflow gradually decreases with increasing intracavernous pressure. Rapid expansion and elongation of the penis with increasing turgidity are observed in this phase.
4. The full erection phase. Maximal expansion and elongation are seen in this phase. The intracavernous pressure increases to about 100 mm Hg and the inflow decreases to only slightly above that of the flaccid phase.

5. The rigid erection phase. Stimulation of the pudendal nerve during the full erection phase results in rigid erection of the penis with intracavernous pressure rising to several times higher than systolic blood pressure. Because blood is not compressible and the venous channels are compressed, contraction of the ischiocavernous muscles compresses the proximal corpora and results in high pressure and rigidity of the mid- and distal portion of the penis. This phase is commonly seen during nocturnal erection [19], masturbation, and sexual intercourse from either spontaneous bulbocavernous activity or bulbocavernous reflex.
6. The detumescence phase. During this phase, venous flow increases [49] and arterial flow decreases until the flaccid state is achieved. The penis usually shows pulsatile decrease in length and girth till it is completely flaccid.

Mechanism of Penile Erection

Various theories have been proposed to explain the erection process. These include arterial polsters [48, 20], arterial and venous polsters [9], sluice theory [11], arteriovenous shunt [31, 32, 50], and contraction of the intrinsic cavernous smooth muscles [15]. Conti's hypothesis of arterial and venous polsters regulating the inflow and outflow of the penis is the most commonly cited theory. By fixing the penile tissue in the flaccid state and during erection, researchers have been able to visualize the anatomic changes during this vascular event. Scanning electron microscopic examination of corrosion penile cast obtained by injecting Batson's solution into the internal pudendal artery, corpus cavernosum, and the glans penis confirms the changes of arterial, venous, and sinusoidal systems seen under light microscope. In addition, intracavernous injection of various pharmacological agents known to contract or relax smooth muscles further clarifies the role of the intrinsic cavernous and arterial smooth muscles in erection and detumescence.

Scanning Electron Microscopic Studies [13]. In the flaccid state, the arterioles are constricted and empty directly into the partially collapsed, contracted sinusoids. The terminal portion of the arteries is spiral-shaped. In the erect corpus, the arteries and arterioles become straight and larger, leading to markedly distended smooth appearing sinusoids. The venous system appears as an extensive network of subtunical venules arising from the most peripheral sinusoidal spaces. These venules join to form intermediary venules of about 100 μm in diameter. After traveling in the trabeculae between the sinusoids and the tunica albuginea for some distance, these larger venules join to form the emissary veins which then exit through the tunica albuginea. During erection, the sinusoids are markedly distended, the interconnections among the sinusoids are much larger, and the spaces between the sinusoids, which are occupied by the cavernous erectile tissues, are much thinner. The small venules are no longer identifiable and the larger ones appear flattened.

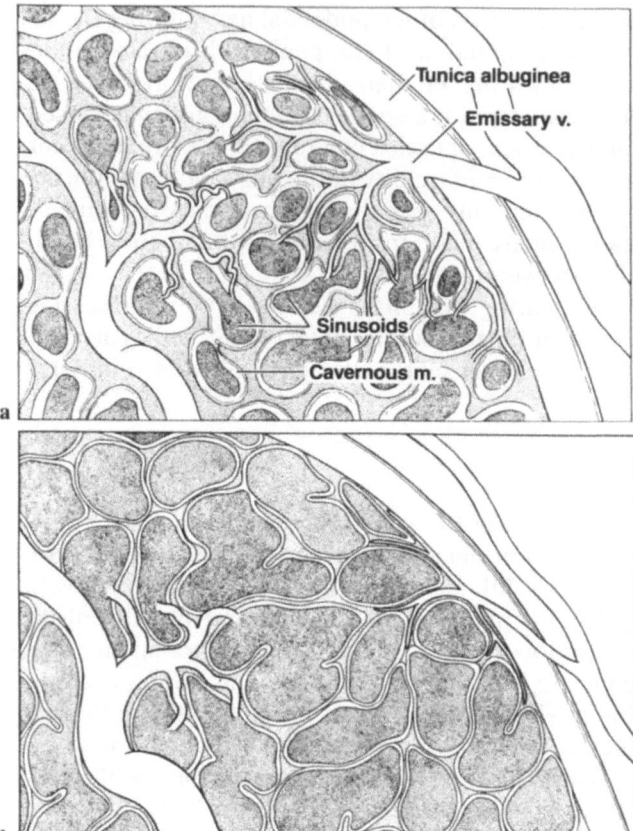

Fig. 2a,b. Mechanism of penile erection. **a** In the flaccid state, the arteries, arterioles and sinusoids are contracted. The intersinusoidal and subtunical venules are open with free flow to the emissary veins. **b** During erection, the muscles of the sinusoidal wall and the arterioles relax, allowing maximal flow to fill the now compliant sinusoidal spaces. The small venules are compressed between sinusoids. The larger intermediary venules are sandwiched and compressed between the distended sinusoidal wall and the noncompliant tunica albuginea thus restrict the venous flow to a minimum. (From [28])

These findings strongly indicate that the subtunical venules are compressed between the sinusoidal walls and the tunica albuginea, thus restricting the venous flow to a minimum during erection (Fig. 2). In addition, the uneven stretching of the layers of the tunica albuginea also contributes to the closure of the emissary veins.

    The sinusoids of the glans penis connect directly to numerous large and small veins, which form the origin of the deep dorsal vein. Due to the lack of tunica albuginea, the glans acts as a large arteriovenous fistula during erection. However, the deep dorsal vein does become partially compressed between the three expanded corpora and the Buck's fascia and contribute to the lesser degree of pressure rise in the dorsal vein and the glans during erection.

Neuroanatomy and Neurophysiology

Neuroanatomy

Autonomic Nervous System

The central erection centers include the septal portion of the hippocampus, the anterior cingulate gyrus, the anterior thalamic nuclei, the mamillothalamic tract, and the mamillary bodies. More specifically, the medial part of the medial dorsal nucleus of the thalamus and the medial preoptic area (MPOA) are probably the most important areas controlling penile erection and sexual drive [29, 41]. There are two spinal centers that are responsible for penile erection: the thoracolumbar and the sacral erection centers. The thoracolumbar center (sympathetic) is located in the intermediolateral gray matter at the T12–L3 levels, whereas the sacral (parasympathetic) center is at the S2–S4 levels [24]. From these nuclei, axons issue ventrally to join the inferior hypogastric and the pelvic plexuses. Nerve bundles from these plexuses innervate the bladder, prostate, rectum, and the penis [24, 51]. The fibers innervating the penis (the cavernous nerves) travel along the posterolateral aspect of the seminal vesicle and the prostate, then penetrate the genitourinary diaphragm. These fibers are located near the lateral aspect of the membranous urethra and ascend gradually to the 1 and 11 o'clock positions to enter the corpora cavernosa with the cavernous arteries and veins. Some of the fibers penetrate the tunica albuginea of the corpus spongiosum. The remaining fibers innervating the distal portion of the corpora cavernosa and spongiosum and glans penis either penetrate the tunica albuginea directly or join the dorsal nerve to be distributed distally. The autonomic nervous system is responsible for the vascular event of penile erection and detumescence.

Somatic Afferent and Efferent Pathways

The sensory component originates in the nerve endings of the glans and penile skin and possibly the corpora cavernosa. These nerve bundles join to form the paired dorsal nerve of the penis. After passing through the genitourinary diaphragm, the dorsal nerve of the penis joins the perineal nerve to form the pudendal nerve. It then travels with the branches of S2–S4 to enter the dorsal roots and the respective spinal segments. The messages from the sensory receptors may pass to the sacral or thoracolumbar erection center to induce reflexogenic erection or travel through the ascending spinal tracts to the thalamus and the brain for sensory perception. This sensory input is also the afferent arm of the bulbocavernous reflex.

The somatic efferent pathway originates in the motor cortex. The impulses are carried via the corticospinal tract to the anterior horn of the S2–S4 segments. The messages are relayed via the anterior sacral roots to the pudendal nerve to innervate the ischiocavernous and bulbocavernosus muscles. Contraction of the ischiocavernous muscle after the corpora have filled with blood produces rigidity of the penis, with the pressure in the corpora cavernosa rising well above the systolic pressure [27]. Rhythmic contraction of the bulbocavernous muscle helps expel the semen from the urethra during ejaculation.

Neurophysiology

Penile erection and detumescence are controlled by smooth muscles of the cavernous trabeculae and the arterioles; this event is probably regulated by the impulses from both the sympathetic and parasympathetic nervous systems. However, the exact neurotransmitters responsible for erection and detumescence are still under investigation. The new concept of noncholinergic and nonadrenergic transmitters that can be synthesized, stored, and released from the same neurons releasing acetylcholine or norepinephrine (cotransmission) makes the issue even more complicated [7, 17].

Cholinergic Mechanism. Acetylcholine is a known transmitter in autonomic ganglia and postganglionic neuroeffector junctions. Recent studies suggest that exogenous acetylcholine may act on vascular endothelium to release the endothelium-derived relaxing factor (EDRF), nitrous oxide (NO), which then acts on the smooth muscles to induce vasodilation [14, 35, 36]. Histochemical studies have identified the existence of cholinergic nerves in the penis of humans and several species of animals. Ultrastructural studies on human penile tissue also confirm neural varicosities containing small, clear vesicles, typical of cholinergic terminals [3]. A recent study by Andersson and coworkers suggested that cholinergic transmission may be responsible for the volume increase of the penis and that a noncholinergic mechanism contributes to the vasodilation. The present literature suggests that acetylcholine may act in concert with other vasodilator transmitters such as EDRF or vasoactive intestinal polypeptide (VIP) and may inhibit the sympathetic transmission (cross talk) [7], thereby effecting smooth muscle relaxation, vasodilation, and penile erection.

Adrenergic Mechanism. Numerous studies have demonstrated the presence of α- and β-adrenergic receptors in penile blood vessels and cavernous smooth muscles [16]. In addition to the α_1-receptors, which mediate the response to norepinephrine released from postganglionic nerve endings, the α_2-receptors, which mediate inhibition of transmitter release from prejunctional nerves, are also shown to exist in the penile tissues. Recent pharmacological studies of inducing penile erection by intracavernous injection of α-adrenergic blocking agents and detumescence by injection of α-adrenergic agents suggest that the adrenergic impulses may be important in detumescence.

Peptidergic Mechanism. Noncholinergic and nonadrenergic input may play an important role in erection and detumescence. Several neuropeptides including VIP [1, 22, 43, 52], substance P, somatostatin, peptide histidine-isoleucine (PHI), enkephalins, calcitonin gene-related peptide (CGRP) [44], and neuropeptide Y [NPY] have been identified in nerves supplying the penile vessels and penile tissue. Due to its prominent vasodilator action, VIP has been studied extensively in recent years. It has been suggested that its relaxation effect on the smooth muscles may be mediated through an increase in cyclic adenosine monophosphate (cAMP), which leads to a reduction in cytosolic calcium concentration and decreased contractility. Acetylcholine and VIP also appear to be localized in the same parasympathetic pathways in the rat penis; they may act as cotransmitters in the penis to promote erection. An other peptide that may have some function in the erectile process is NPY. This is localized in the same nerve endings as norepinephrine, and may be involved in the detumescence process.

Central Neurotransmitters. In the central nervous system, the dopaminergic and adrenergic receptors are responsible for enhancing and the serotoninergic receptors for inhibiting sexual drive [43]. Several substances have been shown to influence sexual behavior in animals or humans. Among these, dopamine, apomorphine (a dopamine agonist), α_2-blocker, yohimbine, and oxytocin are known to enhance sexual activity or induce erection. On the other hand, 5-hydroxytryptamine (5-HT), γ-aminobutyric acid (GABA), and endogenous opioid peptides are inhibitors of sexual activity.

Hormonal Factors

Hormones are essential to regulate the development of male sexual maturity such as gonadotropin secretion, muscle pattern, spermatogenesis, hair growth, acne, and male pattern baldness. In adults, androgen regulates male sexual interest, seminal emission, and possibly frequency and magnitude of nocturnal penile erection. Recent studies have shown that erection in response to visual sexual stimulation is not affected by androgen withdrawal in hypogonadal men, suggesting that androgen enhances but is not essential for penile erection [2, 21].

In animals, loss of libido, erection and ejaculation due to castration can be restored by systemic testosterone administration or injection of testosterone into the medial preoptic anterior hypothalamic area [23, 18]. Autoradiographic studies have also shown that these brain sites accumulate large quantities of testosterone following systemic administration [34, 37]. Hormonal modulation may act in peripheral genital organs as well as nerve cells to affect neuronal activities such as transmitter synthesis, storage, release, re-uptake, and receptor sensitivity [10, 30]. Androgen receptors are also present on neurons in the sacral parasympathetic nucleus and at sites of penile afferent termination in the spinal cord [37] as well as on supraspinal neurons in the hypothalamus and limbic system [34, 37]. It is very likely that these substances may act physiologically at various sites to regulate sexual drive, penile erection, and ejaculation.

Pharmacology of Erection

Recent in vitro and in vivo studies of the effect of pharmacological agents on the penile tissue have revolutionized the diagnosis and treatment of erectile impotence. Agents which have proved to have a relaxing effect on the penile smooth muscle tissues in vitro studies such as papaverine, nitroglycerine, calcium channel blockers, and VIP all induce penile erection when injected into the corpora cavernosa. In addition, the α-blockers such as phentolamine and phenoxybenzamine also induce penile erection after intracavernous injection. On the contrary, the α-adrenergic agonists such as epinephrine, norepinephrine dopamine, metaraminol, phenylephrine, and ephedrine, which contract penile smooth muscles in vitro studies, all cause detumescence when injected into the corpora cavernosa. These pharmacological studies are summarized in Tables 1 and 2 [27].

Of interest is the application of this knowledge to clinical problems in urology. Besides using relaxing agents and α-blockers to induce penile erection for diagnosis and treatment of erectile impotence [6, 25, 26, 40, 46, 47, 53], one can also use these agents to assess the penile deformity and curvature

Table 1. Erection-inducing drugs

Smooth muscle relaxant	papaverine, nitroglycerine
α-Blockers	phentolamine, phenoxybenzamine, moxisylyte
Calcium channel block	verapamil
Peptides	vasoactive intestinal polypeptide
Antidepressant	trazodone
Prostaglandin (PGE)	PGE 1

Table 2. Detumescence-inducing drugs.
(Modified from Lue and Tanagho [27])

Epinephrine
Norepinephrine
Phenylephrine
Dopamine
Metaraminol

in Peyronie's disease and to reassure psychogenic impotent patients of their normal erectile ability. In addition, α-adrenergic agonists such as epinephrine, norepinephrine, phenylephrine, and metaraminol have been used to counteract the priapism induced by papaverine or phenoxybenzamine [27]. These agents are also increasingly being used to treat spontaneously occurring priapisms and unwanted erections during transurethral resection of the prostate under anesthesia. Further study of various pharmacological agents known to cause impotence such as antihypertensives, antipsychotics, and antidepressants is currently underway in some research centers, and will certainly advance our knowledge of the pharmacology of impotence.

Summary

The recent interest and progress in the research of penile physiology has significantly advanced our understanding of this essential human function. Neurologically, neurotransmitters released after stimulation of the cavernous nerves relax the cavernous and arteriolar smooth muscles to initiate the vascular event. Hemodynamically, erection involves increased sinusoidal compliance, arterial inflow, and venous resistance. Expansion of the entire sinusoidal system in a space limited by the tunica albuginea eventually compresses the subtunical venular plexuses and reduces the outflow to a minimum. A few equilibrium is then established with intracavernous pressure of about 100 mm Hg (full erection). Spontaneous or reflex contraction of the ischiocavernous muscle further increases the intracavernous pressure to several times higher than the systolic blood pressure (rigid erection). Meanwhile, the recent research in pharmacology and the introduction of intracavernous injection of vasoactive agents have also revolutionized the diagnosis and treatment of erectile impotence.

Continuing research into the central mechanism, oral medications, and changes of the nerves, arteries, and cavernous erectile tissues in aging patients and in patients with various diseases may further change our understanding of the pathophysiology and improve treatment for millions of impotent men in the not so distant future.

References

1. Andersson PO, Bloom SR, Mellander S (1984) Haemodynamics of pelvic nerve induced penile erection in the dog: possible mediation by vasoactive intestinal polypeptide. J Physiol 350:209
2. Bancroft J, Wu FCW (1983) Changes in erectile responsiveness during androgen therapy. Arch Sex Behav 12:59
3. Benson GS, McConnell J, Lipschultz LI et al. (1980) Neuromorphology and neuropharmacology of the human penis. J Clin Invest 65:506
4. Bochdalex V (1854) Ergebnisse über einen bis jetzt übersehenen Teil des Erektionsapparates des Penis und der Clitoris. Vierteljahrschr Prakt Heilkunde 43:115
5. Breza J, Aboseif SR, Orvis BR, Lue TF, Tanagho EA (1989) Detailed anatomy of penile neurovascular structures: surgical significance. J Urol 141:437–443
6. Brindley GS (1983) Cavernosal alpha-blockade: a new technique for investigating and treating erectile impotence. Br J Psychiat 143:332
7. Burnstock G (1986) The changing face of autonomic neurotransmission. Acta Physiol Scand 126:67
8. Christensen GC (1954) Angioarchitecture of the canine penis and the process of erection. Am J Anat 95:227
9. Conti G (1952) L'erection du penis humain et ses bases morphologico-vasculaires. Acta Anat 14:217
10. Crowley WR, Zelman FP (1981) The neurochemical control of mating behavior. In: Adler NT (ed) Neuroendocrinology of reproduction, physiology and behavior. Plenum Press, New York
11. Deysach LJ (1939) Comparative morphology of erectile tissue of penis with especial emphasis on probable mechanism of erection. Am J Anat 64:111
12. Dorr L, Brody M (1967) Hemodynamic mechanisms of erection in the canine penis. Am J Physiol 213:1526
13. Fournier GR Jr, Juenemann KP, Lue TF et al. (1987) Mechanism of venous occlusion during canine penile erection: an anatomic demonstration. J Urol 137:163
14. Furchgott RF (1984) The role of endothelium in the responses of vascular smooth muscle to drugs. Ann Rev Pharm Toxicol 24:175
15. Goldstein AMB, Meehan JP, Zakhary R et al. (1982) New observations on the microarchitecture of the corpora cavernosa in man and possible relationship to mechanism of erection. Urology 20:259
16. Hedlund H, Andersson KE (1985) Comparison of the responses to adrenoceptor and muscarinic receptor active drugs in isolated human corpus cavernosum and cavernous artery. J Auton Pharmacol 5:81
17. Hokfelt T (1979) Nonadrenergic, noncholinergic autonomic neurotransmission mechanisms. Neurosci Res Prog Bull 17:424
18. Johnston P, Davidson JM (1972) Intracerebral androgens and sexual behavior in the male rat. Horm Behav 3:345
19. Karacan I, Aslan C, Hirschkowitz M (1983) Erectile mechanism in man. Science 220: 1080
20. Kiss F (1921) Anatomisch-histologische Untersuchungen über die Erektion. Z Anat 61:455
21. Kwan M, Greenleaf WJ, Mann J et al. (1983) The nature of androgen action on male sexuality: a combined laboratory and self report study in hypogonadal man. J Clin Endocrinol Metab 57:557
22. Larsen JJ, Ottesen B, Fahrenkrug J et al. (1981) Vasoactive intestinal polypeptide (VIP) in male genitourinary tract, concentration and motor effect. Invest Urol 19:211
23. Lisk RD (1967) Neural localization for androgen activation of copulatory behavior in the male rate. Endocrinology 80:754
24. Lue TF, Zeineh SJ, Schmidt RA et al. (1984) Neuroanatomy of penile erection: its relevance to iatrogenic impotence. J Urol 131:273

25. Lue TF, Hricak H, Marich KW et al. (1985) Vasculogenic impotence evaluated by high-resolution ultrasonography and pulsed Doppler spectrum analysis. Radiology 155:777
26. Lue TF, Hricak H, Schmidt RA et al. (1986) Functional evaluation of penile veins by cavernosography in papaverine-induced erection. J Urol 135:479
27. Lue TF, Tanagho EA (1987) Physiology of erection and pharmacologic management of impotence. J Urol 137:829
28. Lue TF (1988) Male sexual dysfunction. In: Tanagho EA, McAninch JW (eds) Smith's General Urology, 12th edn. Appleton & Lange, Norwalk, Conn, Chap 37, pp 663–678
29. MacLean PD, Denniston RH, Dua S (1963) Further studies on cerebral representation of penile erection: caudal thalamus, midbrain, and pons. J Neurophysiol 26:274
30. McEwen BS (1981) Neural gonadal steroid actions. Science 211:1303
31. Newman HF, Northrup JD, Devlin J (1964) Mechanism of human penile erection. Invest Urol 1:351
32. Newman HF, Northrup JD (1981) Mechanism of human penile erection: an overview. Urology 17:399
33. Polak JM, Gu J, Mina S et al. (1981) Vipergic nerves in the penis. Lancet II:217
34. Rees HD, Michael RP (1982) Brain cells of the male rhesus monkey accumulate ^{3}H-testosterone or its metabolites. J Comp Neurol 206:273
35. Saenz de Tejada I, Blanco R, Goldstein I et al. (1985) Cholinergic neurotransmission in human penils corpus cavernosum smooth muscle. Fed Proc 236:454
36. Saenz de Tejada I, Cohen RA (1987) Human corpus cavernosum smooth muscle relaxation to acetylcholine is an endothelium mediated response. J Urol 137:184A
37. Sar M, Stumpf WE (1977) Androgen concentration in motor neurons of cranial nerves and spinal cord. Science 197:77
38. Shirai M, Ishii N, Mitsukawa S et al. (1978) Hemodynamic mechanism of erection in the human penis. Arch Androl 1:345
39. Shirai M, Ishii N (1981) Hemodynamics of erection in man. Arch Androl 6:27
40. Sidi AA, Cameron JS, Duffy LM et al. (1986) Intracavernous drug-induced erections in the management of male erectile dysfunction: experience with 100 patients. J Urol 135:704
41. Slimp JC, Hart BL, Goy RW (1978) Heterosexual, autosexual and social behavior of adult male rhesus monkeys with medial preopticanterior hyothalamic lesions. Brain Res 142:105
42. Steers WD, McConnell J, Benson G (1984) Anatomical localization and some pharmacological effects of vasocative intestinal polypeptide in human and monkey corpus cavernosum. J Urol 132:1048
43. Steers WD (1990) Neural control of penile erection. Semin Urol 8:66–79
44. Stief CG, Benard F, Bosch RJLH, Aboseif SR, Lue TF, Tanagho, ET (1990) A possible role of calcitonin-gene-related peptide in the regulation of the smooth muscle tone of the bladder and penis. J Urol 143:392–397
45. Tanagho EA, Lue TF (1990) Physiology of penile erection. In: Chisholm G, Fair WR (eds) Scientific foundations in urology, 3rd edn. Year Book, Chicago, pp 420–426
46. Virag R (1982) Intravenous injection of papaverine for erectile failure. Letter to the Editor. Lancet II:938
47. Virag R, Frydman D, Legman M (1984) Intravenous injection of papaverine as a diagnostic and therapeutic method in erectile failure. Angiology 35:79
48. Von Ebner V (1900) Über klappenartige Vorrichtungen in den Arterien der Schwellkörper. Anat Anz 18:79
49. Wagner G (1981) Erection, physiology and endocrinology. In: Wagner G, Green R (eds) Impotence: physiological, psychological, and surgical diagnosis and treatment. Plenum Press, New York, Chap 2, pp 25–26
50. Wagner G, Bro-Rasmussen F, Willis EA et al. (1982) New theory on the mechanism of erection involving hitherto undescribed vessels. Lancet 1:416
51. Walsh PC, Donker PJ (1982) Impotence following radical prostatectomy: insight into etiology and prevention. J Urol 128:492

52. Willis E, Ottsen B, Wagner G et al. (1981) Vasoactive intestinal polypeptide (VIP) as a possible neurotransmitter involved in penile erection. Acta Physiol Scand 113:547
53. Zorgniotti AW, Lefleur RS (1985) Auto-injection of the corpus cavernosum with a vasoactive drug combination for vasculogenic impotence. J Urol 133:39

Neuropharmacology of Penile Erection In Vitro

G. Wagner

Introduction

In vitro studies are defined as studies of biologic processes made to occur outside the body in an artificial environment. This may involve cultivating cells, metabolic and/or kinetic studies, or recording electrical and mechanical activity. The clear advantage of having a piece of isolated tissue is that a series of naturally occurring humoral factors can be ruled out and a controlled situation obtained. However, the natural activity of the tissue may only be *assumed* to be present, as acute denervation and sudden disappearance of normal circulation are difficult factors to evaluate. It is well known that tissue which has been removed and placed in an artificial medium needs a certain time to recover or equilibrate to the new situation. Often, one medium is used for transportation and a second for the actual study of the functions.

Compared with other tissues in the body, few in vitro studies have been performed using penile tissue. In those that have been performed, mechanical activity of the trabecular smooth muscle of animals and man has been most widely studied and the trabecular tissue of the corpus spongiosum has been studied to a lesser extent. Even fewer in vitro studies have been devoted to the penile artery. Studies of individual cells and their membrane potential and of the functional connection between cells do not seem to have been undertaken, most attention having been paid to pharmacological intervention and the effect of given substances on mechanical activity. There have also been very few kinetic and metabolic studies.

Regulation of Muscle Activation

The degree of activation (or deactivation) of a smooth muscle cell is related to a series of stimuli, quite unlike striated muscle, which is solely controlled by nervous regulation. These regulatory mechanisms include:

1. *Neural regulation* functions due to the release of chemical transmitters which are intimately related to the cells at the nerve terminals (Fig. 1). Not all cells, but rather groups of cells are innervated.

U. Jonas et al. (Eds.) Erectile Dysfunction
© Springer-Verlag Berlin Heidelberg 1991

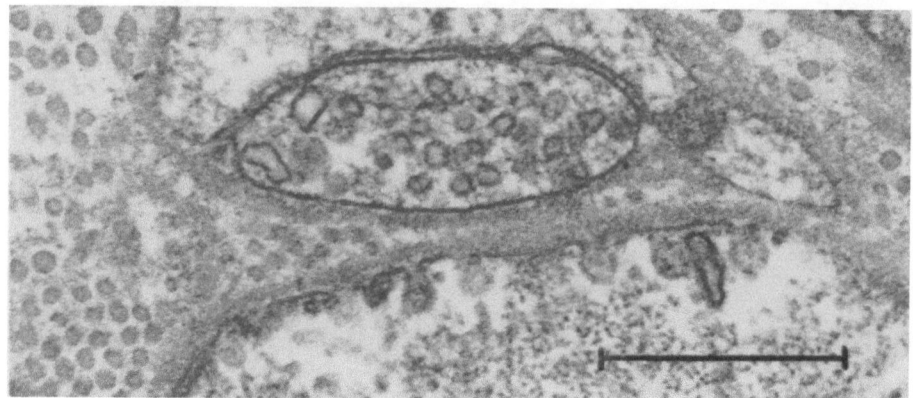

Fig. 1. Electron micrograph showing small nerve terminal adjacent to a smooth muscle cell of corpus cavernosum. Bar: 0.5 µm. (From Schmalbruch & Wagner [27])

2. *Various hormones* activate smooth muscles in general, but it does not seem to be a physiological regulatory mechanism of any importance in penile smooth muscle.
3. *The ionic composition* of the fluid phases surrounding the smooth muscle cells exerts an influence upon them.
4. *Myogenic tonus* is a characteristic feature of smooth muscle. It can be seen when the muscle is loaded, thereby developing more force, or when it responds with a contraction if a fast pull is exerted. The spontaneous activity (which may be regular or irregular) is another characteristic of most smooth muscles.

Calcium

As in striated muscle, the cytoplasmic concentration of free calcium (Ca_i^{2+}) is the key mechanism of contraction within the cells of smooth muscle. Unlike striated muscle, however, the smooth muscle is also dependent on the presence of external calcium, as an induced contraction can only be maintained for a few minutes in a calcium-free medium. The quick, contractile response (1 ms) of striated muscle cells is due to a fast delivery of calcium to the contractile filaments, exclusively from the sarcoplasmic reticulum. By contrast, smooth muscle cells have to transport calcium across the cell membrane and thereby have a considerably slower response (several seconds).

The control of intracellular calcium is undertaken by several different processes, not all of which are completely understood. Figure 2 shows in schematic form that two major pathways for calcium influx exist; one channel system is sensitive to changes in the membrane potential (potential sensitive

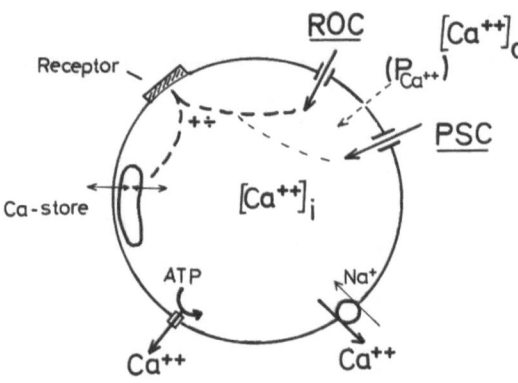

Fig. 2. Schematic presentation of smooth muscle cell with calcium pathways. *POC*, receptor operated channel; *PSC*, potential sensitive channel

channel, PSC) and another channel system is operated by the receptor systems (receptor operated channel, ROC). If depolarization of the membrane occurs, the PSC will open and allow an influx of calcium, which, in turn, initiates a contraction. Conversely, if hyperpolarization occurs, this will prevent calcium from entering the cell. The receptor activation, when initiated by a transmitter, may act in either an enhancing or an inhibitory way on the calcium influx through the ROC, but it may also be able to activate calcium directly from the intracellular calcium stores. A third way in which the receptor complexes may act is by changing the permeability of other ion channels, thereby creating a depolarization, and thus activating the ROC.

Intracellular mechanisms can prevent the tendency of the intracellular concentration to increase, by uptake partly into the sarcoplasmic reticulum and partly into the mitochondria. The most important mechanism in most vascular smooth muscle tissue seems to be a calcium efflux across the plasma membrane, primarily by means of a calcium pump running on ATP hydrolysis and to a lesser extent by means of a sodium-calcium exchange system.

Methods of In Vitro Studies

From these considerations, it is clear that there are many different possible approaches of interfering with the contractile state of the smooth muscle, but also that isolated tissue will lose its natural external controls. This phenomenon has to be accepted when attempting to extrapolate from in vitro experimental results to an in vivo situation.

Mechanical Activity

In vitro *mechanical activity* is recorded by preparing a muscle strip and extending it between two points, one of which is connected to a recording

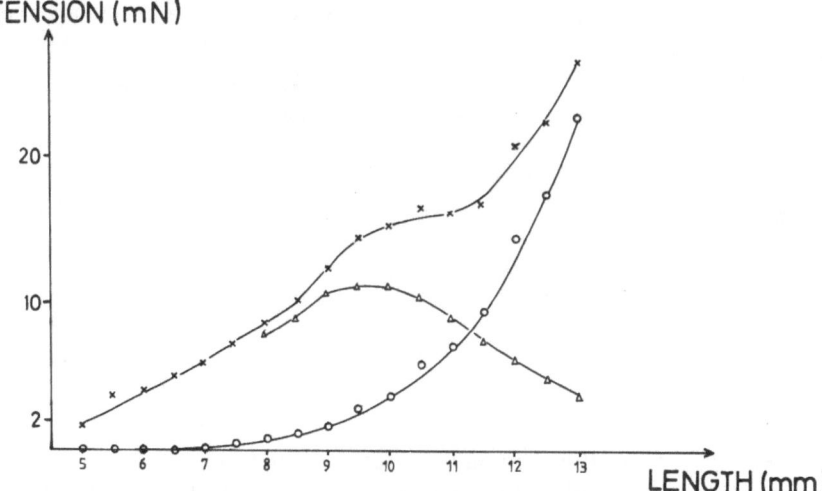

Fig. 3. Length-tension diagram of smooth muscle tissue strip from porcine corpus cavernosum. *Crosses* indicate tension during maximum contraction elicited by supramaximal electrical field stimulation. *Circles* indicate tension developed by stretching the unstimulated tissue, and *triangles* indicate the calculated tension developed by active contraction of the tissue at different lengths

device for isotonic or isometric contractions. The feasibility of using either of these two types of contraction for pharmacological evaluation has only been discussed in one publication, which maintains that the results of both methods are similar [1]. It is not easy to decide which state is the most natural for the muscle cell. In situ the cells most likely alternate between a relaxed, unloaded state and a contracted, shortened state during flaccidity, while the state during erection would be a loaded (passively stretched), relaxed one, changing to isometric contraction during the early phase of detumescence.

These different situations may produce quite different results in induced tension of the muscle when maximally provoked by a chemical substance. Figure 3 shows the result of an experiment performed with a muscle strip from porcine corpus cavernosum to establish curves for resting and maximally contracted states at different lengths. As the length is increased, passive tension gradually develops from zero. At each length increment, a supramaximal electrical stimulus was applied to obtain a contraction, and the actively developed tension was established. From such studies the optimal length of a given strip can be determined and expressed as the length to which the muscle has to be stretched in order to give maximum tension when stimulated. The length will correspond to a degree of tension which is dependent on the cross-sectional area of the muscle strip. Most investigators stretch their preparations to a length which provides a passive tension of 5–10 mN, which would be quite close to the optimal length shown in the example in Fig. 3.

Spontaneous rhythmic activity is quite often recorded when human corporeal tissue is placed in organ bath solution. Adaikan notes that 50% of his specimens exert this activity [1], while other authors note less [2] or more [3] frequency in this respect. In bovine tissue, spontaneous activity is almost always present. It is of interest to note that Sjöstrand and Klinge described rhythmic oscillations in penile volume with the same periodicity as the rhythmic contractions in isolated tissue [4].

Electrical Activity

Applying the sucrose gap method to bovine tissue, phasic penile retractor muscle contractions were associated with electrical firing [5]. Similarly, in vitro studies using cavernous tissue and external wires to record, electrical potential changes occurred during spontaneous contractions [6, 7].

In vivo recording in animals as well as in human [8–10], also points in this direction, although it is not possible to determine what is myogenic activity and what is due to nervous regulation in the intact organism. Both in vitro and in vivo, the electrical activity is abolished by smooth muscle relaxing compounds [9, 11].

Adrenergic Regulation

Extensive basic pharmacological studies of the retractor muscle and penile artery in bulls and of the corpus cavernosum in a series of other domestic animals were undertaken in the 1970s by Klinge and Sjöstrand [3, 4, 12]. In the late 1970s, the human corpus cavernosum was thoroughly described by Adaikan [1], and Hedlund and coworkers contributed with elegant experimentation in studies of human cavernosal tissue and human penile artery conducted from 1983 to 1985, in which they also applied the newly described and synthesized neurotransmitters [2, 13–16]. All these comprehensive and other individual studies [17–19] substantiate the adrenergic system as the principal system controlling contraction. As clear a dose-dependent, contractile response is evoked by norepinephrine in doses of 10^{-7}–10^{-5} M as is prevented by α-adrenoceptor blocking agents. The density of α-receptors has been evaluated as ten times that of the β-receptors. Only 10% of the total α-receptor population was of the α_2-type [20].

The α_1-adrenoceptor agonist, phenylepiphrine, and the α_2-adrenoceptor agonist, clonidine, both have a contractile effect as well, but their relative potency varies among studies by different authors [2, 21, 22] (Wagner, unpublished results; Fig. 4). However, when these compounds were tested with human cavernous artery, Hedlund and Andersson found clonidine to be more potent than norepinephrine and that the α-adrenoceptor blocking agents prazosin (α_1) and rauwolscine (α_2) had about the equal relaxant effects on norepinephrine stimulation, indicating that α_2-adrenoceptors dominate

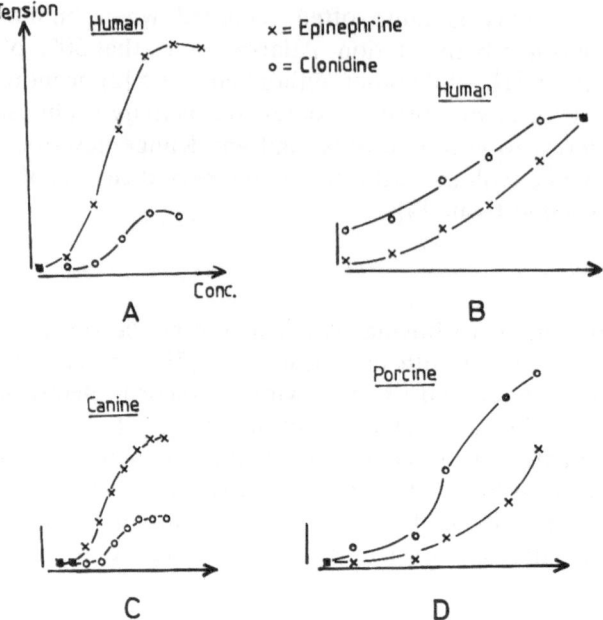

Fig. 4. Four dose-response curves from four different authors (*A*, [16]; *B*, [21]; *C*, [22]; *D*, [23]) comparing the contractile effect of noradrenline (*crosses*) and clonidine (*circles*)

in the cavernous artery [2]. It is obviously important to appreciate these differences as the development of a rational clinical treatment for a pharmacologically induced, prolonged erection is based on the knowledge acquired from in vitro studies, as indicated above.

A newly developed α_1-adrenoceptor antagonist (YM 12617) has been shown to have a more potent blocking action than prazosin and to be more selective for α_1- than for α_2-adrenoceptors in mesenteric and pulmonary arteries and in the lower urinary tract and prostate of rabbits [23, 24]. YM 617, which is an isomer of YM 12617, had been found to be even more potent and selective. This compound was tested in porcine and human cavernosal tissue and found to be effective in blocking norepinephrine response and in relaxing tissue which had been precontracted with norepinephrine at concentrations of 10^{-6}–10^{-8} *M* and even as low as 10^{-17} *M* in a few specimens [23]. Spontaneous activity was not influenced by YM 617 as is the case when other α-blocking agents are administered (Fig. 5).

Cholinergic Regulation

Although in vivo experiments stimulating nerves to provoke erections have been performed since the nineteenth century, the transmission system and

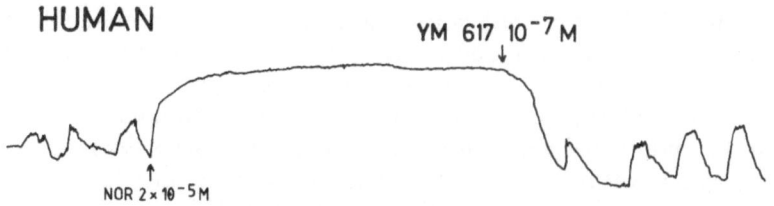

Fig. 5. Isolated human corpus cavernosum strip exhibits spontaneous contractions, contracts when noradrenaline is applied, and relaxes when YM 617 is added to the bath. Spontaneous activity is not effected

the chemical substances involved in this process are still under debate. The traditional hypothesis that acetylcholine (Ach) is the transmitter has been challenged by many reports and indeed disproved by in vivo experiments on animals and humans. These experiments demonstrated that atropine (local or systemic) is ineffective in preventing normal or electrically induced erection.

Klinge and Sjöstrand found that the penile retractor muscle and the penile artery (both from bulls) gave three different responses to Ach: contraction, suppression of nerve stimulation, or contraction followed by pronounced relaxation [12]. Adaikan found that 60% of the strips tested slowly relaxed, while 25% of the strips tested contracted [1]. In later experiments, neither Benson et al. nor Hedlund and Andersson could confirm these findings [18, 2]. The latter demonstrated that in muscle precontracted with norepinephrine Ach had a potent relaxant action which could be blocked by scopolamine. This provided evidence that the effect was mediated by muscarinic receptors. Furchgott's observation that the endothelial cells lining the lumen of vascular structures act as intermediates to a relaxatory response was an important contribution to the understanding of Ach's possible effect as a neuroeffector of the release of a postulated endothelial-derived relaxatory factor (EDRF) [25]. It has since been suggested that this factor is NO. When the endothelial cells were removed, Ach was rendered ineffective in vascular tissue. This observation led Saenz de Tejada and coworkers to study whether similar mechanisms were present in the corpus cavernosum and to repeat some of Hedlund's experiments [26].

In their study, the cavernosal muscle strips were mechanically rubbed between two fingers for 20 s and thereby denuded of their endothelial lining. Such strips responded normally to norepinephrine, but the relaxation effect caused by Ach disappeared. This observation was interpreted to demonstrated that, as with other vascular structures, the endothelium lining of the lacunar spaces is required for the relaxation induced by exogenous Ach. One might assume that if this were to occur as part of a normal physiological process, a system to regulate it would be necessary. The observation by Schmalbruch and Wagner of nerve terminals very close to the endothelial cells might indicate the morphological basis of such a nervous regulation of

the endothelium [27]. Further studies by Blanco et al. on Ach metabolism revealed that human corporeal tissue incubated with labeled choline could synthesize Ach [28]. It cannot be deduced from these experiments whether both the synthesis and the release of Ach during field stimulation were derived from the endothelial lining or from the smooth muscles themselves.

Endothelin is a novel family of endothelium derived peptides [29] which seem to be predominantly of vasoconstrictor nature (see [30] for review). A recent study by Saenz de Tejada et al. indicates that endothelin mRNA is expressed in cultures of endothelial cells derived from human corpus cavernosum [31]. A high receptor affinity to plasma membranes was found and a dose-dependent contraction of human corpus cavernosal muscle strips was demonstrated. The effect was long lasting, but could be reversed by Ach. These findings have been confirmed by Holmquist et al., who also demonstrated that vasoactive intestinal polypeptide (VIP) was able to relax strips precontracted with endothelin. [32].

The observations that the endothelium may be intimately involved in the contractile regulation of the smooth muscle of the penis give rise to speculations as to pathological developments affecting the normal function of these cells lining the smooth muscles. It seems extremely complicated to solve, as most in vitro studies using human tissue are undertaken either on completely normal tissue (rarely) or on tissue which is supposedly damaged. Moreover, these studies are not conducted in any well-defined manner, whether from cadavers or from biopsies taken during surgery directed at restoring erectile function. Hence studies of animal models creating lesions of the endothelium in a well-defined way seem to be of utmost importance if the development of local pathology preventing normal function of the penile smooth muscle is to be understood.

VIP and neuropeptide Y (NPY) have both been identified in cavernosal smooth muscle and in the vasculature inside and outside the tunica albuginea [33, 34]. In vitro studies of the effect of VIP show a decrease in tone, abolition of spontaneous activity, and a reduction in the amplitude of cell tissue which has been precontracted with norepinephrine tissue cell at concentration levels of 10^{-8}–10^{-6} M, clearly indicating a relaxatory postsynaptic effect, since it is not affected by the neurotoxin tetrodotoxin (TTX) [6, 14, 35, 36].

Both NPY and VIP have recently been shown to be localized in the cavernous tissue and in the helicine arteries [27]. The physiological significance of NPY in erection has not been clearly defined, since the studies of Hedlund and Andersson on human smooth muscle and in penile artery as well as our own observations in porcine smooth muscle could not demonstrate any effect of NPY in concentrations of up to 10^{-3} M [14, 23]. In a recent study, Kirkeby et al. found that at a concentration of at 10^{-6} M two of eight test strips taken from normal human corpus cavernosum contracted by up to 20% of the tension developed in contractions induced by a high potassium concentration, while the other six strips were unaffected [37]. Thus the role of NPY in relation to erectile function seems obscure.

Histamine

In their early study on the effect of histamine in the penile artery and retractor muscle of bulls, Klinge and Sjöstrand [12] found histamine to contract the tissue, while Adaikan and Karim [38] and Adaikan [1] were able to demonstrate a varied response: either contraction, relaxation, or contraction followed by relaxation. By applying specific H_1- or H_2-receptor agonists, it was demonstrated that stimulating H_2-receptors mainly caused relaxation, and stimulating H_1-receptors always caused contraction. The H_2-receptor blocking agent, cimetidine, prevented the relaxation, a phenomenon which has also been reported clinically. Kirkeby et al. saw no effect of histamine in unstimulated preparations, but demonstrated a relaxatory effect in norepinephrine precontracted tissue [39]. This effect was not blocked by cimetidine. Again, the results of in vitro experiments with a naturally occurring compound are conflicting.

Prostanoids

Different prostaglandins (PG) were tested by Klinge and Sjöstrand demonstrating a contractile effect of $PGF_{2\alpha}$ and a relaxatory effect of PGE_1 [3]. These findings were confirmed in studies on human tissue by Adaikan, who also showed that the PG synthetase inhibitors produced inhibition of spontaneous activity and decreased the resting tone [1]. In 1984, Roy et al. showed that human corpus cavernosum muscle could generate PG and thromboxanes in vitro, suggesting that arachidonate cascade products might be of importance in controlling erectile function [40]. Hedlund and Andersson found that $PGF_{2\alpha}$ contracted human penile artery and corpus cavernosum, and that PGE_1 was an effective relaxatory agent in both tissues [15]. PGI_2 exerted a contractile response in the smooth muscle of the trabecular tissue, but markedly relaxed arterial segments precontracted by norepinephrine or $PGF_{2\alpha}$. PGI_2 was later tested in an animal model in vivo and was found not to increase cavernosal arterial blood flow [41]. However, the clinical usefulness of PGE_1, which was shown to be effective in vitro, is now widespread [42].

Calcium Channel Blockers and Potassium Channel Openers

Studies of calcium channel blockers on isolated corpus cavernosum tissue have shown that nifedipine, verapamil, and diltiazam could all abolish the contractions induced by a high external potassium concentration, and, to a certain extent, a blocking effect of the electrically induced contractions was observed [43]. A new series of compounds called potassium channel openers (pinacidil or chromakalin) are effective vasodilators and used clinically in the treatment of hypertension [44]. Two studies have shown them to have a clear depressant effect upon spontaneous activity and that tissue precontracted with norepinephrine is relaxed by potassium channel blockers [45, 46].

The variety of compounds which are effective in altering the mechanical state of the penile smooth muscle gives ample opportunity for intellectual exercises in search of a way that clinically leads to a rational and secure way of pharmacological intervention.

References

1. Adaikan PG (1979) Pharmacology of the human penis. PhD Thesis, University of Singapore, Singapore, pp 1–213
2. Hedlund H, Andersson K-E (1985) Comparison of the responses to drugs acting on adrenoceptors and muscarinic receptors in human isolated corpus cavernosum and cavernous artery. J Auton Pharm 5:81
3. Klinge E, Sjöstrand NO (1977) Comparative studies of some isolated mammalian smooth muscle effectors of penile erection. Acta Physiol Scand 100:354
4. Sjöstrand NO, Klinge E (1979) Principal mechanisms controlling penile retraction and protrusion in rabbits. Acta Physiol Scand 106:199
5. Samuelson U, Sjöstrand NO, Klinge E (1983) Correlation between electrical and mechanical activity in myogenic and neurogenic control of the bovine retractor penis muscle. Acta Physiol Scand 119:335
6. Wagner G (1989) Vasoactive polypeptide et erection. Contracept Fert Sexualite 17:1049
7. Wagner G, Sjöstrand NO (1988) Autonomic pharmacology and sexual function. In: Sitsen JMA (ed) The pharmacology and endocrinology of sexual function. Elsevier, Amsterdam, p 32 (Handbook of sexology, vol 6.)
8. Wagner G, Gerstenberg T (1988) Human in vivo studies of electrical activity of corpus cavernosum (EACC). J Urol 139:327A
9. Wagner G (1988) Electrical activity of the corpus cavernosum: Functional and pharmacological perspectives. In: Proceedings of the Third Biennial World Meeting on Impotence. International Society of Impotence Research, Boston, p 7
10. Wagner G, Gerstenberg T, Levin RJ (1989) Electrical activity of corpus cavernosum during flaccidity and erection of the human penis: a new diagnostic method? J Urol 142:723
11. Stief CG, Bischoff WF, Thon U, Wetterauer A, Kramer E, Seidl E, Jonas U (1990) The diagnosis of neurogenic (autonomic) impotence; single potential analysis of cavernous electrical activity. J Urol 143:246A
12. Klinge E, Sjöstrand NO (1974) Contraction and relaxation of retractor penis muscle and the penile artery of the bull. Acta physiol Scand [Suppl] 420:1–88
13. Andersson K-E, Hedlund H, Mattiasson A, Sjögren C, Sundler F (1983) Relaxation of isolated human corpus spongiosum induced by vasoactive intestinal polypeptide, substance P, carbachol and electrical field stimulation. World J Urol 1:203
14. Hedlund H, Andersson K-E (1985) Effects of some peptides on isolated human erectile tissue and cavernous artery. Acta Physiol Scand 134:1245–1250
15. Hedlund H, Andersson K-E (1985) Contraction and relaxation induced by some prostanoids in isolated human penile erectile tissue and cavernous artery. J Urol 134:1245

16. Hedlund H (1985) Receptor functions in human prostate, vas deferens and penile erectile tissues. Doctoral thesis, University of Lund, Lund, Sweden, pp 1–155
17. Melman A, Henry D (1979) The possible role of the catecholamines of the corpora in penile erection. J Urol 121:419
18. Benson GS, McConnell JA, Lipschite LI (1980) Neuromorphology and neurophysiology of the human penis. J Clin Invest 65:506
19. Wein AJ, Arsdalen KV, Levin RM (1983) Adrenergic corporal receptors. In: Krane RJ, Siroky MB, Goldstein I (eds) Male sexual function. Little Brown, Boston, p 33
20. Levin RM, Wein AJ (1979) Quantitative analysis of alpha and beta adrenergic receptor densities in the lower urinary tract of the dog and the rabbit. Invest Urol 17:75
21. Kimura K, Kawanishi Y, Tamura M, Imagawa A (1989) Assessment of the alpha-adrenergic receptors in isolated human and canine corpus cavernosum tissue. Int J Impotence Res 1 [3/4]:189
22. Lin JS-N, Yu P-C, Yang MCM, Kuo J-S (1989) Detumescent effect of clonidine on penile erection. Int J Impotence Res 1 [3/4]:201
23. Fujii K, Kuriyama H (1985) Effects of YM-12617, an *alpha* adrenoceptor blocking agent, on electrical and mechanical properties of the guinea-pig mesenteric and pulmonary arteries. J Pharmacol 235:764
24. Honda K, Nakagawa C (1986) *Alpha*-1 adrenoceptor antagonist effects of the optical isomers of YM-12617 in rabbit lower urinary tract and prostate. J Pharmacol 239:512
25. Furchgott FR (1983) Role of endothelium in response of vascular smooth muscle. Circ Res 5:557
26. Saenz de Tejada I, Blanco R, Goldstein I, Azadzoi K, de las Morenas A et al (1988) Cholinergic neurotransmission in human corpus cavernosum. I. Responses of isolated tissue. Am J Physiol 254:459
27. Schmalbruch H, Wagner G (1989) Vasoactive intestinal polypeptide (VIP)- and neuropeptide Y (NPY)-containing nerve fibres in the penile cavernous tissue of green monkeys (Cercopithecus aethiops). Cell Tissue Res 256:529
28. Blanco R, Saenz de Tejade I, Goldstein I, Krane RJ, Wotiz HH, Cohen RA (1988) Cholinergic neurotransmission in human corpus cavernosum, II. Acetylcholine synthesis. Am J Physiol 254:468
29. Yanagisawa M, Kurihara H, Kimura S, Tomobe Y, Kobayashij N, Mitsui Y et al. (1988) Nature 332:411–415
30. Le Monnier de Gouville A-C, Lippton HL, Cavero I, Summer WR, Hyman AL (1989) Endothelin – A new family of endothelium-derived peptides with widespread biological properties. Life Sci 45:1499
31. Saenz de Tejada I, Carson MP, Traish A, Eastman EH, Goldstein I (1989) Role of endothelin, a novel vasoconstrictor peptide in the local control of penile smooth muscle. J Urol 141:222A
32. Holmquist F, Andersson K-E, Hedlund H (1900) The effect of endothelin on isolated penile erectile tissue from rabbit and man. J Urol 143:144A
33. Larsen JJ, Ottesen B, Fahrenkrug J, Fahrenkrug L (1981) Vasoactive intestinal polypeptide (VIP) in the male genitourinary tract, concentration and motor effect. Invest Urol 19:211
34. Ottesen B, Wagner G, Sundler F, Fahrenkrug J (1981) Vasoactive intestinal polypeptide (VIP) as a possible neurotransmitter involved in penile erection. Acta Physiol Scand 113:545
35. GU J, Polak JM, Probert KN, Islam PJ, Marangos PJ, Mina S, Adrian TE et al (1983) Peptidergic innervation of the human male genital tract. J Urol 130:386
36. Willis EA, Ottesen B, Wagner G, Sundler F, Fahrenkrug J (1983) Vasoactive intestinal polypeptide (VIP) as a putative neurotransmitter in penile erection. Life Sci 33:383
37. Kirkeby HJ, Jörgensen J, Ottesen B (1990) Neuropeptide Y (NPY) in human penile corpus cavernosum tissue and circumflex veins. Occurrence and in vitro effects. J Urol (in press)
38. Adaikan PG, Karim SMM (1977) Effects of histamine on the human penis muscle in vitro. Eur J Pharmacol 45:261

39. Kirkeby HJ, Forman A, Sörensen S, Andersson K-E (1989) Effects of noradrenaline, 5-hydroxytryptamine and histamine on human penile cavernous tissue and circumflex veins. Int J Impotence Res 1:181
40. Roy AC, Tan SM, Kottegoda ST, Ratnam SS (1984) Ability of human corpora cavernosa muscle to generate prostaglandins and thromboxanes in vitro. IRCS Med Sci 12:608
41. Bosch RJLH, Benard F, Aboseif SR, Stief CG, Stackl W, Lue TF et al (1989) Changes in penile hemodynamics after intracavernous injection of prostaglandin E_1 and prostaglandin I_2 in pigtailed monkeys. Int J Impotence Res 1:211
42. Jünemann K-P, Alken P (1989) Pharmacotherapy of erectile dysfunction: a review. Int J Impotence Res 1/2:71
43. Fovaeus M, Andersson K-E, Hedlund H (1987) Effects of some calcium channel blockers on isolated human penile erectile tissues. J Urol 138:1267
44. Weston AH, Abbot A (1987) New class of antihypertensive acts by some opening K^+-channels. Trends Pharmacol Sci 8:283
45. Holmquist F, Andersson K-E, Fovaeus M, Hedlund H (1988) K^+ channel openers for relaxation of penile erectile tissue. In: Proceedings of the Third Biennial World Meeting on Impotence. International Society of Impotence Research, Boston, p 148
46. Giraldi A, Wagner G (1988) The effect of K^+-channel opener pinacidil upon porcine, simian and human corpus cavernosum. In: Proceedings of the Third Biennial World Meeting on Impotence. International Society of Impotence Research, Boston, p 159

Investigations into the Innervation
of the Corpora Cavernosa Penis

J. Staubesand

The introduction of pharmacological agents into the corpora cavernosa penis (CCP) for the treatment of erectile dysfunction, which was started a few years ago, has now become a generally accepted procedure. It has also led to a great deal of physiological and pharmacological research [1, 3, 10], the results of which have shown that an extremely complicated interplay between the autonomic nervous system and smooth muscle cells in the CCP is necessary to produce an erection. In this paper I wish to describe two new additional characteristics of the innervation of the CCP.

The above-mentioned (primarily pathomorphologically motivated) examination of operative material has revealed that nerve fibers – either singly or lying together to form plexuses – are to be found in the immediate neighborhood of the endothelium both of the vascular spaces and of the blood vessels supplying the erectile tissue. Generally speaking, the autonomic fibers, with few exceptions, reach only to the outer border of the tunica media [5, 11, 13]. We could confirm this neuroendothelial contact, first observed in human material (Fig. 2), in other species; namely, the monkey (Fig. 1), rabbit, and rat.

The short distance from the endothelial cells (Figs. 1, 2) may either influence the interaction between the endothelium and myocytes, or carry impulses to the latter directly, or both [6, 10, 12, 14]. Certain morphological peculiarities of these nerve fibers and their occasionally plexiform appearance might also suggest that they are afferent. The majority of axon terminals contain cholinergic (and sometimes also adrenergic and peptidergic [7]) vesicles, many of these are agranular and some granular in appearance (Figs. 1b, 2b). However, the actual nature of the neural transmitter [1, 9, 10] can only be unequivocally established by immunohistochemistry.

The second departure from the expected relationships concerns the innervation of the smooth muscles of the CCP. The neural effectors of smooth muscle cells are usually between 100 nm and 2 µm from the cell, noticeably further than the synaptic distance of the motor endplates of striated muscle. Most of the exceptions which have been described (and which remind one of true synaptic distance; i.e., between 40 and 100 nm) are found in the smooth muscle of the iris [4], vas deferens, bladder, and certain blood vessels [8]. The majority of distances significantly below 100 nm seen in the CCP were found in monkeys (Fig. 3). Not so many neuromyocytic

U. Jonas et al. (Eds.) Erectile Dysfunction
© Springer-Verlag Berlin Heidelberg 1991

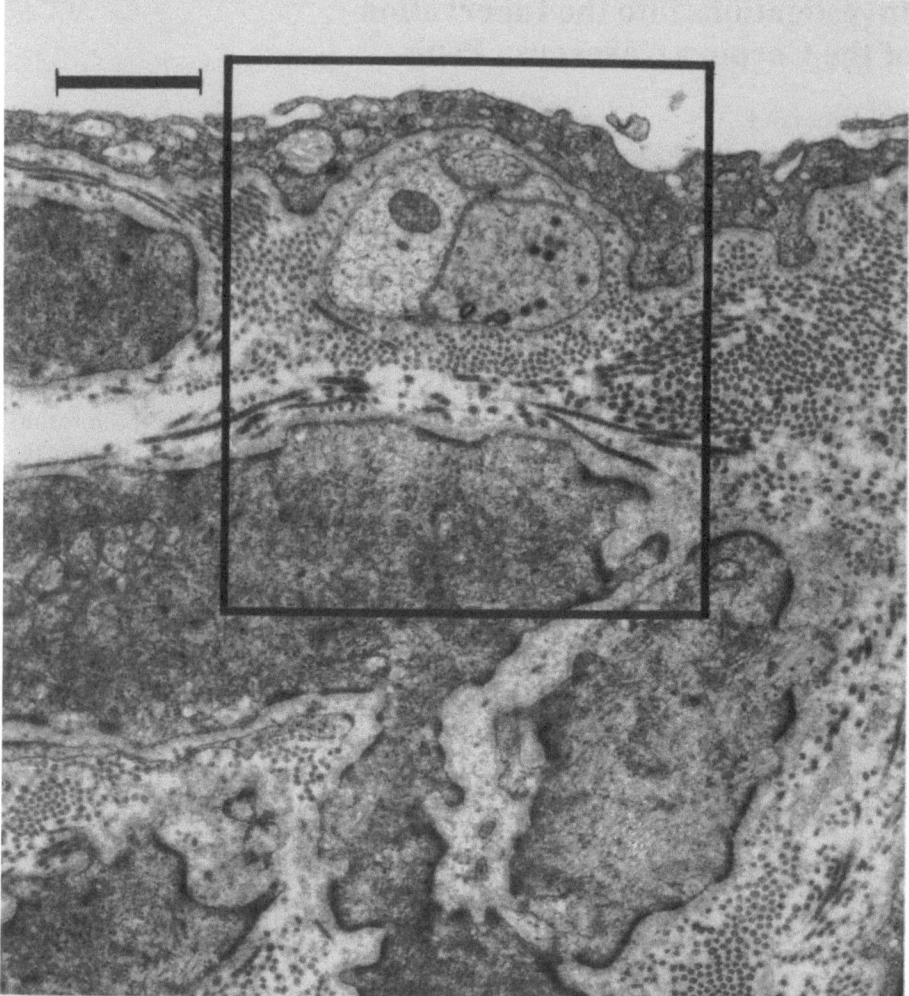

Fig. 1a. Perfusion-fixed CCP of a monkey (*Cercopithecus aetheops*) aged 4 years. The lumen of a vascular space is seen at the top of the figure, showing the typically flat edge of the endothelial cells; in the subendothelium, three axons can be seen, and, below these, smooth muscle cells. Primary magnification ×4800; for final enlargement see scale (= 1 μm)

contacts could be demonstrated in human tissue (Fig. 4). This difference in frequency is not necessarily due, however, to any species difference; for obvious reasons, the human tissue specimens came from the periphery of the CCP, whereas the animal material included the central part of the erectile tissue.

Although it may be accepted that the predominant type of innervation found in the CCP is concerned with the musculature, and therefore relatively widespread and representing a slow path, there are grounds [3] for assuming

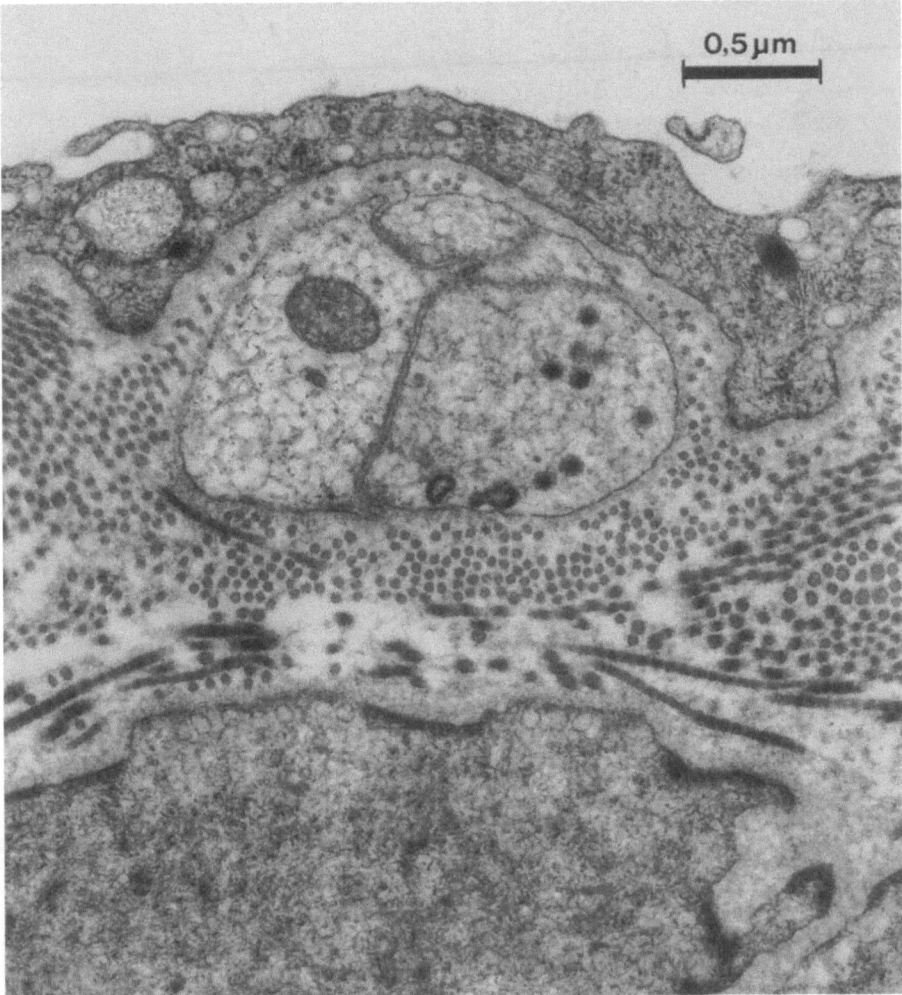

Fig. 1b. Enlargement of area marked in Fig. 1a. Endothelial cell with basement membrane near upper border of figure; notice axons with many small agranular vesicles (probably cholinergic), a few granular vesicles (probably adrenergic) and one mitochondrion. Primary magnification ×13 000; for final enlargement see scale

that the "faster" myocytes are essentially significant as "pacemakers" during the initial phase of erection. The observed coincidence of neuroendothelial and neuromuscular contacts seems to be somewhat unusual.

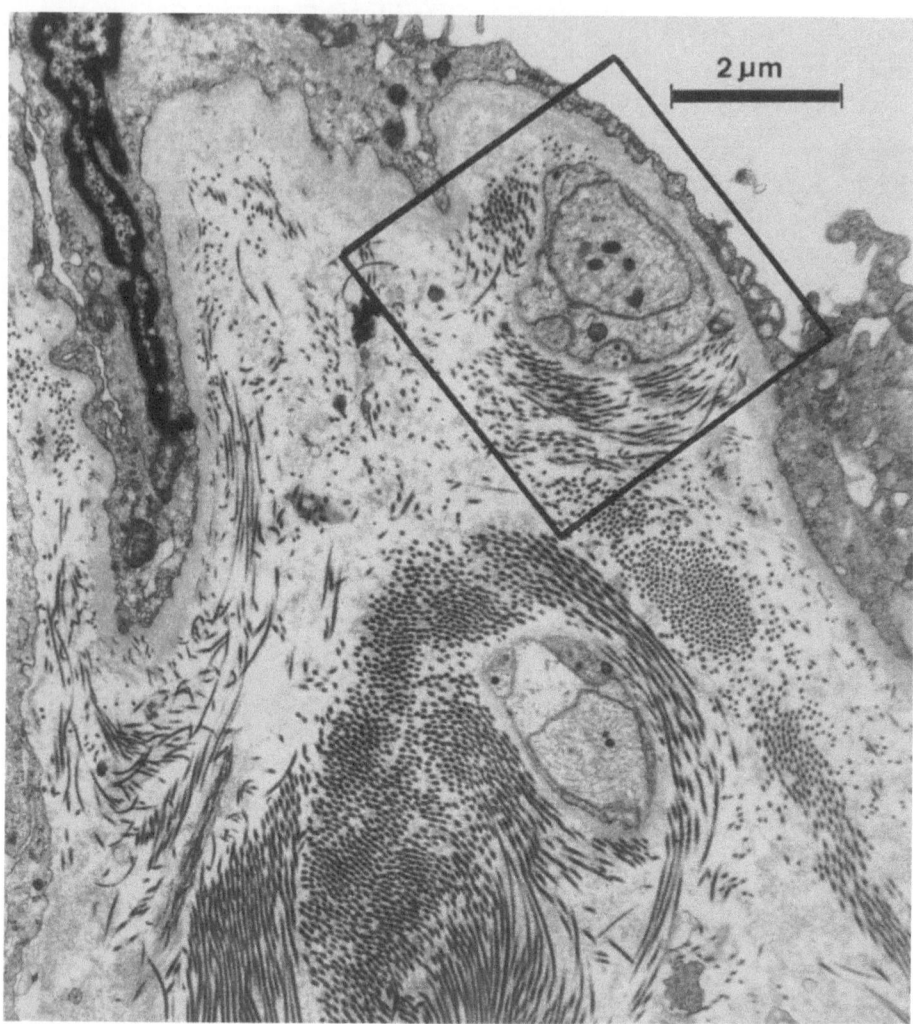

Fig. 2a. Immersion-fixed biopsy of a patient (N.G.) aged 19 years (clinical diagnosis was venous leak). Three unmyelinated nerve fibers lying together within a single Schwann cell can be seen beneath the endothelium of a blood sinus. The outline of the enlargement (see Fig. 2b) is indicated. Primary magnification ×3700; for final enlargement see scale

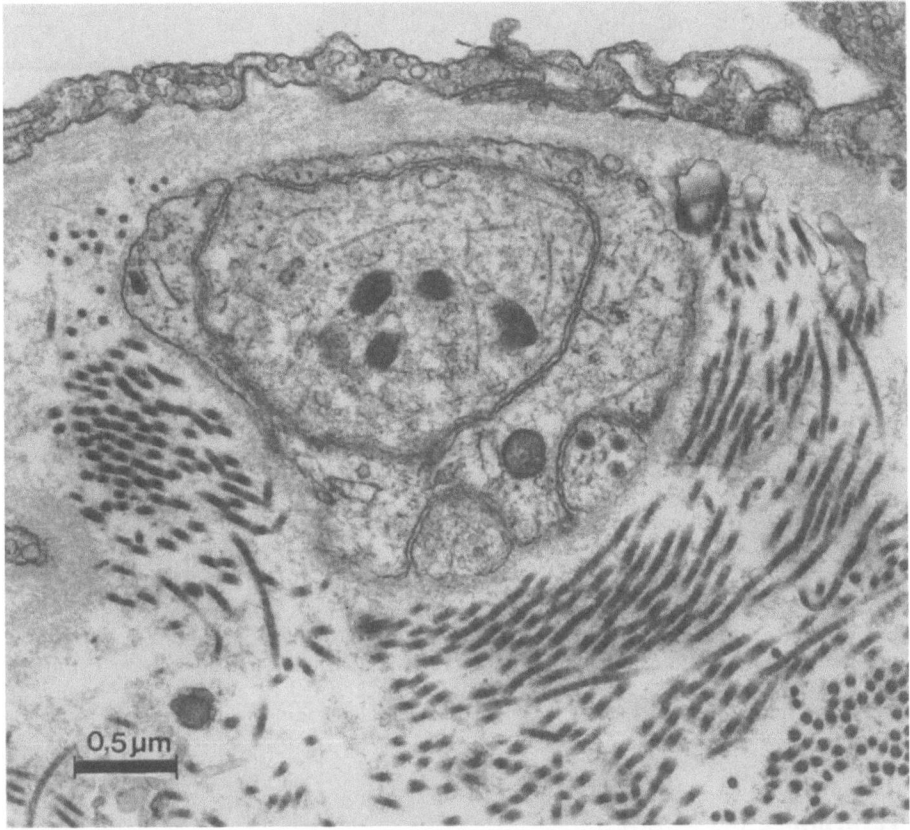

Fig. 2b. Enlargement of area marked in Fig. 2a. Primary magnification × 1300; for final enlargement see scale

Summary

With a view to clarifying the problem of erectile dysfunction, the CCP have been examined in man, the rabbit, the rat, and the monkey (Cercopithecus aetheops). Subendothelial autonomic nerve fibers, either single or lying together in a plexiform arrangement, have been found near the endothelium of the vascular spaces of the CCP. Many agranular and some granular vesicles containing the neurotransmitters can be seen in the axon terminals. Direct short-distance connections can be observed lying in gutters formed by the plasma membranes of some of the interstitial muscle cells, and it is suggested that these cells may be "pacemakers" which come into play during the early stages of erection.

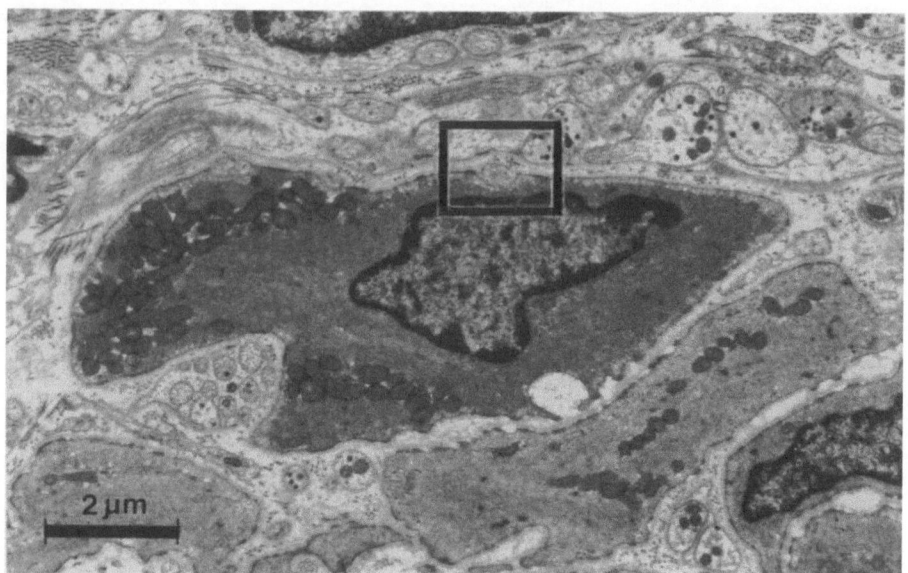

Fig. 3a. Perfusion-fixed CCP in a monkey (*Cercopithecus aetheops*) aged 4 years. In the center, a mitochondrion-rich, strikingly osmiophilic smooth muscle cell. The myocyte is surrounded in a very unusual manner by nerve fibers on nearly all sides. Near the upper boundary of the cell, three exceptionally closely packed naked axons can be seen. The outline of the enlargement (see Fig. 3b) is indicated. Primary magnification × 3700; for final enlargement see scale

References

1. Adaikan PG, Karim SMM, Kottegoda SR, Ratnam SS (1983) Cholinoreceptors in the corpus cavernosum muscle of the human penis. J Auton Pharmacol 3:107–111
2. Colquhoun D, Ogden DC, Mathie A (1987) Nicotinic acetylcholine receptor of nerve and muscle: functional aspects. TIPS 8:465–472
3. Dail WG, McGuffee L, Minorsky N, Little S (1987) Responses of smooth muscle strips from penile erectile tissue to drugs and transmural nerve stimulation. J Auton Pharmacol 7:287–293
4. Dietrich HJ, Fischer G, Hiller U (1988) The smooth muscle of the iris of the gray parrot. Z Mikrosk Anat Forsch 102:239–250
5. Flöel H, Staubesand J (1978) Neuroendotheliale Kontakte in der Wand großer Venen bei Ratte und Katze; elektronenmikroskopische Befunde. VASA 7:114–118
6. Furchgott RF, Zawadzki JV (1980) The obligatory role of endothelial cells in the relaxation of arterial smooth muscle by acetylcholine. Nature 288:373–376
7. Geiger SR (ed) (1980) The cardiovascular system. Vascular smooth muscle. Oxford University Press, Oxford, p 571 (Handbook of physiology, sect 2, vol II)
8. Luff SE, McLachlan EM (1980) Frequency of neuromuscular junctions on arteries of different dimensions in the rabbit. Guinea pig and rat. Blood Vessels 26:95–106
9. Rand MJ, McCulloch MW, Story DF (1980) Catecholamine receptors on nerve terminals. In: Szekeres L (ed): Adrenergic activators and inhibitors, Springer, Berlin Heidelberg New York (Handbook of experimental pharmacology, vol 54, part 1)
10. Saenz de Tejada I, Blanco R, Goldstein I, et al. (1988) Cholinergic neurotransmission in human corpus cavernosum. Responses of isolated tissue. Am J Physiol 254:459–467

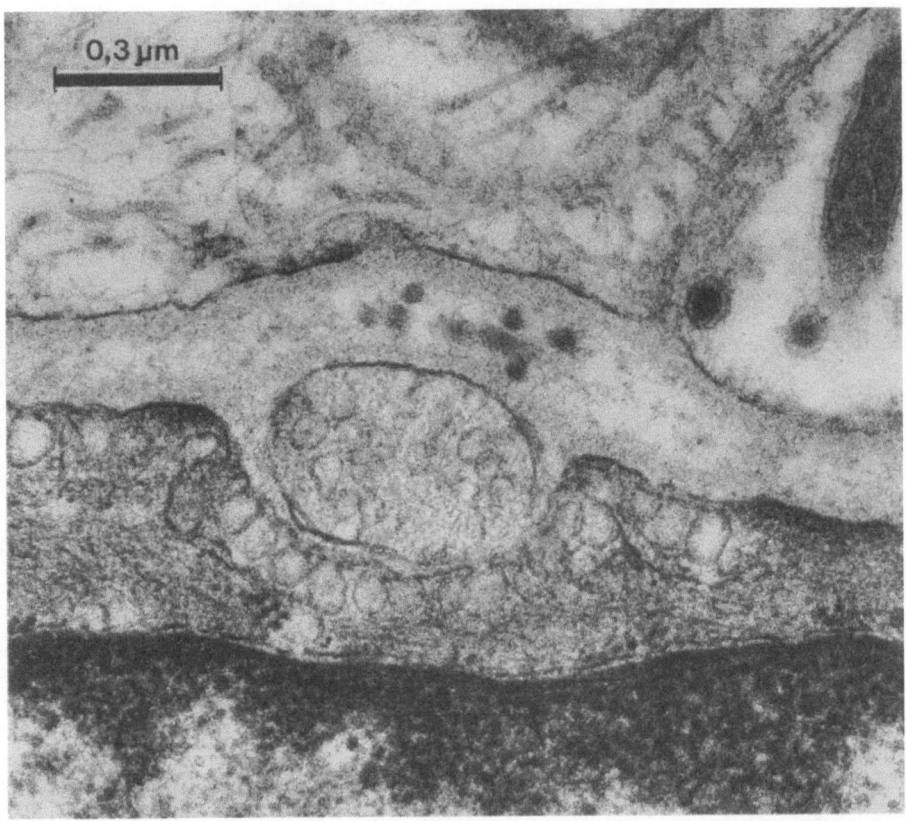

Fig. 3b. Enlargement of area marked in Fig. 3a. In the center, a very close synapse-like neuromuscular connection can be seen. The axon – containing small, agranular (probably cholinergic) vesicles – in a gutter formed by the infolding of the cytoplasmic membrane of the myocyte. Primary magnification × 24 000; for final enlargement see scale

11. Staubesand J (1977) Intimale Axone und Transmittersegment in der Mündungsstrecke der V. saphena magna. VASA 6:208–210
12. Sütsch G, Saeed M, Bing RJ (1988) Uncertain role of endothelium-derived relaxing factor in mesenteric arterioles of cats and rabbits. Artery 15:176–191
13. Van der Zypen E (1974) Über die Ausbreitung des vegetativen Nervensystems in den Vorhöfen des Herzens. Acta Anat 88:363–384
14. Vane JR, Gryglewski RJ, Botting RM (1987) The endothelial cell as a metabolic and endocrine organ. TIPS 8:491–496

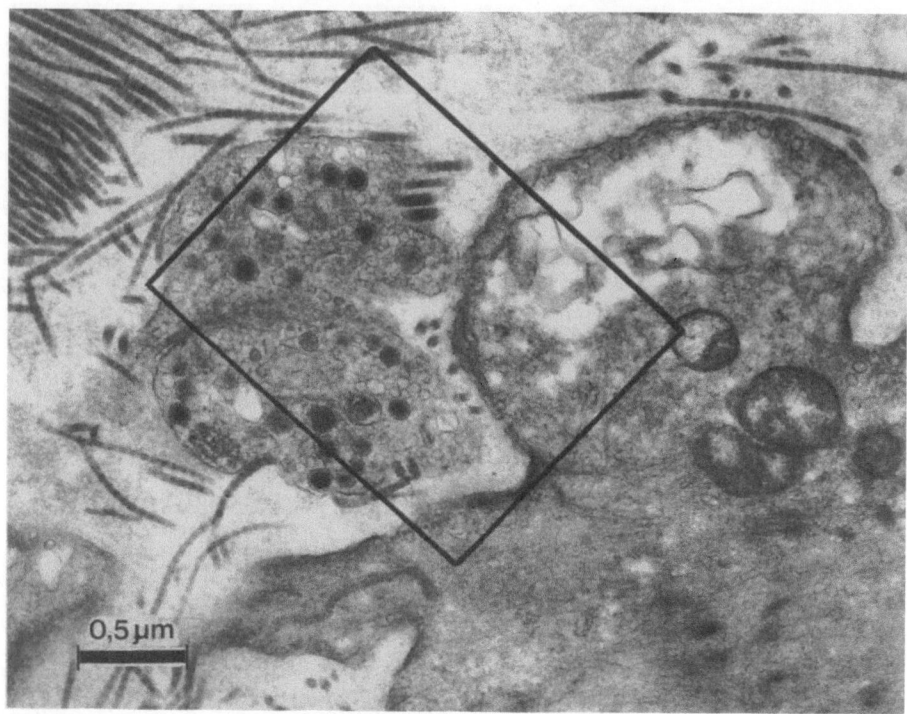

Fig. 4a. Immersion-fixed biopsy from CCP of a two axons reach out (*above left*) towards a smooth muscle cell (*below right*). As in Figs. 2b and 3b, two types of vesicle (probably cholinergic and adrenergic) can be seen. Primary magnification × 13 100; for final enlargement see scale

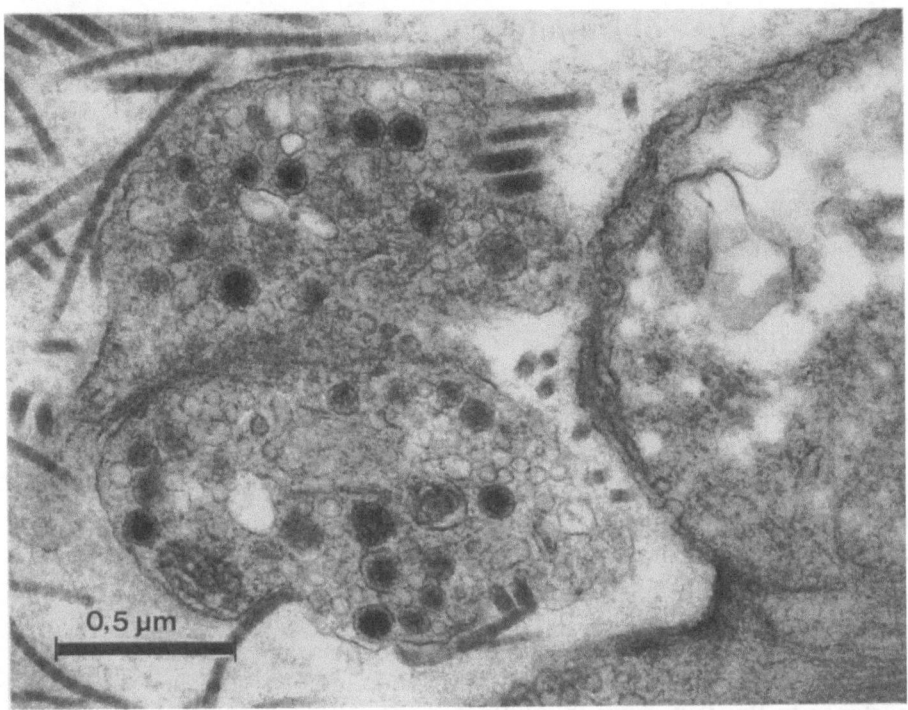

Fig. 4b. Enlargement of area marked in Fig. 4a. Primary magnification × 24 000; for final enlargement see scale

Endocrinology of Impotence

T.H. Schürmeyer and R.D. Hesch

Introduction

Endocrine disturbances can be observed in only a minor group of patients with erectile dysfunction. However, the high success rate of endocrine therapy in these patients and the impact of endocrine disease on their metabolic homeostasis (apart from erectile dysfunction) make the diagnosis of endocrine disturbances an integral part of the total diagnostic approach to impotence.

Endocrine influences throughout the fetal period, the first weeks of life, and puberty not only create the anatomical prerequisites of erectile function by controlling the evolution of the sexual organs, but also affect the sex-specific development of the brain. The endocrinologist attaches special importance to this fact, since in adults it is not reflexogenic erections, but the psychogenic facilitation of these reflexes which seem to be under endocrine control.

Sexual Differentiation

Following the sexual differentiation of the gonads induced by genetic information on the Y chromosome, steroidogenesis starts in a small number of Leydig's cells at week 6 of embryonic development. Together with a gonadal glycoprotein produced by Sertoli's cells, the müllerian inhibiting substance (MIS), gonadal steroids control the further development of the sex-specific phenotype. MIS is necessary for regression of the müllerian ducts [46, 65], while testosterone and its main metabolite 5α-dihydrotestosterone (DHT) are responsible for the growth of the internal and external male sexual organs [38, 47, 72, 96]. A genetic defect causing inadequate metabolization of testosterone to DHT results in incomplete sexual differentiation in men (testicular feminization) similar to the X-chromosomal genetic disorders of androgen receptor function (androgen resistance; for review see 105).

Marked structural sex differences can be demonstrated within the brain. The structural dimorphism of the brain seems to be caused by high concentrations of androgens and estrogens circulating throughout the period of fetal

U. Jonas et al. (Eds.) Erectile Dysfunction
© Springer-Verlag Berlin Heidelberg 1991

Plasma testosterone (ng/ml)

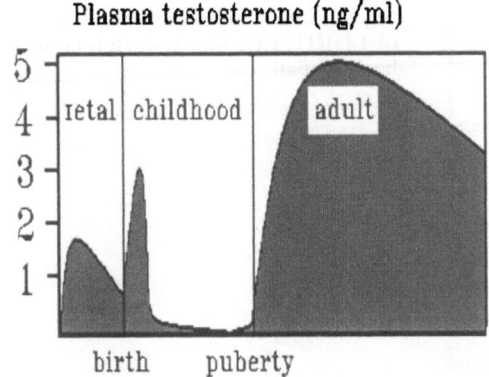

Fig. 1. Changes in plasma testosteron levels during development

and early postpartal development [17, 20, 28, 29, 42–44, 71, 76, 78, 95, 102; Fig. 1]. In animals, adult sexual behavior seems to be dependent to some degree on the imprinting effects of these estrogens and androgens on the developing brain [9, 22, 23, 30, 36, 74]. In humans, however, the evolution of sex-dependent differences in central nervous system (CNS) functions seems to be based on the dimorphism in brain structure [12, 14, 18, 19, 34, 54, 55, 59, 63, 64]. Though behavior is a function of the CNS system, reports concerning the influence of pre- and early postpartal exposure to sex steroids on sexual behavior in humans are inconsistent and speculative (for review see 74, 106). In humans, not only the impact of the sex-dependent development of the brain on sexual behavior and function, but also the importance of the actual function of the hypothalamic-pituitary-gonadal (HPG) axis in erectile function are uncertain.

Physiology of the HPG Axis

In men, testosterone (5–10 mg/day) is synthesized within the Leydig's cells of the testes under the influence of Lutieinizing hormone (LH), a glycoprotein hormone secreted by the anterior lobe of the pituitary in an episodic fashion. For the initiation and maintenance of spermatogenesis, both testosterone and Follicle-stimulating hormone (FSH), a second gonadotropin secreted by the pituitary, seem to be necessary. Sexual function, on the other hand, depends only on the level of circulating testosterone. The typical LH secretion pattern is believed to result from episodic secretion of a decapeptide, Luteinizing hormone-releasing hormone (LHRH), by hypothalamic cells (Fig. 2). LHRH secretion is modulated by various neuroendocrine systems. On the hypothalamic level, neuronal information on the environmental and metabolic situation of the subject is integrated to a single digital signal. This is enforced

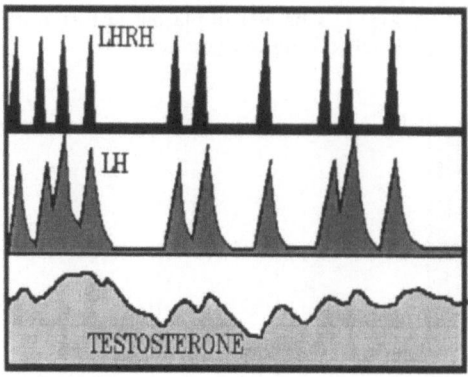

time -->

Fig. 2. Schematized secretion patterns of LHRH, LH, and testosterone in a healthy man

on the pituitary level and translated to an analog endocrine signal of circulating testosterone within the testes.

Within the circulation, testosterone is transported bound to sex hormone-binding globulin (SHBG), a binding protein with an affinity and specifity lower than that of the intracellular androgen receptor, but far higher than that of albumin, the second carrier of testosterone in the blood stream. Only 2%–3% of testosterone is available for free transport into the target cell. In many tissues, it is transformed to DHT or estradiol before being bound to a specific receptor. Aromatization of testosterone to estradiol has to occur within the structures of the CNS (2), where both receptors for androgens and estrogens are found [68, 79, 86]. This enzymatic conversion seems to be required for most central functions of androgens, e.g., feedback inhibition of the HPG axis, and probably some psychological effects also [56, 62, 67].

The reduction of testosterone to DHT occurs in most androgen-responsive tissues outside the blood-brain barrier, namely the prostate, penis, hair follicles, sebaceous glands, and seminal vesicles. The activated steroid-receptor complex causes transcription of DNA within the nucleus of the cell. The resultant messenger RNA is translated into proteins and peptides, which are responsible for the androgen-induced effects. Receptors for androgens are also localized in the sacral parasympathetic nuclei [87] that are involved in erectile function in man.

Apart from the well-documented role of steroid receptors in feedback regulation of the HPG axis, binding sites for androgens and estrogens within the CNS also link the HPG axis to other endocrine systems and to psycho-neurologic functions of the CNS itself. Thus, various endocrine, neurologic, and psychiatric disturbances may result in sexual days functions with or without a disorder of the HPG axis, namely erectile impotence. Equally, disorders of HPG function can enforce pre-existing metabolic, neurologic, or psychiatric diseases.

Pathophysiology of the HPG Axis

The effect of hypogonadism and testosterone substitution therapy on libido and sexual behavior is well established, but the influence of androgen substitution therapy on erectile function is unclear. Erections occur in prepubertal boys, and men with plasma testosterone concentrations in the range of castrates can achieve normal reflexogenic and psychogenic erections. The number of nocturnal erectile activities seems to be decreased in the latter and can be normalized by androgen substitution [8, 53].

Male hypogonadism may be of testicular origin (primary hypogonadism) or may result from pituitary or hypothalamic disturbances (secondary hypogonadism). The determination of plasma testosterone concentrations allows correct diagnosis of hypogonadism, and the measurement of plasma gonadotropin concentrations permits differentiation between primary (hypergonadotropic) and secondary (hypogonadotropic) hypogonadism. Pituitary LH secretion response to intravenously given LHRH (100 µg) in a 30 min test or, if there was no response with this test, to intranasal LHRH administered over several days, revealed a hypothalamic rather than a pituitary cause of secondary hypogonadism. Whatever disturbance of the HPG axis is detected, the clinician must aim for a clear-cut diagnosis such as Klinefelter's syndrome (see Tables 1 and 2). If causal therapy of the hypogonadism is not feasible, in most patients androgen substitution therapy will be necessary, not only to achieve normal sexuality, but also to curtail the negative effects of androgen deficiency on metabolism and organ function of, e.g., the muscle, bone, and bone marrow (for review see 66).

Androgens that cannot be transformed either by aromatization, e.g., mesterolone, drostanolone and oxymetholone [40, 58], or by 5α-reduction are inadequate for androgen substitution therapy. Androgens that are methylated at position 17α, e.g., methyltestosterone, fluoxymesterone, methandrostenolone, and stanozolol are obsolete due to their unpredictable and possibly life-threatening, hepatotoxic side effects [4, 11, 21, 26, 32, 33, 45, 89, 103]. Adequate androgen substitution therapy is afforded by the administration of testosterone esters, e.g., testosterone enanthate, cypionate, or

Table 1. Normal range of plasma hormone concentrations

Hormone	Normal range of plasma concentration
Testosterone	> 3 ng/ml
LH	3–15 mU/ml
FSH	2–10 mU/ml
Prolactin	< 25 ng/ml
Thyroxine	4.5–12.5 µg/dl
Triiodothyronine	0.5– 2.0 ng/ml
Thyroid-stimulating hormone	0.2– 4.0 ng/ml

Table 2. Differential diagnosis of endocrine disorders causing erectile impotence

---

1   Hypogonadism
1.1 Primary hypogonadism
    – Anorchia, castration, trauma
    – Klinefelter's syndrome, XYY- or male XO- or XX-syndrome
    – Kryptorchism
    – Orchitis
1.2 Secondary hypogonadism of pituitary origin
    – Pituitary tumor (adenoma, germinoma, meningioma)
    – Meningoencephalitis or local infection
    – Pituitary ischemia/infarction (e.g., Sheehan's syndrome)
    – Pituitary irradiation, trauma, neurosurgery
1.3 Secondary hypogonadism of hypothalamic origin
    – Kallmann's syndrome, Prader-Willi's syndrome, Laurence-Moon syndrome
    – Idiopathic delayed puberty
    – Hypothalamic tumor (craniopharyngioma, histiocytosis X)
    – CNS trauma or irradiation
    – Drugs (estrogens, morphine, neuroleptics, sedatives)
2   Hyperprolactinemia
    – Prolactinoma
    – Uremia
    – Drugs (neuroleptics, sedatives, antiemetics, reserpine)
3   Stress disorders and endogenous hypercortisolism
    – Malnutrition (anorexia, cachexia)
    – Physical or psychic stress
    – Cushing's syndrome
    – Psychiatric disease (depression, anxiety disorders)
4   Hyperthyroidism/hypothyroidism

---

cyclohexanecarboxylate as an intramuscular depot every 3–4 weeks at a
dose of 200–250 mg [88, 90, 100]. The effect of the shorter ester testosterone
propionate is inadequate, since it lasts for not longer than 5 days. Where
intramuscular administration of androgens is prohibited, e.g., in patients
under cumarin therapy, testosterone undecanoate may be prescribed. As this
ester bypasses in part the first pass of the liver, the administration of 120 mg
of it results in an elevation of hypogonadal plasma testosterone concentrations into the normal range for several hours; the androgen thus has to be
taken 2–3 times a day [91, 98]. In the near future, percutaneous testosterone
substitution therapy by means of transdermal delivery devices may prove to
be a promising and safe modality for the treatment of male hypogonadism
[6, 7, 35].

Nongonadal Endocrine Disorders Causing Erectile Dysfunction

Since, in humans, psychogenic stimuli seem to be of greater importance in
elicting penile erection than reflexogenic stimuli, the various afore-mentioned

metabolic, endocrine, neurogenic, and psychogenic interactions within the CNS account for a multitude of disturbances that may result in erectile dysfunction. In metabolic disturbances such as hyperthyroidism or hypothyroidism, in critically ill patients such as poorly controlled diabetics [107], and in severe psychiatric disease, e.g., depression, a decline in libido rather than the consistent inability to achieve erections comes to the fore as an impairment of sexual function [77].

During stress, catecholamine is secreted by sympathetic nerves and the adrenal medulla and the hypothalamic-pituitary-adrenal axis is activated. Animal experiments suggest that an increase in circulating epinephrine may oppose the relaxation of smooth muscle tone necessary for erection and may even cause detumescence of the erected penis [10, 27]. In contrast to these experimental findings, clinical experience shows that impotence does not usually result from high levels of circulating catecholamines, but can be caused by sympatholytics (methyldopa, guanethidine, clonidine) and α- or β-receptor blocking agents [94, 99].

The hypothalamic-pituitary-adrenal system and the HPG axis are linked on more than one level. Neurons containing corticotropin-releasing hormone (CRH) have a direct synaptic connection to LHRH secreting cells [60] and seem to induce a decrease in LHRH secretion in vitro [70] and in animals in vivo [69, 73, 75, 80, 81]. In humans, hypercortisolism resulting from a continuous infusion of CRH for 24 h [93] was found not to interfere with the normal secretion pattern of testosterone (unpublished data). In female rats, CRH is a potent inhibitor of sexual receptivity [97], but its effect on sexual behavior in male animals is unknown. Endocrine and behavioral data obtained in rodents may not be of any significance for the interaction of CRH with behavior and sexual functions in primates, since in rodents CRH generally seems to induce a behavioral activation, e.g., an increase in novelty [49, 101], whereas in primates under CRH, arousal rises and behavioral inhibition occurs [48]. Data on the effect of CRH on libido and erectile function in humans are not available.

Both LHRH secretion and sexual function are influenced by endorphins and enkephalins. Continuous activation of the endogenous opioid system, e.g., in long-distance runners or during psychological stress [5, 15, 16, 51, 52, 82], results in a disturbance of LH-RH secretion [39, 57]. By this mechanism, CRH may indirectly interfere with reproductive and sexual functions, since the hypothalamic dynorphin and β-endorphin secretion seem to be regulated by CRH-containing neurons [1]. In humans, physical stress for 20 days results in a lasting decrease of testosterone secretion [92] and even a short-term physical strain like a 100-km run effects a drop in plasma testosterone concentrations into the hypogonadal range in most subjects (Fig. 3). This endocrine finding can be explained by the inhibitory influence of activated endogenous opioid secretion on episodic LHRH secretion [3, 25, 41, 57] and correlates with the loss of libido and the occurrence of impotence in male heroin addicts [13, 24].

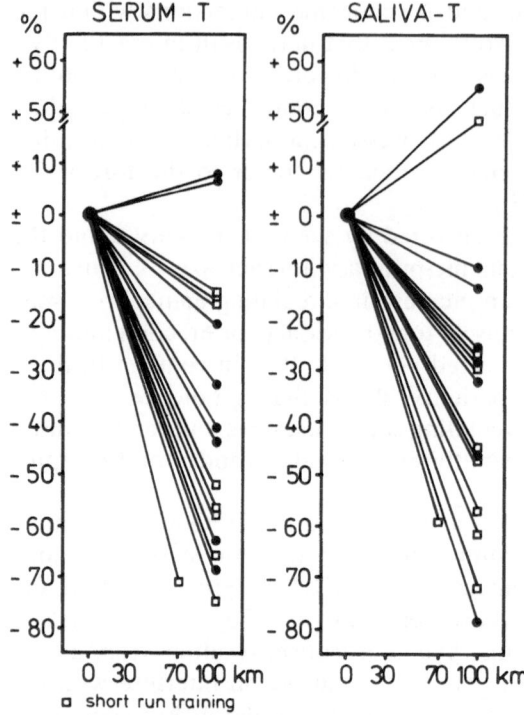

Fig. 3. Influence of a 100-km run on serum and saliva testosterone in 17 healthy athletes. The changes are shown as percentages of the starting values. *Open squares* indicate volunteers trained for short runs, *closed circles* indicate those trained for long runs

In social groups of primates, the close interactions between the stress-responsive, sympathicoadrenomedullary and hypothalamic-pituitary-adrenal systems and the HPG axis may regulate social balance, and the effect of social stress on sexual functions and endocrine changes seems to be dependent on the social rank of the male animal [84, 85]. This clearly suggests that a social situation may result in endocrine disorders, which lead to disturbed function of systems under endocrine regulation such as the reproductive system. However, a direct analogy of these observations in animals to the psychological and social situation of humans in our far more complex industrial social environment seems inappropriate.

In patients with hyperprolactinemia, secondary hypogonadism and a decrease in libido and erectile capacity may result from an invasive growing pituitary prolactinoma. In most hyperprolactinemic patients, the occurrence of impotence associated with low, normal, or decreased plasma testosterone concentrations cannot be explained on the basis of a local pituitary destruction by the adenoma. Prolactin seems to stimulate hypothalamic dopamine and endorphin turnover, and thus indirectly influences LHRH secretion [31, 83]. The administration of naloxone, an opioid antagonist, results in normalization of LH-RH secretion in hyperprolactinemia [31]. Since testosterone substitution therapy does not restore potency in about 50% of the hyperprolactinemic patients [37], prolactin may cause a disturbance in sexual functions directly via antagonism to the peripheral actions of testosterone [61], or indirectly by its effects on endorphin and CNS catecholamine secretion. The etiology of hyperprolactinemia has to be clarified in all hyperprolactinemic patients with erectile dysfunction (see Table 2). In most patients, treatment of hyperprolactinemia with bromocriptine will be the therapy of choice [50].

Summary

Primary and secondary hypogonadism and hyperprolactinemia are endocrine disorders that have to be excluded in patients with erectile dysfunction by determining plasma testosterone and prolactin concentrations (Fig. 4). Testosterone substitution therapy or treatment of hyperprolactinemia with bromocriptine have a high rate of therapeutic success only if a decreased secretion of androgens or an increased secretion of prolactin can be demonstrated. Links between other endocrine systems and the CNS seem to play an important role in the development of impotence and/or hypogonadism in patients with metabolic or psychiatric disorders, even if the decrease in erectile function is actually caused by the psychic or social situation of the subject.

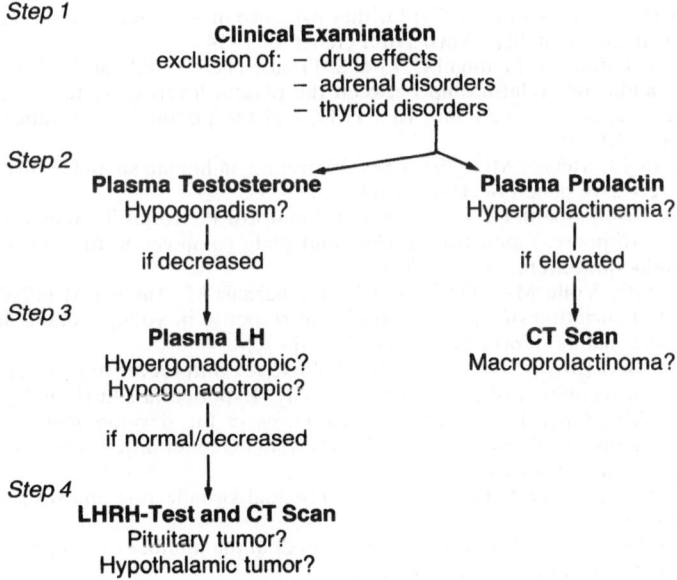

Fig. 4. Diagnostic procedure for identifying possible endocrine cause of impotence

References

1. Almeida OFX, Nikolarakis KE, Herz A (1988) Evidence for the involvement of endogenous opioids in the inhibition of luteinizing hormone by corticotropin-releasing factor. Endocrinology 122:1034–1041
2. Attardi B, Geller LN, Ohno S (1976) Androgen and estrogen receptors in brain cytosol from male, female and testicular feminized mice. Endocrinology 98:864
3. Azizi F, Vagenakis AG, Longcope C, Ingbar SH, Braverman LE (1973) Decreased serum testosterone concentration in male heroin and methadone addicts. Steroids 22:467–472
4. Bagheri SA, Boyer SL (1974) Peliosis hepatis associated with androgenic-anabolic steroid therapy. Ann Intern Med 81:610–619.
5. Baker ER (1981) Menstrual dysfunction and hormonal status in athletic women: a review. Fertil Steroil 36:691
6. Bals-Pratsch M, Knuth UA, Yoon YD, Nieschlag E (1986) Transdermal testosterone substitution therapy for male hypogonadism. Lancet II:943–946
7. Bals-Pratsch M, Langer K, Place VA, Nieschlag E (1988) Substitution therapy of hypogonadal men with transdermal testosterone over one year. Acta Endocrinol (Copenh) 118:7–13
8. Bancroft J, Wu FC (1983) Changes in erectile responsiveness during androgen replacement therapy. Arch Sex Behav 12:59–66
9. Baum MJ (1976) Effects of testosterone propionate administered perinatally on sexual behavior of female ferrets. J. Comp Physiol Psychol 90:399–410
10. Benard F, Stief GC, Bosch R et al. (1988) Systemic infusion of epinephrine: its effect on erection. Proc 6th Int Symp for Corpus Cavernosus Revascularization & 3rd World Meeting on Impotence 1988, October 6, p 16 (Abstract)
11. Bernstein MS, Hunter RL, Yanchnim S (1971) Hepatoma and peliosis in Fanconi's anemia. N Engl J Med 184:1135–1136
12. Bock RD, Kolakowski D (1973) Further evidence of sex-linked major gene influence on human spatial ability. Am J Hum Genet 25:1–14
13. Bolelli G, Lafiscia S, Flamigni C, Lodi S, Franceschetti F, Filicori M, Mosca R (1979) Heroin addiction: relationship between the plasma levels of testosterone, dihydrotestosterone, androstenedione, LH, FSH, and the plasma concentration of heroin. Toxicol 15:19–29
14. Bouchard TJ, McGee MG (1977) Sex differences in human spatial ability: Not a sex-linked recessive gene effect. Soc Biol 24:332–335
15. Boyden TW, Pamenter RW, Grosso D, Stanforth P, Rotkis T, Wilmore JH (1982) Prolactin responses, menstrual cycles, and body composition of women runners. J Clin Endocrinol Metab 54:711–714
16. Brisson GR, Volle MA, DeCarufel D, Desharnais M, Tanaka M (1980) Exercise-induced dissociation of the blood prolactin response in young women according to their sports habits. Horm Metab Res 12:201–205
17. Bubenik GA, Brown GM (1973) Morphologic sex differences in primate brain areas involved in regulation of reproductive activity. Experientia 29:619–621
18. Buffery AW, Gray JH (1972) Sex differences in the development of spatial and linguistic skills. In: Ounstead C, Taylor DC (eds) Gender differences: their ontogeny and significance. Churchill, London
19. Burnett SA, Lane DM, Dratt LM (1979) Spatial visualization and sex differences in quantitative ability. Intelligence 3:345–354
20. Calaresu FR, Henry JL (1971) Sex differences in the number of sympathetic neurons in the spinal cord of the cat. Science 173:343–344
21. Carbone JV, Grodsky GM, Hjelte V (1959) Effect of hepatic dysfunction on circulating levels of sulphobromopthalein and its metabolites. J Clin Invest 38:1989–1996
22. Carter CS, Clemens LG, Hoekema DJ (1972) Neonatal androgen and adult sexual behavior in the golden hamster. Physiol Behav 9:89–95

23. Clarke IJ, Scaramuzzi RJ, Short RV (1976) Sexual differentiation of the brain: endocrine and behavioural responses of androgenized ewes to oestrogen. J Endocrinol 71:175–176
24. Cushman P (1972) NY State J Med 72:1261
25. Delitalia G, Giusti M, Mazzocchi G, Granziera L, Tarditi W, Giordano G (1983) Participation of endogenous opiates in regulation of the hypothalamic-pituitary-testicular axis in normal men. J Clin Endocrinol Metab 57:1277–1281
26. DeLorimer AA, Gordan Gs, Löwe RC, Carbone JV (1965) Methyltestosterone, related steroids and liver function. Arch Intern Med 116:289–194
27. Diederichs W, Stief CG, Lue TF, Tanagho EA, et al. (1988) Sympathetic inhibition of papaverine-induced erection. Proc 6th Int Symp for Corpus Cavernosus Revascularization & 3rd World Meeting on Impotence 1988, October 6, p 79 (Abstract)
28. Dörner G, Staudt J (1968) Structural changes in the preoptic anterior hypothalamic area of the male rat, following neonatal castration and androgen substitution. Neuroendocrinology 3:136–140
29. Dörner G, Staudt J (1969) Structural changes in the hypothalamic ventromedial nucleus of the male rat, following neonatal castration and androgen treatment. Neuroendocrinology 4:278–281
30. Edwards DA, Burge KG (1971) Early androgen treatment and male and female sexual behavior in mice. Hormon Behav 2:49–58
31. Evans WS, Cronin MJ, Thorner MO (1982) Hypogonadism in hyperprolactinemia: Proposed mechanisms. In: Ganong WF, Martini L (eds) Frontiers in neuroendocrinology. Raven Press, New York
32. Falk H, Thomas LB, Popper H, Ishak KG (1979) Hepatic angiosarcoma associated with androgenic-anabolic steroids. Lancet II:1120–1123
33. Farrell GC, Uren RF, Perkins KW, Joshua DE, Baird PJ, Kronenburg H (1975) Androgen induced hepatoma. Lancet I:430–432
34. Fennema E, Sherman J (1977) Sex-related differences in mathematics achievement, spatial visualization, and affective factors. Am Educ Res J 14:51–71
35. Findlay JC, Place VA, Snyder PC (1987) Transdermal delivery of testosterone. J Clin Endocrinol Metab 64:266–268
36. Ford JJ (1981) Differentiation of sexual behavior in swine. Biol Reprod (Suppl 1) 24:95A
37. Franks S, Jacobs HS, Martin N, Nabarro JD (1978) Hyperprolactinaemia and impotence, Clin Endocrinol 8:277–287
38. Gillman J (1958) The development of the gonads in man, with a consideration of the role fetal endocrines and the histogenesis of ovarian tumors. Contrib Embryol Carnegic Inst 210:83–131
39. Gold MS, Redmond De, Donabedian RK (1979) The effects of opoate agonist on serum prolactin in primates: possible role for endorphins in prolactin regulation. Endocrinology 105:284–289
40. Gordon RD, Thomas MJ, Poynting JM, Strocks AE (1975) Effect of mesterolone on plasma LH, FSH and testosterone. Andrologia 7:287–296
41. Grossman A, Moult PJA, Gaillard RC, Delitalia G, Toff WD, Rees Lh, Besser GM (1981) The opioid control of LH and FSH release: effects of a met-enkephalin analogue and naloxone. Clin Endocrinol 14:41–47
42. Gurney ME (1981) Hormonal control of cell form and number in the zebra finch song system. J Neurosci 1:658–673
43. Jacobson CD, Gorski RA (1981) Neurogenesis of the sexually dimorphic nucleus of the preoptic area in the rat. J Comp Neurol 196:519–529
44. Jacobson CD, Shryne JE, Shapiro F, Gorski RA (1980) Ontogeny of the sexually dimorphic nucleus of the preoptic area. J Comp Neurol 193:541–548
45. Johnson FL, Feagler JR, Lerner KG, Majerus PW, Siegel M, Hartmann JR, Thomas Ed (1972) Association of androgenc anabolic steroid therapy with development of hepato-cellular carcinoma. Lancet II:1273–1276
46. Josso N, Picard JY (1986) Anti-Müllerian hormone. Physiol Rev 66:1038–1090

47. Jost A (1972) A new look at the mechanism controlling sex differentiation in mammals. John Hopkins Med J 130:38
48. Kalin NH (1985) Behavioral effects of ovine corticotropin-releasing factor administered to rhesus monkeys. Fed Proc 44:249–253
49. Koob GF, Bloom FE (1985) Corticotropin-releasing factor and behavior. Fed Proc 44:259–263
50. Krane RJ, Goldstein I, Saenz de Tejada I (1989) Impotence. N Engl J Med 321: 1648–1659
51. Kreuz LE, Rose RM, Jennings JR (1972) Suppression of plasma testosterone levels and psychological stress. Arch Gen Psychiat 26:479–482
52. Kuoppasalmi K, Näveri H, Härkönen M, Adlercreutz H (1980) Plasma cortisol, androstenedione, testosterone and luteinizing hormone in running exercise of different intensities. Scand J Clin Lab Invest 40:403–409
53. Kwan M, Greenleaf WJ, Mann J, Crapo L, Davidson JM (1983) The nature of androgen action on male sexuality: a combined laboratory-self-report study on hypogonadal men. J Clin Endocrinol Metab 57:557–562
54. Lake dA, Bryden MP (1976) Handedness and sex differences in hemispheric asymmetry. Brain and Language 3:266–282
55. Landsdell H (1962) A sex difference in effect of temporal lobe neurosurgery on design preference. Nature (London) 194:852–854
56. Larsson K, Söderstein P, Beyer C (1973) Introduction of male sexual behavior by oestradiol benzoate in combination with dihydrotestosterone. J Endocrinol 57:563
57. Lightman SL, Jacobs HS, Maguire AK, McGarrick G, Jeffcoate SL (1981) Constancy of opioid control of lueinizing hormone in different pathophysiological states. J Clin Endocrinol Metab 52:1260–1263
58. Luisi M, Franchi F (1980) Double blind group comparative study of testosterone undecanoate and mesterolone in hypogonadal male patients. J. Endocrinol Invest 3:305–308
59. Maccoby EE, Jacklin CN (1974) The psychology of sex differences. Stanford University Press
60. MacLusky NJ, Naftolin F, Leranth C (1988) Immunocytochemical evidence for direct synaptic connections between corticotropin releasing factor (CRF) and gonadotropin-releasing hormone (GnRH) containing neurons in the preoptic area of the rat. Brain Res 439:391–395
61. Margrini G, Ebiner JR, Burckhardt P, Felber JP (1976) Study on the relationship between plasma prolactin levels and androgen metabolism in man. J Clin Endocrinol Metab 43:944
62. McEwen BS, Lieberburg K, Chaptal C, et al. (1977) Aromatization: important for sexual differentiation of the neonatal rat brain. Hormon Behav 9:249
63. McGee MG (1979) Human spatial abilities: Psychometric studies and environmental, genetic, hormonal, and neurological influences. Psychol Bull 86:889–918
64. McGlone J (1978) Sex differences in functional brain asymmetry. Cortex 14:122–128
65. Miller WL (1990) Editorial: Immunoassays for human Mullerian inhibitory factor (MIF): New insights into the physiology of MIF. J Clin Endocrinol Metab 70:8–10
66. Mooradian AD, Morley JE, Korenman SG (1987) Biological actions of androgens. Endocr Rev 8:1–28
67. Muttge WG (1975) Effects of antiestrogens on testosterone stimulated male sexual behavior and peripheral target tissues in the castrated male rat. Physiol Behav 14: 839
68. Naftolin F, Ryan KJ, Petro Z (1971) Aromatization of androstenedione by the diencephalon. J Clin Endocrinol Metab 33:368
69. Nikolarakis KE, Almeida OFX, Sirinathsinghji DJS, Herz A (1988) Concomitant changes in the in vitro and in vivo release of opioid peptides and luteinizing hormone releasing hormone from the hypothalamus following blockade of receptors for corticotropin releasing factor. Neuroendocrinology 47:545–550

70. Nikolarakis KE, Almeida OFX, Herz A (1986) Stimulation of hypothalamic β-endorphin and dynorphin release by corticotropin-releasing factor (in vitro). Brain Res 399:152–155
71. Nottebohm F, Arnold AP (1976) Sexual dimorphism in vocal control areas of the songbird brain. Science 194:211–213
72. Ohno S, Christian LC, Wachtel SS, et al (1976) Hormone-like role of H-Y antigen in bovine freemartin gonad. Nature (London) 261:597–599
73. Ono N, Lumpkin MD, Samson WK, McDonald JK, McCann SM (1984) Intrahypothalamic action of corticotropin-releasing factor (CRF) to inhibit growth hormone and LH release in the rat. Life Sci 35:117
74. Pardridge WM, Gorski RA, Lippe BA, Green R (1982) Androgens and sexual behavior. Ann Intern Med 96:488–501
75. Petraglia F, Sutton S, Vale W, Plotsky P (1987) Corticotropin-releasing factor decreases plasma luteinizing hormone levels in female rats by inhibiting gonadotropin-releasing hormone release into hypophysial-portal circulation. Endocrinology 120: 1083–1088
76. Pfaff DW (1966) Morphological changes in the brain of adult male rats after neonatal castration. J Endocrinol 36:415–416
77. Pogach LM, Vaitukaitis JL (1983) Endocrine disorders associated with erectile dysfunction. In: Krane RJ, Siroky MB, Goldstein I (eds) Male sexual dysfunction. Little & Brown, Boston, pp 63–76
78. Raisman G, Field PM (1973) Sexual dimorphism in neuropil of the preoptic area of the rat and its dependence on neonatal androgen. Brain Res 54:1–29
79. Rees HD, Michael RP (1982) Brain cells of the male rhesus monkey accumulate 3H-testosterone or its metabolites. J Comp Neurol 206:273–277
80. Rivier C, Vale W (1984) Influence of corticotropin releasing factor on reproductive functions in the rat. Endocrinology 114:914–921
81. Rivier C, Rivier J, Vale W (1986) Stress-induced inhibition of reproductive functions: role of endogenous corticotropin-releasing factor. Science 231:607
82. Rose RM, Kreutz LE, Holaday JW et al. (1968) Androgen responses to stress: excretion of testosterone, epitestosterone, androsterone and eticholanolone during basic combat training and under threat of attack. Psychosom Med 30:721–732
83. Sakar DK, Yen SC (1985) Hyperprolactinaemia decreases the luteinizing hormone releasing hormone concentration in pituitary portal plasma: A possible role for β-endorphin as a mediator. Endocrinology 116:2080–2084
84. Sapolsky RM (1982) The endocrine stress-response and social status in the wild baboon. Hormon Behav 16:279
85. Sapolsky RM (1986) Stress-induced elevation of testosterone concentrations in high ranking baboons: role of catecholamines. Endocrinology 118:1630–1635
86. Sar M, Stumpf WE (1977) Distribution of androgen target cells in rat forebrain and pituitary after (3H)-dihydrotestosterone administration. J Steroid Biochem 8:1131–1135
87. Sar M, Stumpf WE (1977) Androgen concentration in motor neurons of cranial nerves and spinal cord. Science 197:77–79
88. Schulte-Beerbühl M, Nieschlag E (1980) Comparison of testosterone, DHT, LH and FSH in serum after injection of testosterone enanthate or testosterone cypionate. Fertil Steril 33:201–203
89. Schürmeyer TH, Nieschlag E (1983) The clinical pharmacology and toxicology of androgens. In: Briggs M, Corbin A (eds) Progress in hormone biochemistry and pharmacology. Eden Press, Quebec London, pp 439–462
90. Schürmeyer TH, Nieschlag E (1984) Comparative pharmacokinetics of testosterone enanthate and testosterone cyclohexanecarboxylate as assessed by serum and salivary testosterone levels in normal men. Int J Androl 7:181–187
91. Schürmeyer TH, Wickings EJ, Freischem CW, Nieschlag E. (1983) Saliva and serum testosterone following oral testosterone undecanoate administration in normal and hypogonadal men. Acta Endocrinol (Copenh) 102:456–462

 92. Schürmeyer TH, Jung K, Nieschlag E (1984) The effect of an 100 km run on testi-
     cular, adrenal and thyroid hormones. Int J Androl 7:276–282
 93. Schürmeyer TH, Avgerinos PC, Gold PW, Chrousos GP (1989) Effects of 24 h con-
     tinuous oCRH infusion on ACTH and cortisol secretion patterns in man. Acta En-
     docrinol (Copenh) (Suppl 1) 120:219
 94. Segraves RT, Madsen R, Carter CS (1985) Erectile dysfunction associated with
     pharmacological agents. In: Segraves RT, Schoenberg HW (eds) Diagnosis and treat-
     ment of erectile disturbances: a guide for clinicians. Plenum Press, New York, pp
     22–63
 95. Short RV (1974) Sexual differentiation in the brain of the sheep. In: Forest MG,
     Bertrand J (eds) Endocrinologie sexuelle de la periode perinatale. INSERM, Paris,
     pp 121–142
 96. Siiteri PK, Wilson JD (1974) Testosterone formation and metabolism during male
     sexual differentiation in the human embryo. J Clin Endocrinol 38:113–125
 97. Sirinathsinghji DJS, Rees Lh, Rivier J, Vale W (1983) Corticotropin-releasing factor
     is a potent inhibitor of sexual receptivity in the female rat. Nature (London) 305:
     232–235
 98. Skakkebaek NE, Bancroft J, Davidson DW, Warner P (1981) Androgen replacement
     with oral testosterone undecanoate in hypogonadal men: a double blind controlled
     study. Clin Endocrinol 14:49–61
 99. Slag MF, Morley JE, Elson MK (1983) Impotence in medical clinic outpatients.
     JAMA 249:1736–1740
100. Sokol RZ, Palacios A, Campfield LA, Saul C, Swerdloff RS (1982) Comparison of
     the kinetics of injectable testosterone in eugonadal and hypogonadal men. Fertil
     Steril 37:425–430
101. Sutton RE, Koob GF, Le Moal M, Rivier J, Vale W (1982) Corticotropin releasing
     factor produces behavioral activation in rats. Nature (London) 297:331–333
102. Toran-Allerand CD (1981) Gonadal steroids and brain development. Trends Neurosci
     4:118–121
103. Werner FC, Hamger FM, Kritzler RA (1950) Jaundice during methyl-testosterone
     therapy. Am J Med 8:325–331
104. Wilson JD (1987) Disorders of androgen action. Clin Res 35:1–12
105. Wilson JD, George FW, Griffin JE (1981) The hormonal control of sexual develop-
     ment. Science 134:1149–1151
106. Young WC, Goy RW, Phoenix CH (1964) Hormones and sexual behavior. Science
     143:212–218
107. Zeidler A, Gelfand R, Draus R, Tauscher JK, Chopp RT (1981) Circadian variation
     in plasma prolactin, gonadotropins, and testosterone in diabetic male patients with
     and without impotence. Fertil Steril 35:653–656

Diagnostic Procedures

Psychological Evaluation and Psychometry

U. Hartmann

Psychological diagnosis and evaluation is of major importance within the multidisciplinary examination of erectile dysfunction. In many cases, the significance of psychogenic versus organic pathogenic factors, the existence and intensity of psychopathological symptoms, and relevant relationship factors are more crucial to therapeutic considerations than the medical aspects of evaluation.

The rapidly spreading propagation of intracavernous self-injection of vasoactive drugs has brought together patients and medical practitioners in their demand for a supposed pat solution to erectile problems. Since possible long-term complications cannot be completely ruled out today and – judging by high drop-out rates [2, 28] – patient acceptance seems ambivalent, a critical point of view remains necessary.

Indisputably, the last decade has led to an enormous increase in our understanding of the fundamental somatic processes of human erection and to considerable progress in diagnostic instruments by which organic factors have become determinable with formerly unknown precision. However, an identifiable organic anomaly does not automatically constitute a relevant or even the *crucial* causal factor, a statement which equally holds for psychological factors and which qualifies both today's figures about the incidence of organogenic impotence and older figures about psychogenically caused impotence. Beyond that, we still do not know how many organic or psychosexual factors could be found in men who do *not* complain of erectile problems.

The inappropriate and fruitless controversy about the proportion of organic versus psychogenic erectile dysfunctions should be replaced by a clear look at some of the fundamentals of male impotence.

Impotent men represent an extremely heterogeneous group of patients. The inability to achieve or maintain erections during coitus is the end result of a variety of possible etiological patterns. At the extreme points of an imagined normal distribution, there is a presumably relatively small number of *purely* psychogenic and *purely* organic erectile dysfunctions, but for the majority of impotent men both sources of causal factors are involved in a quantitatively, qualitatively, and, relating to their development over time, highly individualized combination.

A rigid dichotomization into somatic and psychological pathogenesis fails to meet the complex clinical reality, since a meaningful subpartitioning of

U. Jonas et al. (Eds.) Erectile Dysfunction
© Springer-Verlag Berlin Heidelberg 1991

this heterogeneous group is impossible if the border line is inflexible. The subgrouping not only has to identify the various etiological factors, but must understand their dynamic interaction in order to come to accurate decisions pertaining to therapeutic interventions. True psychosomatic reasoning – already established in cases of female sexual disorders – still remains rare for male sexual dysfunctions.

In spite of all efforts to set up a rational and standardized diagnostic algorithm there is no *single* biological marker for an organic erectile dysfunction [22]. In a well-designed study [22], 30%–40% of those carefully diagnosed to be organically impotent were able to show erections adequate for coitus. In a French investigation on 43 impotent men, all presenting certified vascular factors, anxious neurotic symptoms could be identified in 65% of cases [9]. On the other hand, we know from various studies that primarily psychogenically impotent men can show poor nocturnal penile tumescence (NPT) monitoring results and an insufficient response to intracavernous injection of vasoactive drugs. Many patients of this group also have a tendency to underestimate the quality of their erections and to respond in the same way as men with organic impotence [24]. These examples illustrate the growing complexity of diagnostic classification which not only has to assess the erectile capacity under various stimuli and situational conditions, but should also take into account the quality of erotic stimuli, able to elicit sexual excitement in the individual patient.

Erectile dysfunctions should be evaluated in a multiaxial frame of reference in which psychological examination must assume an important function and should not be handled superficially. Publications from German urologic centers are primarily marked by a tendency – compared to studies from France for example – to practically dismiss the psychological aspects of the evaluation by referring only to a (frequently not exactly specified) questionnaire or to an interview, whereas the increasingly subtle and differentiated somatic aspects are dealt with in great detail. In other centers, a psychological evaluation is conducted only after a positive response to an intracavernous injection [15]. Such a procedure is not in accordance with current knowledge and deprives the patient of the opportunity to present his problem in all its facets.

The psychological evaluation of erectile dysfunction rests on two principal methods, namely (a) psychometric tests, and (b) the diagnostic interview.

Psychometry

The psychometric instruments employed in the assessment of erectile impotence can be divided into three groups:

1. Standardized personality questionnaires such as the Minnesota Multiphasic Personality Inventory (MMPI), the California Psychological In-

ventory (CPI), the Eysenck Personality Questionnaire (EPQ), or the Freiburger Persönlichkeits – Inventar (FPI) in German speaking countries
2. Questionnaires that have been more specifically designed for assessing sexual dysfunctions such as the Derogatis Sexual Functioning Inventory (DSFI)
3. Questionnaires compiled only for classifying erectile problems

The MMPI and other standardized personality questionnaires were mainly examined with respect to their ability to differentiate psychogenic from organic impotence. The design of these studies was very similar. On the basis of NPT monitoring, the patients were allocated to organic and psychogenic criterion groups and the test scores of the two groups were compared. The discriminative validity of the MMPI seemed promising after a study in the 1970s reported a 70%–80% likelihood of psychogenic impotence by using a specific decision rule [4]. In a series of cross – validation studies, however, this result could not be replicated and the other personality questionnaires proved to be equally disappointing with regard to their discriminative validity, which in some cases was not significantly greater than chance [11, 17–20, 23, 27].

Of those questionnaires belonging to group two, the DSFI developed by Derogatis et al. [8] created the most interest. By using the DSFI an acceptable discrimination seemed to be possible initially, but this result could not be replicated either [8, 25].

Thus, it can be concluded with a high degree of certainty that neither standardized personality inventories nor more general sexual questionnaires are able to differentiate psychogenic from organic impotence. This result is a consequence of the afore-mentioned heterogeneity of this group of patients, which renders it highly unlikely that *any* personality questionnaire would be able to differentiate a heterogeneous group of psychogenically impotent patients from an equally heterogeneous group of organically impotent men [25]. Standardized personality inventories can be of some use in the psychological evaluation of erectile dysfunctions, but only when used according to their original intention, i.e., to diagnose and classify psychopathologically relevant personality traits or profiles. Even here the employment of these time-consuming instruments is probably limited, since the interpretation requires profound psychodiagnostic skills.

The only psychometric instruments which have some validity in this field are those in group three, i.e., questionnaires specifically developed for assessing erectile dysfunction. However, these are not yet standardized, and in most cases are compiled by the various clinical centers or research groups for their individual purposes. The few relevant publications have again focused on differentiating psychogenic from organic impotence. As expected, the results are highly specific for the different samples and for the set of questions used. Accordingly, the items which significantly contributed to discrimination in two older studies [1, 16] could not be confirmed in a replication study, which in turn reported discriminant validity for different items [24]. In a more recent investigation all patients were classified correctly by means of a discriminant function analysis of the responses to a specifically developed questionnaire [10].

All things considered, the use of psychometric assessment instruments in the evaluation of erectile dysfunction appears rather limited. Only those questionnaires specifically designed for the assessment of erectile dysfunction seem to permit a discrimination between organic and psychogenic impotence, but they are in desperate need of standardization of items and scales. Future efforts should not be primarily directed towards improving the discriminative validity, but should instead put more emphasis on the clinical usefulness of these instruments. They should provide the clinician with advance information regarding problem areas that are to be focused on during the interview, and priorities for therapeutic interventions and should also assess progress in sexual functioning [26]. To this end, a questionnaire developed at our center (IFB 3.1)[1], which contains 127 items referring to desire, sexual activity, masturbation, morning erections, partnership, history of erectile dysfunction, somatic risk factors, and age-related changes, has proved capable of providing a good general view of the main characteristics of the erectile problem. According to a preliminary analysis of 70 patients, it also has adequate discriminative validity, since 84% of the carefully diagnosed and assigned subjects were correctly classified.

Stripped to its essentials, this questionnaire, too, is nothing more than a structured extract of a thorough anamnesis. Thus, for both the psychological evaluation of erectile disturbances and the differentiation between organic and psychogenic etiological factors, subtle and skillful inquiry into the psychosexual history and careful assessment of the specific pattern of complaints remains of central importance.

The Diagnostic Interview

The clinical interview forms the main component of the psychological evaluation of erectile impotence. In addition to comprehensive knowledge of sexual medicine it requires at least a fundamental familiarity with prevalent psychological concepts about the etiology of sexual dysfunctions.

Psychological Aspects in the Etiology of Sexual Dysfunctions

We do yet not have a comprehensive and widely accepted model of the psychic causation of sexual dysfunction. According to traditional psychoanalytic

---

[1] Available from the author

theories, a sexual disability is the symptomatic expression of an underlying neurotic conflict – in most cases related to unresolved oedipal problems. The sexual disorder represents a compromise between anxiety-inducing impulses and specific defense mechanisms, and the "renunciation" of (coital) sexual activities allows a certain personal stabilization. An erectile problem could thus be characterized as a neurotic inhibition of the normal sexual response cycle.

With good reason, the advocates of the new sex therapy, based mainly on the work of Masters and Johnson [21], criticized that not all sexual dysfunctions are symptomatic of deeper neurotic conflicts, but are often caused rather "superficially" (in extreme cases by a single stressful episode, e.g., alcohol, new partner) since sexual dysfunctions tend to persist and become chronic even if the initial cause of the symptom no longer exists. This phenomenon is due to the circle of causation and aggravation that consists of performance anxiety, fear of failure, and avoidance behavior, a mechanism that is of central importance in the etiology and maintenance of sexual disorders. Lack of sexual knowledge or experience and – especially in the case of erectile problems – exaggerated expectations regarding sexual performance are other prominent factors. Finally, an important innovation of the new sex therapy lies in the now widely accepted view that psychosexual disturbances not only emerge as intrapsychic problems but, in many cases, constitute a partnership problem as well. For this reason, the female partner should be involved in the evaluation and treatment of erectile dysfunctions.

As a result of recent research, a future model of psychogenic impotence will have to consider the interaction of at least three components, namely (a) a constitutionally predetermined *vulnerability* of the sexual response system; (b) the effects of certain *risk factors* arising from the sexual biography, the partnership, and also organic pathologies; and (c) the individual *coping strategies*.

What is needed is a comprehensive theory of sexual arousal that accounts for both functional and dysfunctional subjects. Drawn from several lines of psychological research, Barlow and associates [3, 5, 6] have proposed a cognitive-affective model of sexual dysfunction that tries to highlight the differential response of sexually functional and dysfunctional men with regard to anxiety and cognitive interference. Two of the major findings of their experiments are that: (1) cognitive distraction reduces sexual arousal in functional subjects but has no effect on dysfunctionals, and (2) performance demand and anxiety induction either have no effect, or increase sexual arousal in functional men. In dysfunctional men they decrease sexual arousal [7]. These studies suggest that sexually dysfunctional men typically experience a negative affect specific to the sexual situation, while sexually functional men endorse a positive affect under the same conditions. A more recent study further suggests that the nature of the dysfunctionals' response can be described as largely "depressive" as opposed to "anxious", since the sexually dysfunctional men experienced a perceived lack of control, negative expectancies of themselves and the outcome of their efforts, and other cognitive features of clinical depressives [5]. The theoretical implications of these findings seem promising, but are in need of further empirical support.

For the purposes of clinical practice and research, the etiological concept of Kaplan [12–14] has proved useful as a working model of psychogenically caused sexual dysfunctions. According to this concept, the determinants of psychogenic impotence operate on different layers of causation ranging from rather superficial and mild factors to problems deeply rooted in the personal and early biography. Whereas the immediate antecedents – above all performance anxiety and fear of failure – are instrumental in *all* psychosexual dysfunctions and are rather specific for the particular type of disorder, deeper intrapsychic conflicts and relationship problems can be operative in various degrees of severity and acuity, but are unspecific for the particular dysfunction. As for erectile dysfunctions, it can be concluded from this concept that the loss of erection originates from an interaction of specific, immediate pathogenic factors (i.e., the invasion of performance anxiety and interfering cognitions) with the particular physiological stage of the sexual response cycle. If defenses against performance anxiety break down at an early stage no erection will build up; if the destructive anxiety is evoked at a later stage, a loss of the existing erection will result. As can be seen below, this concept might also serve as a useful guideline for the diagnostic interview.

Content Areas of the Diagnostic Interview

In evaluating psychological factors relating to erectile impotence, the diagnostic interview should focus mainly on the current sexual problem and its immediate causation and pay less attention to more general personality traits. The clinical interview should be conducted in an open and supportive atmosphere and be structured only insofar as the interviewer should attain information about the areas discussed in the following four sections.

1. The Current Sexual Problem and Its History

This topic covers important and essential information for diagnostic classification. The duration and chronicity of the erectile disorder and its formal descriptors can be assessed by the following questions:

- Has the erectile dysfunction existed since the first sexual experiences (primary disorder)?
- Has it developed after a longer symptom-free phase (secondary disorder)?
- Has there been an alternation of symptom-free and symptomatic intervals (phasic disorder)?
- Is the disorder bound to specific conditions (situational disorder)?

– Is the dysfunction confined to a specific partner or type of partner (partner related disorder)?

If the erectile dysfunction is *not* primary, it must be assessed whether its onset has been insidious or acute, after an identifiable life event like loss of partner, occupational problems, or excessive stress. It must also be established whether the erectile disturbance has developed secondary to an ejaculatory dysfunction. In evaluating erectile problems one often detects a long-lasting history of premature ejaculation, but frequently a loss of ejaculatory control emerges *after* an erectile dysfunction has developed. In a few patients, the erectile disorder is associated with a retarded ejaculation, which in most cases reveals deep-seated intrapsychic problems.

An area even more important than the foregoing is the evaluation of the *immediate causes* according to the etiological concept of Kaplan. For that it is advantageous to ask the patient for a detailed description of the "typical" course of sexual interaction with his partner and its possible variants. In the clinical assessment the focus should be on sexual functioning as well as the subjective experience and emotional aspects. Important questions are:

– What kind of feelings and cognitions emerge at the beginning of the sexual contact and what course do they run?
– In which stage do performance anxiety and other interfering thoughts (e.g., spectatoring) come up and which are the most critical phases that normally lead to a loss of erection (frequently the intromission phase)?
– In which way are subjective arousal and the degree of erection related (dissociated versus parallel)?
– Does the sexual excitement of the partner influence the sexual functioning? A sexually indifferent and unaroused partner can put a damper on the man's excitement but on the other hand, a sexually responsive and highly aroused woman can be anxiety inducing for many men with erectile problems.
– Does the man receive enough stimulation by his partner (particularly important for older patients with a physically higher need for genital stimulation)?
– How do both partners react to a loss of erection?

A final complex of the current sexual problems relates to the incidence and extent of noncoital erections, sexual desire, and the sexual self concept of the patient. The interviewer should try to establish whether the erectile dysfunction is global or if the patient can achieve erections during masturbation or spontaneously (nocturnal or morning erections). At this point, the afore-mentioned tendency of psychogenically impotent men to underestimate their erections and to answer in the same way as men with organic impotence must be taken into account. The interviewer should bear this in mind and inquire critically, what the patient understands by a semi or fully rigid erection.

The relationship between the various aspects of sexual desire and erectile impotence is complex and cannot be dealt with in detail here. The interviewer should attempt to clarify if there is a reduction of sexual desire and loss of sexual pleasure *secondary* to erectile problems or if the sexual desire has not been affected by the functional problems. If desire is reduced it should be assessed if the reduction of libido – or a constitutionally low desire – has preceded the erectile problems or has developed secondary to it.

Regarding sexual self concepts, the interviewer must be aware of excessive expectations regarding genital functioning and penile rigidity that are still typical for the sexual scripts of many men. Some of the most prevalent sexual myths have been compiled by Zilbergeld [29]: "In sex, as elsewhere, it's performance that counts; the man must take charge of and orchestrate sex; a man always wants and is always ready to have sex; all physical contact must lead to sex; sex equals intercourse; sex requires an erection." Severely distorted demands for performance can often be found in young and rather inexperienced patients, but also in older patients who cannot accept an age-related reduction of sexual functioning.

2. Deeper Causes of Sexual Dysfunctions

Not all erectile disturbances have deeper intrapsychic or partner-related roots. This fact, however, together with the consequential implications for treatment strategies, renders an evaluation of deep-seated factors even more important. The psychodynamic infrastructure [14] of erectile impotence cannot be assessed or measured directly because psychic processes are involved that operate outside of the patient's conscious awareness. Since the remote causes are unspecific, no questions can be suggested, but the interviewer should keep an eye on the following areas:

– Traumatic experiences
– Cultural or educational indoctrination
– Neurotic processes, in which the sexual symptom serves as a defense against unconscious fears elicited by sexual behavior

3. The Relationship – Dyadic Causes

Although not all sexual dysfunctions are seen as relationship problems today, the assessment of partner-related causal factors remains extremely important. Even if only the male partner has a sexual problem, both partners are affected and often experience considerable marital discord. If possible the couple should be interviewed both together and apart. According to the heterogeneity of male and female sexualities, the spectrum of sexual interactions between the impotent man and his partner is extremely multifarious. The female partner includes the woman who has always been sexually indifferent or even aversive and who is secretly relieved that sexual intercourse has finally subsided, the sexually responsive woman who rejects manual or oral stimulation and clearly demands coital erections of her partner, and the cooperative woman who can cope with the sexual problems for a time, but who is willing and able to join the treatment.

Apart from the basic information, i.e., has the erectile impotence been in existence *before* the current partnership or has it developed *within* it, the interviewer should gain an impression of the specific kind of sexual interaction and should clarify if the sexual disorder only sets the stage for different dyadic problems. Causes of marital discord are, among others, parental transferences, lack of trust, power struggles, and failure of communication.

The term "sexual collusion" depicts a partner constellation, in which the partner who is symptom-free maintains an unconscious interest in the sexual problem of his partner. Frequently these motives have determined the choice of a partner, when for example a vaginistic woman with strong fears of penetration chooses a partner who is not able to have intercourse with her since he himself suffers from premature ejaculation or erectile problems. It is difficult to gain an insight into such subtle dyadic patterns even if both partners can be interviewed. Ignoring constellations like this, however, significantly increases the risk that any therapeutic intervention will fail, because it will be – consciously or unconsciously – sabotaged by the partner.

In summary, some of the most important items to be considered in the differential diagnosis of psychogenic versus organic impotence are as follows:

- Insidious versus acute onset of erectile problems
- Global inability to have erections versus situational inability
- Long history of psychosexual problems versus secondary disorder
- Presence or absence or adequate morning erections, masturbatory erections, and non-coital erections
- Presence or absence of partner-related problems or stressful life events associated with the onset of erectile problems
- History of depression or other relevant psychopathological symptoms
- Performance anxiety and fear of failure primary versus secondary to erectile problems

4. Psychiatric Symptoms

The relationship between psychiatric disorders and sexual dysfunctions is highly complex. On the one hand, many psychiatric illnesses are associated with psychosexual problems. On the other hand, patients with severe psychiatric disorders are capable of having perfectly normal sexual responses. In many cases a psychiatric illness afflicts the sexual desire rather than the genital functioning or the sexual dysfunction is due to the side effects of medication.

The interviewer should inquire if psychopathological symptoms are detectable (the most important ones are alcoholism, depressive syndromes, anxiety disorders, and personality disorders) and if there is a dynamic connection to the erectile dysfunction. The psychiatric illness can be the cause of erectile problems, it can be secondary to them, but it is also possible that the psychopathology is coincidental without being dynamically connected to the psychosexual problem.

Final Remark

The psychological assessment and evaluation of erectile dysfunction should not be confined to statements concerning the discrimination between organic and psychogenic factors or to psychopathological symptoms, but must attempt to take the complexity and the various facets of this highly prevalent psychosexual problem into account. This applies in particular to the interaction of organic and psychological etiological factors: An age-related, nonpathological weakening of erectile rigidity or a relatively "mild" organic factor always interacts with an individual's sexual history, a typical sexual self-concept, and the specific pattern of dyadic relationships. The interplay of these factors determines if an erectile dysfunction will emerge or if a constructive arrangement will be possible. Thus, during both evaluation and treatment, erectile impotence cannot be viewed as an isolated problem, because every therapeutic intervention is going to have a specific impact on the whole system. A thorough and skilful psychological evaluation can spare the patient the financial expense and emotional stress of a full medical assessment if he does not need it, because his problem is primarily caused by intrapsychic or partner-related factors. For this reason, the psychological evaluation should not be degraded to a mere supplier of psychological data, or function as an alibi for an otherwise purely somatic medicine. Only a truly multidisciplinary approach will be successful in adequately treating the impotent patient, but it requires more tolerance from both psychological and medical sides and a partial withdrawal from entrenched standpoints.

References

1. Abel GG et al. (1982) Differential diagnosis of impotence in diabetics. Neurol Urodynamics 1:57–69
2. Althof SE et al. (1989) Why do so many people drop out from auto-injection therapy for impotence? J Sex Marital Ther 15:121–129
3. Barlow DH (1986) Causes of sexual dysfunction: The role of anxiety and cognitive interference. J Consult Clin Psychol 54:140–148
4. Beutler LE et al. (1975) MMPI and MIT discriminators of biogenic and psychogenic impotence. J Consult Clin Psychol 43:899–903
5. Bruce TJ et al. (1989) Differences in anticipatory and situational affective responding between sexually functional and dysfunctional men. Paper presented at the annual

meeting of the Association for the Advancement of Behavior Therapy, Washington, DC

6. Bruce TJ et al. (1989) Differential response to distraction of sexually functional and dysfunctional men. Paper presented at the annual meeting of the Association for the Advancement of Behavior Therapy, Washington, DC

7. Dekker J, Everaerd W (1989) Psychological determinants of sexual arousal: A review. Behav Res Ther 27:353–364

8. Derogatis LR et al. (1976) Discrimination of organic versus psychogenic impotence with the DSFI. J Sex Marital Ther 2:229–240

9. Gellman R, Gellman Barroux C (1986) Réflexions critiques sur les impuissances d'origine vasculaire. Psychologie Médicale 18:399–401

10. Hatch JP et al. (1987) Psychometric differentiation of psychogenic and organic erectile disorders. J Urol 138:781–783

11. Jefferson TW et al. (1989) An evaluation of the Minnesota Multiphasic Personality Inventory as a discriminator of primary organic and primary psychogenic impotence in diabetic males. Arch Sex Behav 18:117–126

12. Kaplan HS (1974) The new sex therapy. Brunner/Mazel, New York

13. Kaplan HS (1979) Disorders of sexual desire. Brunner/Mazel, New York

14. Kaplan HS (1983) The evaluation of sexual disorders. Brunner/Mazel, New York

15. Keuler F, Altwein JE (1989) Diagnostik der erektilen Impotenz. Urologe [A] 28: 241–247

16. Kockott G et al. (1980) Symptomatology and psychological aspects of male sexual inadequacy: results of an experimental study. Arch Sex Behav 9:457–475

17. Lemaire A et al. (1987) Les explorations psychologiques standardisées dans l'exploration de l'impuissance. Psychologie Médicale 19:819–821

18. Levenson H et al. (1986) MMPI evaluation of erectile dysfunction: failure of organic vs. psychogenic decision rules. J Clin Psychol 42:752–754

19. Marshall P (1980) Differentiation of organic and psychogenic impotence on the basis of MMPI decision rules. J Consult Clin Psychol 48:407–408

20. Martin LM et al. (1983) Psychometric differentiation of biogenic and psychogenic impotence. Arch Sex Behav 12:475–485

21. Masters WH, Johnson V (1970) Human sexual inadequacy. Little, Brown, Boston

22. Sakheim DK et al. (1987) Distinguishing between organogenic and psychogenic erectile dysfunction. Behav Res Ther 25:379–390

23. Segraves KA, Segraves RT (1986) Differentiation of biogenic and psychogenic impotence with the Eysenck Personality Questionnaire and the Inventory of Sexual Attitudes. Personality and Individual Differences 7:423–425

24. Segraves KA et al. (1987) Use of sexual history to differentiate organic from psychogenic impotence. Arch Sex Behav 16:125–137

25. Segraves RT et al. (1981) Discrimination of organic versus psychological impotence with the DSFI: A failure to replicate. J Sex Marital Ther 7:230–238

26. Smith AD (1988) Psychologic factors in the multidisciplinary evaluation and treatment of erectile dysfunction. Urol Clin North Am 15:41–51

27. Staples RB et al. (1980) A reevaluation of MMPI discriminators of biogenic and psychogenic impotence. J Consult Clin Psychol 48:543–545

28. Turner LA et al. (1989) Self-injection of papaverine and phentolamine in the treatment of psychogenic impotence. J Sex Marital Ther 15:163–176

29. Zilbergeld B (1978) Male sexuality. Little, Brown, Boston

Pharmacotesting in Erectile Dysfunction

K.-P. Jünemann

The last decade of impotence research and routine workup was dramatically influenced by the introduction of intracavernous pharmacotherapy. It was common practice in the 1970s and early 1980s to treat patients suffering from erectile failure without further exploration of the etiology. Empirical administration of testosterone or extensive psychotherapy often frustrated the patient as well as the physician. More interest was shown in the diagnostic evaluation of erectile dysfunction with the introduction of nocturnal penile tumescence measurements (NPT) [20] to differentiate between organic and psychogenic impotence.

The major breakthrough, however, was accomplished with the discovery of pharmacologically inducible penile erection for diagnostic and therapeutic purposes by Virag in 1982 [41]. He reported on 25 patients evaluated for erectile failure who underwent intracavernous injection of 80 mg papaverine. He found an intracavernous pressure and arterial inflow increase after drug administration. Virag's report was the milestone for later development of advancing progress in the diagnostic workup and classification of male sexual dysfunction. Pharmacological and basic research studies of the erectile tissue took place in the following years. Intracavernous injection and self-injection therapy with papaverine or other vasoactive agents very soon became first-choice treatment alternatives to surgical options such as penile revascularization, venous ligation, or penile prosthesis implantation. By that time, it became obvious that some patients profit from pharmacotherapy and some do not, the latter requiring other treatment modalities. The new situation demanded a more subtle differentiation of the pathogenesis of erectile dysfunction in order to determine the correct treatment regimen for each etiological group (Fig. 1) [17]. Despite difficulties with a number of patients who could not be categorized into one of the etiological groups owing to a combination of several pathological factors, it was determined that only 20%–30% of all impotent men are psychogenic and that 50%–80% belong to the organic group [42, 31, 26]. These data were only attained by an extensive diagnostic workup of erectile failure, which was further improved by incorporating intracavernous injection of vasoactive drugs into classical as well as newly defined diagnostic tests, e.g., pharmaco-Doppler sonography [40] or pharmacocavernosometry and -graphy [45]. Furthermore, intracavernous pharmacotesting for diagnostic purposes became accepted world-

U. Jonas et al. (Eds.) Erectile Dysfunction
© Springer-Verlag Berlin Heidelberg 1991

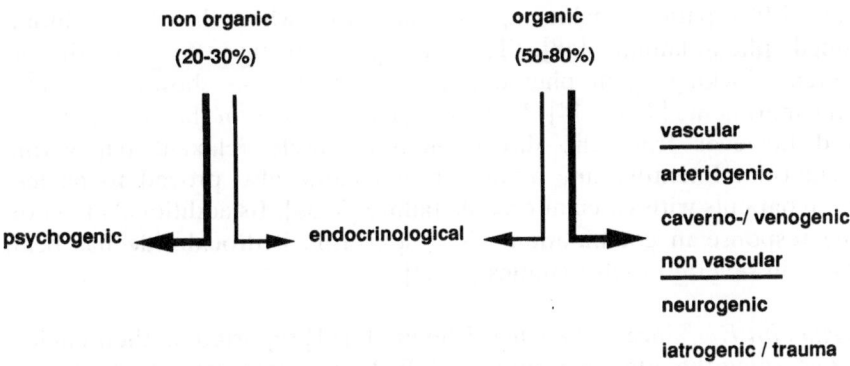

Fig. 1. Pathogenesis of erectile dysfunction

wide as a simple and reliable office procedure to simplify and further improve differentiation between etiological subgroups [2].

Pharmacology

Generally, to date, three different vasoactive agents are used for phar-macotesting as well as pharmacotherapy: papaverine, papaverine/phentolamine and prostaglandin (PGE_1). Other drugs or drug combinations such as (VIP) plus phentolamine, calcitonin gene-related peptide (CGRP) and PGE_1, etc. are under investigation and may, in future, compete with the agents usually administered. For diagnostic purposes, the regimen of pharmacotesting for all three drugs is similar (see below). However, the pharmacokinetics and the resulting side effects are quite different and require more detailed explanation.

Papaverine. An opium alkaloid of papaver somniferum (the opium poppy), papaverine exerts a myotonolytic effect by directly inhibiting phosphodiester-ase, which inactivates cyclic adenosine monophosphate (cAMP), resulting in smooth muscle relaxation of the corporeal tissue and culminating in a full erection [39]. For decades, it was used for intestinal colics and peripheral and cerebral circulatory disorders before being applied intracorporeally for diagnostic and therapeutic purposes in impotent patients by Virag in 1982 [41].

Papaverine/Phentolamine. In 1985, Zorgniotti and Lefleur [47] were the first to introduce the drug combination papaverine/phentolamine (30 mg/1 mg) in the treatment of erectile dysfunction. They demonstrated good results in 250 patients tested for intracavernous pharamacotherapy, with an overall success

---

rate of 71.9% patients achieving normal coitus when the drug solution contained phentolamine [48]. The erection-inducing effect of the α-adrenergic blocking agent phentolamine methylate was shown in several animal experiments [7, 13, 14]. Its hemodynamic effect on the erectile tissue differed however from the direct smooth muscle relaxant papaverine hydrochloride. Phentolamine administration alone also proved to be less potent in patients with vascular erectile failure [3, 38]. Its additional effect on erectile response in combination with papaverine hydrochloride has been described in several in vitro studies [8, 27].

Prostaglandin E₁. Since 1986, when Ishii et al. [11] reported on their clinical data concerning the administration of PGE_1 to impotent patients, PGE_1 has gained more supporters and users for diagnostic and therapeutic purposes in patients with erectile failure. The same group reported an 85% success rate of pharmacologically induced erection sufficient for coitus in 88 patients receiving 10–20 µg PGE_1 [12]. The pharmacological effect of PGE_1 seems to be an α-2 antiadrenergic reaction resulting in pronounced smooth muscle relaxation of the erectile tissue [10]. Almost 90% of the drug is inactivated during one single lung passage and degraded by the liver and kidneys [9, 30].

Practical Dosage

It is very difficult to compare one drug or drug combination with an other, as drug dosage and patient selection vary significantly from author to author, not to mention the learning process experienced by each investigator on commencing impotence work. In his pilot study, Virag [41] administered 80 mg papaverine hydrochloride in pharmacotesting. In 1985, Virag and colleagues [39] reported on 277 patients tested with 80 mg papaverine injection and for diagnostic evaluation. They utilized visual sexual stimulation (VSS) in combination with a tenfold lower dose of 8 mg papaverine, and maintained that they were able to distinguish between vascular and psychogenic impotence. Wagner [43] introduced mechanical penile vibration after administration of 28 mg papaverine as a clinical test for erectile function. Brindley [5], who initially reported on phenoxybenzamin (2–10 mg), administered 5–120 mg papaverine to induce a full erection [4]. Buvat et al. [6] administered up to 160 mg (10–160 mg) papaverine monosubstance to evaluate the erectile response with an initial standard dose of 80 mg. They recommended 20–40 mg of the monosubstance for psycho- and neurogenic cases. Lue and Tanagho [25] recommended 60 mg papaverine in 2–5 ml saline solution and advised adjusting the dosage according to the penile size. Furthermore, Lue placed a rubber band round the base of the penis prior to injection and left it there for 2 min in order to prevent severe systemic side effects from rapid venous outflow.

Papaverine   }   **40 - 80 mg**   **Fig. 2.** The most common drug doses for
                                       (up to 160mg)   corpus cavernosum injection tests (CCIT)

Papaverine / Phentolamine   }   **0.25 to 3 ml**

(15 mg / 0.5 mg per ml)

Prostaglandin E$_1$ }   **5 to 20 µg**
                                       (up to 40 µg)

Summarizing the literature, papaverine hydrochloride is used in doses ranging from 10–160 mg for pharmacotesting, with an initial dose of 40–80 mg (Fig. 2). Up to September 1989, more than 3000 patients were tested in larger series with papaverine hydrochloride [16] and almost 4000 with papaverine/phentolamine (Table 1). The drug combination introduced by Zorgniotti and Lefleur [47] was a mixture of 30 mg papaverine hydrochloride and phentolamine methylate 0.5–1 mg/ml solution. An erection sufficient for intercourse was achieved in 71.9% of 250 patients tested [48]. In the following years, various authors reported on excellent results in pharmacotesting on impotent men with various drug mixture ratios, such as papaverine + phentolamine 30 + 1 mg/ml [46, 22], 15 + 0.5 mg/ml [36, 37, 24], 50 + 1.66 mg/ml [23], 25 + 0.83 mg/ml [34], and 22.5 + 1.25 mg/ml [28]. The quantities applied ranged from 0.25–3 ml of the drug solution. Our own experience showed that a fixed combination of 15 mg/ml papaverine with 0.5 mg/ml phentolamine proved most efficient and safe for rationalizing the differential diagnosis of erectile failure (Fig. 2).

The major advantage of the drug mixture over papaverine mono-substance is the more obvious dose-dependent relationship between responder rate and etiology of impotence. Furthermore, it has been shown in drug surveys that the responder rate to intracorporeal pharmacotesting with papaverine plus phentolamine (65.4%) is superior to papaverine mono-substance (35.7%) (Table 2) [16]. With PGE$_1$, the responder rate was 75.3%. The number of patients tested for pharmacologically induced erection is constantly increasing. Published data exist on 1284 patients enrolled in an intracavernous injection program for diagnostic and therapeutic purposes (Table 1). The most practical dose range appears to be 5–40 µg PGE$_1$ in 1 ml

Table 1. Number of patients (*n*) who underwent pharmacotesting for a diagnostic workup between 08/82 and 09/89. (From Jünemann and Alken [16])

	n
Papaverine	3153
Papaverine/ Phentolamine	3998
Prostaglandin E$_1$	1284

108   K.-P. Jünemann

Table 2. Drug survey. Efficiency and safety of cavernous injection on 408 patients. (From Jünemann et al. [17])

	Erection	Pain	Prol. erection
Papaverine	120/35.7%	0	10/3%
Papaverine/ Phentolamine	257/65.4%	0	9/2.5%
Prostaglandin E_1	238/75.3%	61/19%	0

normal saline [29, 12, 32, 35, 44] with an initial test dose of 20 μg PGE_1 (Fig. 2). The solution employed to dissolve PGE_1 is 1–5 ml saline.

Pharmacotesting

The pharmacological test, corpus cavernosum injection test (CCIT) with vasoactive agents is a fundamental part of our impotence workup. In principle, it is not important which drug is utilized. However, as far as erectile potency is concerned, it has been shown that the combination of papaverine and phentolamine or PGE_1 effects better erection capability than papaverine monosubstance [29]. We prefer the administration of papaverine/phentolamine to that of PGE_1. In accordance with our animal studies [1] and clinical results [16], we no longer utilize papaverine monosubstance owing to its fibrosis-inducing effect and low erection-inducing ability.

Pharmacotesting follows as part of our routine diagnostic program after the patient's psychological and neurological status has been assessed, his case history noted, physical examination performed, and blood samples for evaluation of the hormone and lipid status taken (Fig. 3). NPT measurement and VSS can be utilized alternatively in order to differentiate between psycho- and neurogenic erectile failure.

The next step in our diagnostic build-up is the evaluation of the arterial blood supply of the penis with Doppler sonography in combination with the first injection of our pharmacotesting procedure (pharmaco-Doppler sonography [19]). Once the vascular system of the penis has been assessed, more knowledge must be gained on the corporeal function and the erectile potency of the smooth muscle of the corpora cavernosa themselves. This is the domain of pharmacotesting. Before commencing injection of vasoactive agents into the cavernous bodies, two important points must be taken into consideration:

1. The patient is requested to give his written consent to the pharmacotesting procedure. This is very important, as to date the drugs used for intracavernous pharmacotesting have not yet been approved by any national health authority.

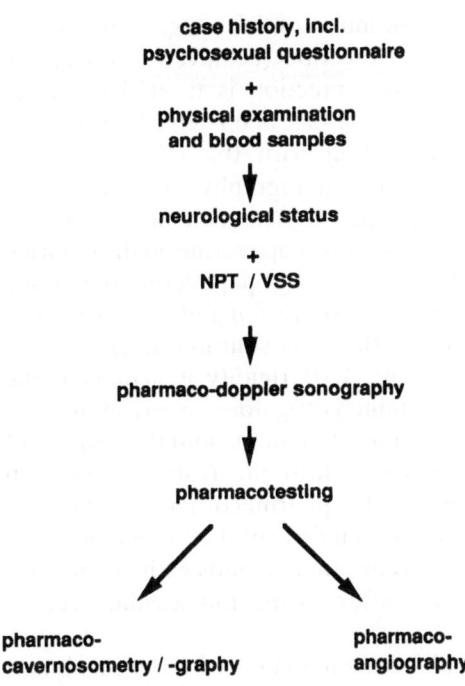

case history, incl.
psychosexual questionnaire

+

physical examination
and blood samples

neurological status

+

NPT / VSS

pharmaco-doppler sonography

pharmacotesting

pharmaco-
cavernosometry / -graphy

pharmaco-
angiography

Fig. 3. Diagnostic pyramid in patients with erectile dysfunction

2. Guarantee must be given that the same drug or drug combination and dosage will be administered to ensure that the results of the erectile response are comparable. Furthermore, a classification system is important to allow an estimation of the erectile response in each patient. We prefer a penrig (penile rigidity) scale [15] similar to that proposed by other authors [36, 21] (E_0, no tumescence; E_1, elongation only; E_2, moderate tumescence; E_3, full tumescence, no rigidity; E_4, rigidity achieved, intercourse possible; E_5, full rigidity).

Testing can be carried out on an in- or outpatient basis. However, we found the former more favorable as it was easier to carry out all examinations within a short period when the patient was hospitalized for 2–3 days. Furthermore, it is safer for the patient should complications arise with pharmacoinjections.

The injection is applied with a 1–5 ml syringe, depending on the volume preferred (we used 2 ml), and a 26 or 27 GA (0.4 × 19) needle. The needle is inserted at a 90° angle into the lateral aspect of *one* corpus cavernosum at the base of the penis with the patient in supine position. For pharmaco-Doppler sonography, the patient's vascular bed is evaluated within 8–10 min after injection: For pharmacotesting, the patient is requested to stand up after 2 min and remain in upright position for 30 min, during which the erectile response is evaluated every 15 min. The result is registered on a specially designed erection flow sheet, which includes the penrig response during the first 30 min has been protocolled, the patient must continue registration every 15 min up to a maximum of 5 h. If an E_4 erection (achieved rigidity) still continues after 5 hours, then the prolonged erection is treated by intra-cavernously injecting a sympathomimetic agent as has been described [18, 33].

Generally, we commence pharmacotesting with 0.5 ml papaverine/ phentolamine in conjunction with Doppler sonography. If there is a possibility of the patient to be tested being either psychogenic or neurogenic, we lower the initial dose to 0.25 ml of 15 mg/ml papaverine hydrochloride plus 0.5 mg/ml phentolamine methylate (3.75 mg papaverine/0.125 mg phentolamine) in order to minimize the risk of prolonged erection. The dosage is gradually increased up to 3 ml of the drug solution in accordance with the erectile response, as shown in Fig. 4. If rigidity is achieved, the patient is classified, together with the determined drug dose, as a responder to pharmacotesting. Injections are performed on a 24-h basis, and the responder dose is administered the following day to confirm the result as this will probably determine the individual drug dose for pharmacotherapy. Should a full erection response ($E_{4/5}$) occur with the initial dose of 0.5 ml, we then test the patient the following day with 0.25 ml. If he still responds with an erection then it can be assumed that the patient suffers from nonvascular erectile dysfunction.

If the patient does not respond to pharmacoinjection with the maximum dosage of 3 ml of the combination, we continue our diagnostic workup with the more invasive procedures (Fig. 3). Furthermore, a final test with 20 µg

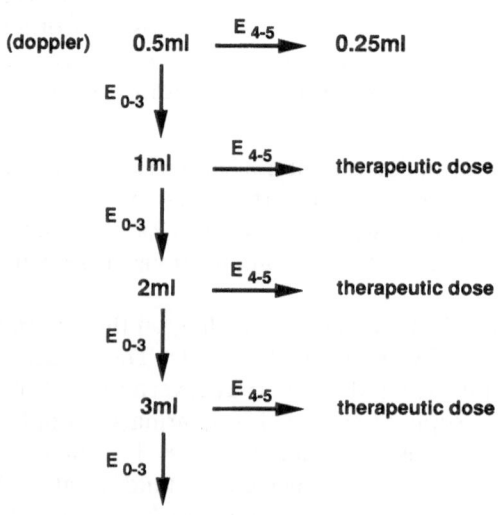

(papaverine / phentolamine - 15mg / 0.5mg)

Fig. 4. Pharmacotesting program with papaverine and phentolamine

PGE$_1$ is carried out. In accordance with our previous results on pharmacotesting with papaverine/phentolamine on 115 patients [15], we were able to classify their erectile dysfunction as follows:

- 0.25–0.5 ml nonvascular
- 0.5–3 ml arterio-/cavernogenic
- Non-responder caverno-/venogenic

Complications

Undesired side effects with pharmacotesting are either limited to the penis itself or are systemic. Possible minor side effects are hematomas occurring at the injection site (2%–10%), a burning sensation on injection, or puncturing of the urethra with subsequent hematuria or subcutaneous injection [16]. In general, these complications resolve within several days. More severe complications derived from incorrect injection such as cavernitis or infections were rarely observed (0.5%); fibrosis-type changes within the corpus cavernosa are unlikely to occur during the diagnostic period.

The most feared and most frequently encountered complication is prolonged erection. The incidence of pharmacologically induced priapism depends on the vasoactive agent and the drug dose utilized (2.4%–9.5%; Table 3). The group most prone to prolonged erection are patients with nonvascular erectile failure. Therefore, the initial dose for pharmacotesting should be lowered in patients with suspected neurogenic or psychogenic erectile failure. An experienced investigator can minimize the risk of prolonged erection to below 3%, as drug survey studies on 408 patients have already shown (Table 2) [16]. Although PGE$_1$ is the safest drug used for pharmacoinjection studies, its limiting factor is the pain-inducing side effect after injection, which may occur in up to 19% [16]. Some patients tested with PGE$_1$ became accustomed to this uncomfortable sensation of pressure, whereas others did not. Therefore, the investigator should decide which drug or drug mixture he prefers to administer to his patients.

Systemic side effects with the injection seldom occur. In our series, blood pressure fluctuation or other cardiovascular complications (e.g., syncopal

Table 3. Patient number (n) and side effects (pain, prol. erection) on pharmacotesting for diagnostic workup between 08/82 to 09/89. (From Jünemann and Alken [16])

	n	Pain	Prol. erection
Papaverine	2134	0	203/9.5%
Papaverine/ Phentolamine	2914	0	153/5.3%
Prostaglandin E$_1$	1284	226/17.6%	28/2.4%

events) were never observed [15]. However, it is of significant importance to make an appropriate patient selection and avoid high-risk patients with other severe ailments such as severe cardiovascular and respiratory complaints, severe hepatopathy or renal insufficiency, glaucoma, or benign prostate hyperplasia with high residual urine. Pharmacotesting is a safe and reliable diagnostic procedure in erectile dysfunction if the above-mentioned recommendations are followed.

References

1. Abozeid M, Jünemann KP, Luo JA, Lue TF, Yen BT, Tanagho EA (1987) Chronic apaverine treatment: the effect of repeated injections on the simian erectile response and penile tissue. J Urol 138:1263–1266
2. Bähren W, Stief C, Scherb W, Gall H, Gallwitz A, Altwein JE (1986) Rationelle Diagnostik der erektilen Dysfunktion unter Anwendung eines pharmakologischen Testes. Akt Urol 17:177–180
3. Blum MD, Bahnson RR, Porter TN, Carter MF (1985) Effect of local alpha-adrenergic blockade on human penile erection. J Urol 134:479–481
4. Brindley GS (1986) Maintenance treatment of erectile impotence by cavernosal unstriated muscle relaxant injection. Br J Psychiatr 149:210–215
5. Brindley GS (1986) Pilot experiments on the actions of drugs injected into the human corpus cavernosum penis. Br J Pharmacol 87:495–500
6. Buvat J, Lemaire A, Marcolin G, Dehaene JL, Buvat-Herbaut M (1987) Intracavernous injection of apaverine (ICIP). Assessment of its diagnostic and therapeutic value in 100 impotent patients. Wld J Urol 5:150–155
7. Domer FR, Wessler G, Brown RL, Charles HC (1978) Involvement of the sympathetic nervous system in the urinary bladder internal sphincter and in penile erection in the anesthetized cat. Invest Urol 15:404–407
8. Goldstein I, Payton TR, de Tejada IS, Krane RJ (1985) Pharmacologic erections: role in the treatment of neurologic impotence. J Urol 133:261A (591)
9. Hamberg M, Samuelsson B (1971) On the metabolism of prostaglandins E_1 and E_2 in man. J Biol Chem 246:6713–6721
10. Hedlund H, Andersson KE (1985) Contraction and relaxation induced by some prostanoids in isolated human penile erectile tissue and cavernous artery. J Urol 134:1245–1250
11. Ishii N, Watanabe H, Irisawa C, Kikuchi Y (1986) Therapeutic trial with prostaglandin E_1 for organic impotence. In: Proceedings of the fifth conference on vasculogic impotence and corpus cavernosum revascularization. Second world meeting on impotence, Prague, Czechoslovakia. International Society for Impotence Research (ISIR)
12. Ishii N, Watanabe H, Irisawa C (1989) Intracavernous injection of prostaglandin E_1 for the treatment of erectile impotence. J Urol 141:323–325
13. Jünemann KP, Lue TF, Abozeid M, Hellstrom WJG, Tanagho EA (1986) Blood gas analysis in drug-induced penile erection. Urol Int 41:207–211
14. Jünemann KP, Lue TF, Fournier GR Jr, Tanagho EA (1986) Haemodynamics of papaverine- and phentolamine-induced penile erection. J Urol 136:158–161
15. Jünemann KP, Jecht E, Müller-Matteis V et al. (1988) Offene Multizenterstudie zur Differentialdiagnostik der erektilen Dysfunktion mit einer Papaverin-Phentolamin-Kombination (BY023). Urologe A 27:2–7
16. Jünemann KP, Alken P (1989) Pharmacotherapy of erectile dysfunction: a review. Int J Impotence Res 1:71–93

17. Jünemann KP, Persson-Jünemann C, Alken P (1990) Pathophysiology of erectile dysfunction. Semin Urol:8:80–93
18. Jünemann KP, Potempa D, Löbelenz M, Alken P (1990) Therapie der prolongierten Erektion. In: Wetterauer U, Stief CG (eds) Diagnostik und Therapie der erektilen Dysfunktion mit vasoaktiven Substanzen. de Gruyter, Berlin New York
19. Jünemann KP, Siegsmund M, Löbelenz M, Alken P (1990) Doppler-Sonographie der Penisarterien. Urologe A 29:113–119
20. Karacan I, Ware JC, Dervent B, Altinel A (1978) Impotence and blood pressure in the flaccid penis: relationship to nocturnal penile tumescence. Sleep 1:125
21. Kiely EA, Ignotus P, Williams G (1987) Penile function following intracavernosal injection of vasoactive agents or saline. Br J Urol 59:473–476
22. Kiely EA, Williams G, Goldie L (1987) Assessment of the immediate and long-term effects of pharmacologically induced penile erections in the treatment of psychogenic and organic impotence. Br J Urol 59:164–169
23. Lakin MM, Montague DK (1989) Intracavernous injections of papaverine and phentolamine: correlation with penile brachial index. Urology 33:383–386
24. Levine S, Althof S, Turner L, Risen C, Bodner D, Kursh E, Resnick K (1989) Side effects of self-administration of intracavernous papaverine and phentolamine for the treatment of impotence. J Urol 141:54–57
25. Lue TF, Tanagho EA (1987) Physiology of erection and pharmacological management of impotence. J Urol 137:829–836
26. Montague DK, James RE Jr, de Wolfe V, et al (1979) Diagnostic evaluation, classification and treatment of men with sexual dysfunction. Urology 14:545
27. Padma-Nathan H, Goldstein K, Azadzoi R, Blanco R, de Tejada IS, Krane RJ (1986) In vivo and in vitro studies on the physiology of penile erection. Semin Urol 4:209–216
28. Padma-Nathan H, Goldstein K, Payton T, Krane RJ (1987) Intracavernosal pharmacotherapy: the pharmacologic erection programme. Wld J Urol 5:160–165
29. Porst H (1989) Prostaglandin E_1 bei erektiler Dysfunktion. Urologe A 28:94–98
30. Rosenkranz B, Fischer C, Boeynaems JM, Frölich JC (1983) Metabolic disposition of prostaglandin E_1 in man. Biochim Biophys Acta 750:231–236
31. Sarramon JP, Rischmann P, Elman B, et al (1986) Within the last five years our experience in impotence vascular surgery. Second world meeting on impotence, Prague Czechoslovakia, June 17–20, 1986
32. Schramek P, Dorninger R, Waldhauser M, Floth A, Porpaczy P (1988) One year clinical experience with prostaglandin E_1 in diagnosis and treatment of erectile dysfunction. In: Proceedings of the sixth biennial international symposium for corpus cavernosum revascularization. Third biennial world meeting on impotence. International Society for Impotence Research (ISIR), Boston
33. Sidi AA, Cameron JS, Duffy LM, Lange PH (1986) Intracavernous drug-induced erections in the management of male erectile dysfunction: experience with 100 patients. J Urol 135:704–706
34. Sidi AA, Chen KK (1987) Clinical experience with vasoactive intracavernous pharmacotherapy for the treatment of impotence. Wld J Urol 5:156–159
35. Stackl W, Hasun R, Marberger M (1988) Intracavernous injection of prostaglandin E_1 in impotent men. J Urol 140:66–68
36. Stief CG, Bähren W, Gall H, Scherb W, Gallwitz A, Altwein JE (1986) Schwellkörper-Autoinjektionstherapie (SKAT): erste Erfahrungen bei erektiler Dysfunktion. Urologe A 25:63–66
37. Stief CG, Bähren W, Gall H, Scherb W. Thon WF, Altwein JE (1986) Preselection, indication and side effects of a therapy with vasoactive drugs (TDV). In: Proceedings of the fifth conference on vasculogenic impotence and corpus cavernosum revascularization. Second world meeting on impotence. Prague, Czechoslovakia. International Society for Impotence Research (ISIR)
38. Tordjman G (1984) Actions des alpha-bloquants sur l'éjaculation prématurée et sur l'érection. Contracep Fert Sex 12:1023–1025
39. Virag R, Bouilly P, Daniel C, Virag H (1985) Intracavernous injection of papaverine

and other vasoactive drugs: new era in the diagnosis and treatment of impotence. In: Virag RH (eds) Proceedings of the first world meeting on impotence CERI, Paris, pp 187–194

40. Virag R, Frydman D, Legman M, Virag H (1984) Intracavernous injection of papaverine as a diagnostic and therapeutic method in erectile failure. Angiology 35:79–87
41. Virag R (1982) Intracavernous injection of papaverine for erectile failure. Lancet II:938
42. Virag R (1986) The screening of impotence by the use of visual sexual stimulation after intracavernous injection of a small (8 mg) dose of papaverine. Second world meeting on impotence, Prague, Czechoslovakia, June 17–20
43. Wagner G (1985) Penile erection provoked by vibration and intracorporeal injection. Nordisk Sexologi 3:113–118
44. Weiske WH (1988) Prolonged erection by vasoactive drugs — its avoidance with PGE_1. In: Proceedings of the sixth biennial international symposium for corpus cavernosum revascularization. Third biennial world meeting on impotence. International Society for Impotence Research (ISIR), Boston
45. Wespes E, Delcour C, Struyven J, Schulmann CC (1986) Pharmacocavernometry-cavernography in impotence. Br J Urol 58:429
46. Williams G, Mulcahy MJ, Kiely EA (1987) Impotence: Treatment by autoinjection of vasoactive drugs. Br Med J 295:595–596
47. Zorgniotti AW, Lefleur RS (1985) Auto-injection of the corpus cavernosum with a vasoactive drug combination for vasculogenic impotence. J Urol 133:39–41
48. Zorgniotti AW (1986) Corpus cavernosum blockade for impotence: Practical aspects and results in 250 cases. J Urol 135:306A (808)

Doppler Ultrasound Investigation of Penile Vessels

H. Gall and G. Holzki

The Doppler ultrasound examination offers a noninvasive method for evaluating a vascular origin of erectile dysfunction. We consider it essential in the interdisciplinary investigation of this disease.

In 1975 Abelson [1] determined for the first time the systolic penile blood pressure by means of Doppler ultrasound. Later, Doppler examination of the penile arteries in the flaccid state was performed by recording the velocity curve. Doppler examination of the superficial and deep penile arteries in the proximal and distal segment was introduced by Jevtich [11] and by Karacan et al. [12]. A further advance was the use of Doppler ultrasound of the penile vessels in combination with the intracavernosal injection of vasoactive drugs (IIVD) [2, 18, 20].

The use of Doppler ultrasound to identify penile venous insufficiency was first suggested by Stief et al. [16], the first study being performed by Gall et al. [6]. Doppler ultrasound makes accessible the following: the deep cavernosal arteries, the superficial dorsal arteries, the deep dorsal vein, ectopic veins, the superficial dorsal veins, and cavernosum-glandular venous shunts (Fig. 1).

Doppler Ultrasound Examination of Penile Arteries

The examination should be performed with the patient lying on his back using directional Doppler flowmeters with an ultrasound probe of 8–10 MHz. The penetration of an 8 MHz probe ranges from 0.25 cm to 3.6 cm [14].

Localisation of Vessels

The superficial dorsal artery is first localized proximally above the root of the penis. The ultrasound probe is placed in the midline dorsally at the root of the penis at an angle of 45° to the horizontal plane. The ultrasound probe is shifted to both sides in order to evaluate the left and the right dorsal penile artery (Fig. 2). The distal positioning occurs proximally of the corona of glans penis at an angle of approximately 45° to the horizontal plane (Fig. 3). If no

U. Jonas et al. (Eds.) Erectile Dysfunction
© Springer-Verlag Berlin Heidelberg 1991

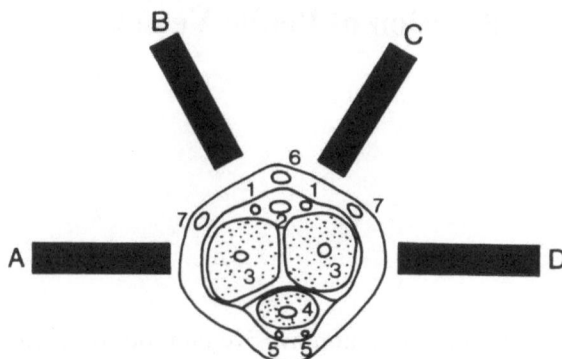

Fig. 1. Cross-section of the penis (scheme). *1*, dorsal artery; *2*, deep dorsal vein; *3*, corpus cavernosum with cavernosal artery; *4*, corpus spongiosum and urethra; *5*, urethral arteries; *6*, superficial dorsal vein; *7*, ectopic veins; *A+D*, position of the Doppler probe for the localisation of the cavernosal arteries; *B+C*, position of the Doppler probe for the localisation of the dorsal arteries

pulse sound can be demonstrated, the course of the dorsal penile artery is followed along the dorsum of the penis. The disappearance of the Doppler signal is recorded as the site of discontinuance. The Doppler signal from the deep cavernosal arteries is localized on both sides proximally at the lateral surface of the root of the penis. At first, the Doppler probe is placed laterally on the dorsum of the penis and is then moved in a dorsal-ventral curve. When the deep artery is reached by the ultrasound cone, the probe is tilted at 45° to the vertical plane (Fig. 4).

The optimal distal recording site for the deep artery was found to be about two-thirds of the distance from the penis root to the corona of glans penis (Fig. 5).

Overall, there are eight localizations for the paired superficial dorsal arteries and the deep cavernosal arteries in the proximal and distal segment.

Assessment of Doppler Signals

With respect to accurate recordings of the flow curves, it is important that the Doppler probe be aimed directly at the center of the vessel to avoid measurement of slower marginal flows instead of the mean instant flow velocity over the vascular cross-section. The clearest Doppler signal is obtained when the ultrasonic waves are directed at an angle of 45° to the vessel.

While searching the vessel slight pressure on the artery by the probe may cause a temporary stenosis with an increased peak velocity. The definitive measurement should be performed without pressure (Figs. 6 and 7).

Doppler Signals over the Flaccid Penis

When the penis is flaccid, the arterial Doppler signal is compared with the velocity curve over the palmar digital artery of the index finger. A strong Doppler signal over the proximal penile arteries shows about the same amplitude as that of the finger artery (Fig. 8). The amplitude normally decreases in the distal vascular segment.

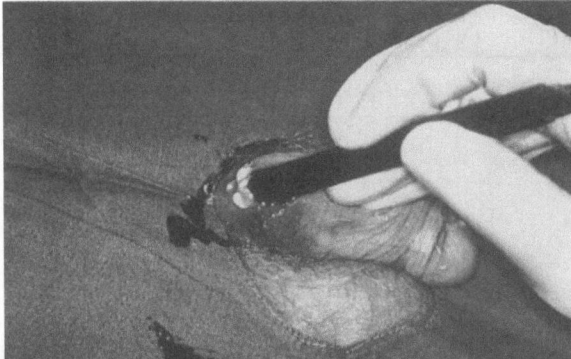

Fig. 2. Position of the Doppler probe for the localisation of the dorsal arteries (proximal segment)

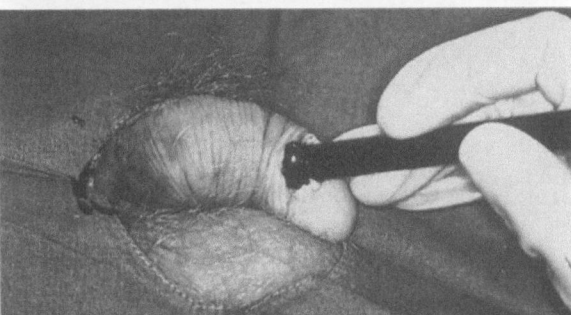

Fig. 3. Position of the Doppler probe for the localisation of the dorsal arteries (distal segment)

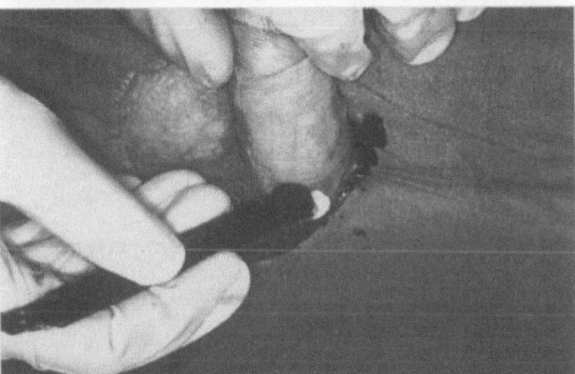

Fig. 4. Position of the Doppler probe for the localisation of the cavernosal arteries (proximal segment)

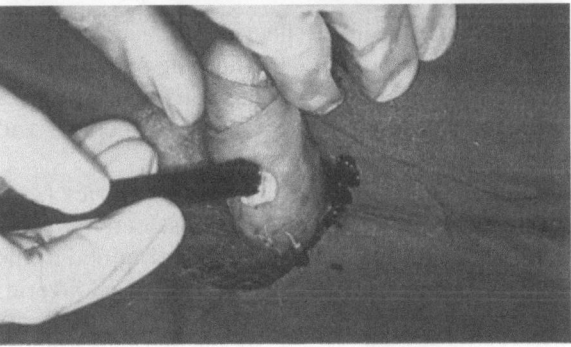

Fig. 5. Position of the Doppler probe for the localisation of the cavernosal arteries (distal segment)

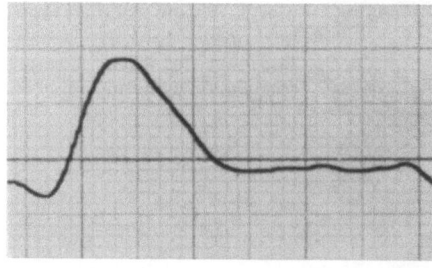

Fig. 6. Doppler signal from a compressed penile artery

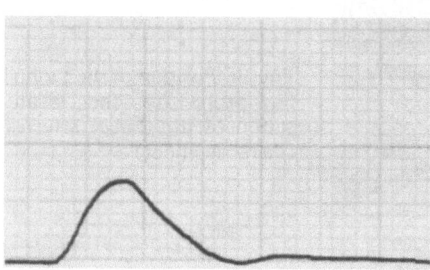

Fig. 7. Doppler signal from a penile artery without compression

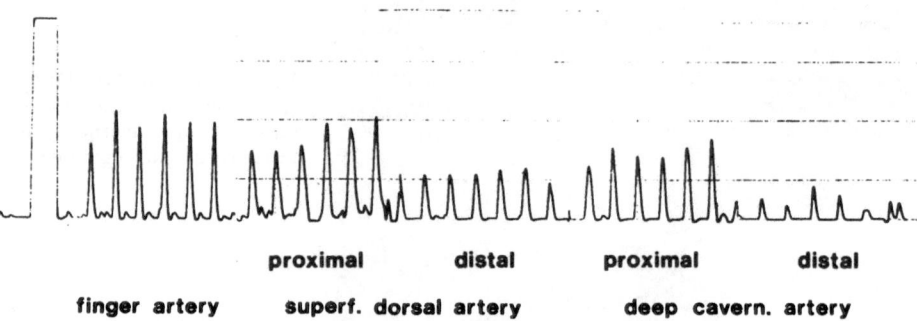

proximal   **distal**   **proximal**   **distal**

finger artery   **superf. dorsal artery**   **deep cavern. artery**

Fig. 8. Doppler signals from all penile arteries in flaccid state (compared with signals of a finger artery)

    The results of the Doppler examination in the flaccid state can be documented as follows: strong signal, +; weak signal, (+); missing signal, 0.

    Compared with arteriography a strong signal reveals a normal artery, a weak signal correlates with a hypoplastic or partially stenosed section, and a missing signal is found in vascular aplasia or total stenosis [4].

    Accuracy of the Doppler examination in localizing penile arteries (performed by a well trained investigator) when compared with selective angiography is higher than 95% [5, 11]. A 100% accuracy is usually obtained in the detection of the superficial penile arteries, while the deep cavernosal arteries are more difficult to detect [4, 10, 17].

Doppler Ultrasonography of Penile Arteries
Following Intracavernosal Injection of Vasoactive Drugs

In this test the Doppler examination of the penile arteries follows the intra-cavernosal injection of small doses of vasoactive drugs like papaverine alone or in combination with phentolamine. Recent publications also propose the use of prostaglandin E1. The technique of the Doppler examination remains unchanged.

For contraindications of diagnostic use of IIVD see the respective chapters. We recommend the following doses, which are approximately equivalent in effect: 12.5 mg papaverine; 0.25 ml of a mixture containing 15 mg/ml papaverine and 0.5 mg/ml phentolamine (SKAT); or 5 µg prostaglandin E1. In patients with a normal penile vascular system injections of these doses may cause full erections [2, 7, 11]. The injection is followed within minutes by maximum perfusion caused by a doubling of the arterial diameter together with maximum systolic blood velocity [13].

The erection obtained by IIVD may be recorded according to this scheme:

E0 – no tumescence
E1 – beginning tumescence
E2 – medium tumescence
E3 – full tumescence
E4 – full tumescence and medium rigidity
E5 – full tumescence and full rigidity

The peak systolic flow in penile arteries following IIVD correlates with the degree of erection and shows a maximum between E2 and E3. The examination should be completed before E4 to avoid incorrect interpretation of a vessel section (missing vessel, arteriosclerosis, dysplasia etc.) (Fig. 9).

In normal penile arteries a biphasic Doppler signal with a significant diastolic flow can be received. The maximum systolic peak velocity increases from approximately 2 cm/s in the flaccid state to more than 13 cm/s in the proximal and more than 6.5 cm/s in the distal segment (measured by directional Doppler Kranzbuehler 762; Figs. 10 and 11).

Hypoplastic arteries often produce monophasic signals revealing markedly reduced systolic peak velocity, a shortened pulse-rising time, and no diastolic flow (Fig. 12). Prepenile or intrapenile partial stenosis causes reduced systolic peak velocity and a rough diastolic decrescendo (Fig. 13). The lack of Doppler signal over a vessel section may be caused by aplasia or complete stenosis [8, 9].

In young potent men hypoplasia or aplasia of one dorsal artery is common and certainly does not lead to primary erectile dysfunction. Further arteriographic investigations have revealed that arterial abnormalities must be severe, bilateral, and involving the deep cavernosal arteries to cause primary erectile dysfunction. We believe that minor abnormalities of the deep cavernosal arteries become more important with increasing age as a cause

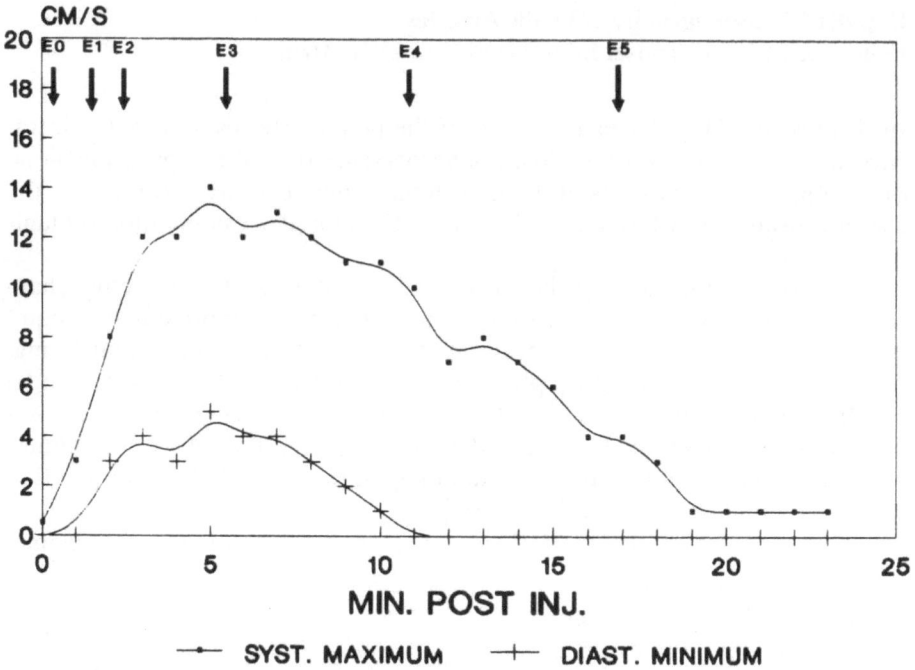

Fig. 9. Course of maximum systolic and minimum diastolic blood velocity following IIVD

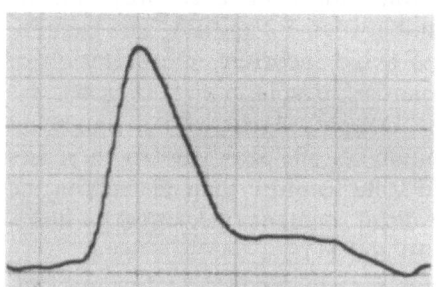

Fig. 10. Doppler signal obtained over a normal dorsal artery (proximal segment)

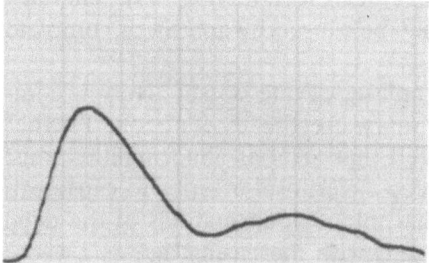

Fig. 11. Doppler signal obtained over a normal dorsal artery (distal segment)

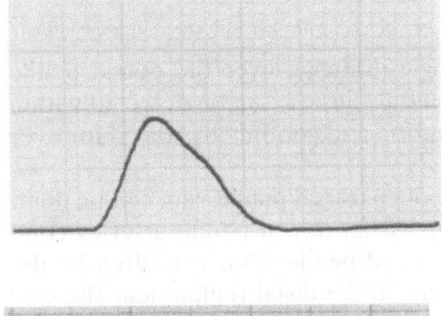

Fig. 12. Monophasic Doppler signal over a dysplastic penile artery

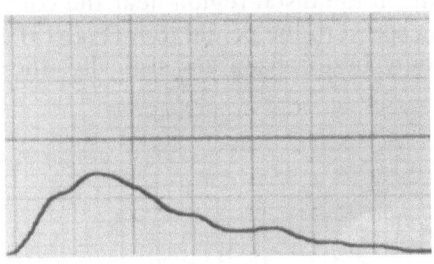

Fig. 13. Doppler signal of an arteriosclerotic penile artery

of secondary impotence, especially when accompanied by risk factors like arteriosclerosis [3, 4].

Comparative investigations with arteriography show that the Doppler method is highly accurate (95%) in the localisation of penile arteries [15]. The primary failure of Doppler ultrasound (with or without IIVD) is that it does not detect a unilateral supply of the corpora cavernosa [4].

Compared with Doppler examination of penile arteries in flaccid state, examination following IIVD is easier, faster, safer, and more reliable because it reflects the hemodynamics in the functional state. The high diagnostic effectiveness of Doppler ultrasound reduces the need for invasive angiography of the internal pudendal artery in the basic examination of erectile dysfunction and in postoperative control [5].

Diagnosis of Venous Incompetence by Doppler Ultrasonography

Doppler examinations of the penile veins should be performed after maximal stimulation of arterial inflow with IIVD (2–3 ml of a standard mixture of papaverine and phentolamine). Routinely we search for pathologic orthograde bloodflow over the dorsal penile veins and for cavernosum-glandular shunts (retrograde bloodflow). The penile anatomy does not allow Doppler localisation of the deep cavernosal veins.

Dorsal Penile Veins

Doppler examination visualizes pathologic drainage over the dorsal penile veins on the dorsum penis. Pathologic venous outflow can be detected within a few seconds after injection of IIVD solution and continually traced for over 30 min.

By means of Doppler ultrasound the deep dorsal penile vein can be demonstrated between the right and left superficial dorsal penile arteries (Fig. 14). Orthograde bloodflow in the deep dorsal penile veins can often be detected over a considerable length; it begins in the distal region near the corona of glans penis and passes at increasing speed to the penile root (Fig. 15). While the deep dorsal penile vein can only be localized accoustically, the superficial venous system is visible.

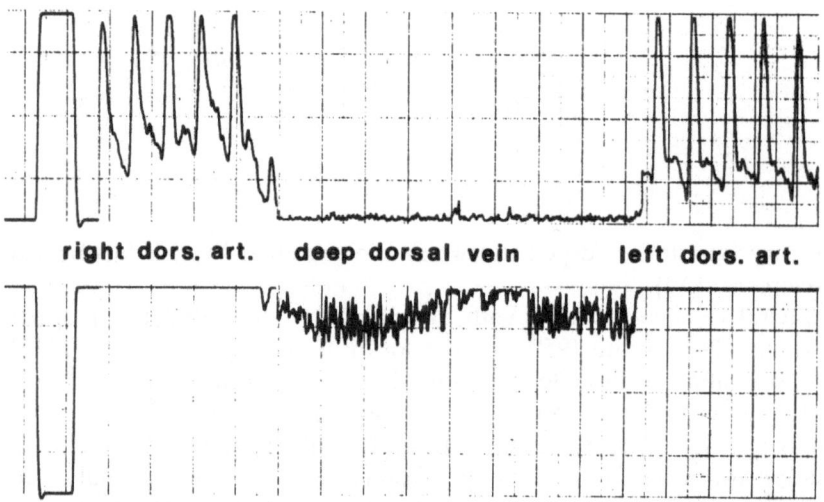

right dors. art.   deep dorsal vein   left dors. art.

Fig. 14. Localisation of the deep dorsal penile vein by means of Doppler ultrasound

distal   **proximal**

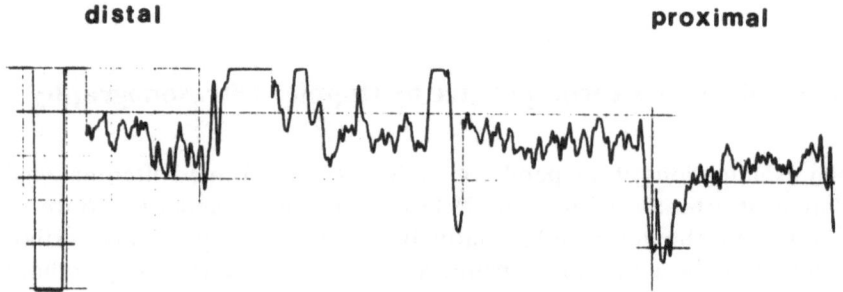

Fig. 15. Course of the deep dorsal penile vein followed by Doppler ultrasound

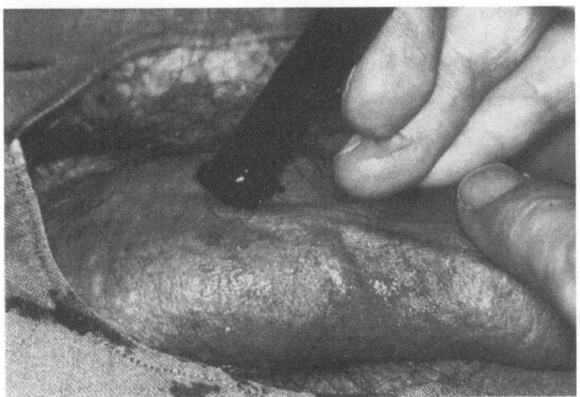

Fig. 16. Clinical illustration of the superficial dorsal vein

distal   **proximal**

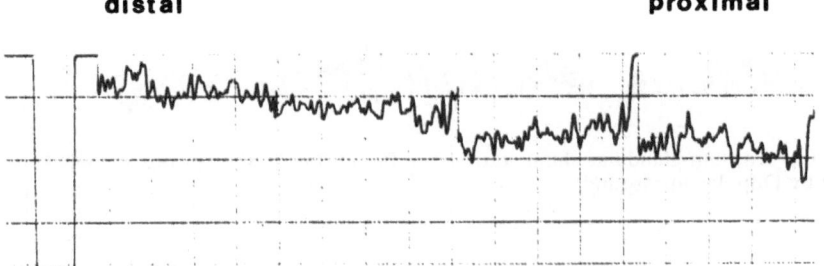

Fig. 17. Course of the superficial dorsal penile vein followed by Doppler ultrasound

Ectopic penile veins and the superficial dorsal vein appear through the skin as subcutaneous veins. The superficial dorsal penile vein originates at the corona of glans penis and continues paramedially to the dorsal penile root (Figs. 16 and 17).

Ectopic penile veins can also be visuallized on the dorsum penis lateral to the superficial penile artery. In the superficial dorsal and ectopic penile veins, the orthograde bloodflow passes from distal to proximal to the penile root (Fig. 18). It is possible to mark the course of the visible superficial dorsal or ectopic penile veins with a coloured pen and then to ligate the vein under local anesthesia [16].

Venous Shunts

A shunt between the corpus cavernosum and corpus spongiosum occurs mainly in association with dorsal vein insufficiency [6]. An example of an isolated shunt is represented by the iatrogenic communication of the corpus cavernosum and glans penis in the priapism operation of Winter [19]. In this case Doppler examination identifies retrograde bloodflow at the cor-

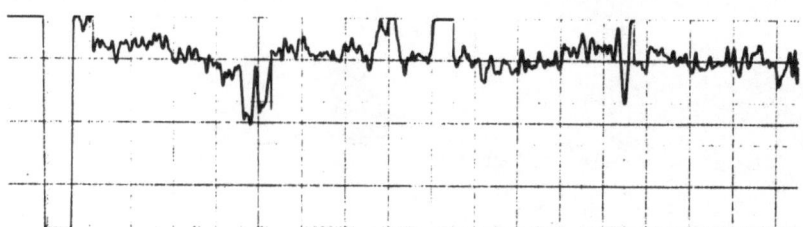

Fig. 18. Course of the right-sided ectopic penile vein followed by Doppler ultrasound

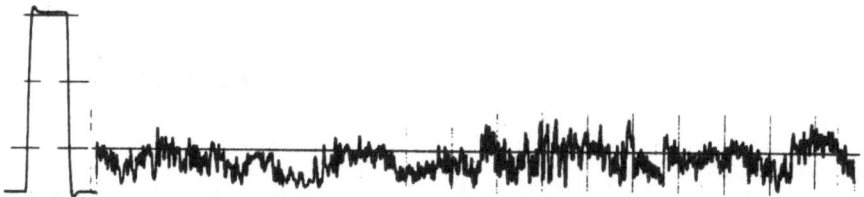

Fig. 19. Cavernosum-glandular shunt: retrograde blood flow at the corona of glans penis detected by Doppler ultrasound

ona of glans penis passing from the corpus cavernosum to the glans penis (cavernosum-glandular shunt) (Fig. 19).

Doppler ultrasound is generally well suited as a non-invasive method of identifying pathologic venous outflow disturbances. In patients with proven venous incompetence, Doppler ultrasound examination compares very favourably with the valid invasive reference method of cavernosography [6].

References

1. Abelson D (1975) Diagnostic value of the penile pulse and blood pressure: A Doppler study of impotence in diabetics. J Urol 113:636–639
2. Bähren W, Stief CG, Gall H, Scherb W, Gallwitz A, Altwein JE (1986) Rationelle Diagnostik der erektilen Dysfunktion unter Anwendung eines pharmakologischen Tests. Akt Urol 17:177–180
3. Bähren W, Gall H, Scherb WH, Stief CG, Thon W (1988) Arterial anatomy and arteriographic diagnosis of arteriogenic impotence. Cardiovasc Intervent Radiol 11: 195–210
4. Gall H, Bähren W, Scherb WH, Stief CG, Gallwitz A (1987) Diagnostik der vaskulären Impotenz: Vergleich Dopplersonographie und Arteriographie. Hautarzt 18: 716–722
5. Gall H, Bähren W, Scherb WH, Stief CG, Thon W (1988) Diagnostic accuracy of Doppler Ultrasound technique of the penile arteries in correlation to selective arteriography. Cardiovasc Intervent Radiol 11:255–231

6. Gall H, Sparwasser Ch, Stief CG, Bähren W, Scherb WH, Holzki G (1990) Diagnosis of venous incompetence in erectile dysfunction: comparative study of cavernosography and Doppler. Urology 35:235–238
7. Hedlund H, Anderson KE (1985) Contraction and relaxation induced by some prostanoids in isolated human penile erectile tissue and cavernous artery. J Urol 134: 1245–1250
8. Holzki G, Gall H, Bähren W, Scherb WH, Beckert R (1988) Identification of dysplastic penile arteries by cw-Doppler ultrasonography. Proc Third World Meeting on Impotence, Boston, p 105
9. Holzki G, Gall H, Bähren W, Scherb WH, Sparwasser Ch (1989) Pharmako-Doppler-Untersuchung der penilen Arterien. Phlebol Proktol 18:196–200
10. Jevtich MJ (1980) Importance of penile arterial puls sound examination in impotence. J Urol 123:820–824
11. Jevtich MJ (1984) Non-invasive vascular and neurologic tests in use for evaluation of angiogenic impotence. Int Angiol 3:225–232
12. Karacan J, Aslan C, Moore C, Aydin H, Sohmen T (1984) Penile blood-pressure index based on NPT monitoring of erectile capacity. Int Angiol 3:233–240
13. Lue TF, Hricac H, Marich KW, Tanagho EA (1985) Vasculogenic impotence evaluated by high-resolution ultrasonography and pulsed Doppler spectrum analysis. Radiology 155:777–781
14. Marshall M (1984) Praktische Doppler-Sonographie. Springer, Berlin Heidelberg New York Tokyo, pp 20–22
15. Porst H, van Ahlen H, Köster O, Schlolaut K-H (1988) Vergleich von Papaverin-induzierter Doppler-Sonographie und Angiographie in der Diagnostik der erektilen Dysfunktion. Urologe(A) 27:8–13
16. Stief CG, Gall H, Scherb WH, Bähren W (1988) Erectile dysfunction due to an ectopic penile vein. Urology 31:300–303
17. Velcek D, Sniderman KW, Vaughan Ed, Sos TA, Muecke EC (1980) Penile flow index utilizing a Doppler pulse wave analysis to identify penile vascular insufficiency. J Urol 124:669–673
18. Virag R, Frydman D, Legman M, Virag H (1984) Intracavernous injection of papaverine as a diagnostic and therapeutic method in erectile failure. Angiology 35:79–87
19. Winter CC (1978) Priapism cured by creation of fistulas between glans penis and corpora caverosa. J Urol 119:227–230
20. Zorgniotti AW, Lefleur RS (1985) Auto-injection of the corpus cavernosum with a vasoactive drug combination for vasculogenic impotence. J Urol 133:39–41

The Penile Blood Flow Study: Evaluation of Vasculogenic Impotence by Duplex Ultrasonography

G.A. Broderick and T.F. Lue

Introduction

Erection is a complex vascular event governed by the integrity of smooth muscle in the arteriolar walls and trabeculae of the corpora cavernosa. In the flaccid state the arteries, arterioles, and sinusoids are contracted with free flow through the emissary veins which exit through the tunica albuginea. Neurotransmitters and local modulators like endothelium-relaxant factor released during sexual stimulation result in smooth muscle relaxation, increase in arterial flow, and sinusoidal compliance. Blood distends the sinusoids, which in turn compress the subtunical venular plexus and reduce the outflow. About 90% of systolic pressure is transmitted to the sinusoidal spaces converting the flaccid shaft into the erect penis [2, 26]. The introduction of intracavernous vasoactive agents by Virag [27] and Brindley [8] has further improved our current understanding of erectile function. Clinical studies based on intracavernous vasoactive agents such as papaverine, phentolamine, prostaglandin E1 (PGE1) and vasoactive intestinal polypeptide (VIP) have revealed that impotence is most often organic in origin and predominantly vasculogenic in etiology [28, 29]. We believe that high resolution ultrasonography and pulsed Doppler spectrum analysis following erection induced by intracorporeal injection is the most reliable and least invasive means of detecting arteriogenic erectile failure and selecting patients for more invasive tests. We have combined our clinical experience with the Doppler penile blood flow study (PBFS) following intracavernous injection of papaverine or prostaglandin E1 in more than 1500 cases, and from this we have generated a set of parameters for diagnosing arteriogenic impotence. The principles, techniques, and criteria of the Doppler PBFS will be reviewed.

Investigating Penile Inflow

In 1971, Gaskell introduced a noninvasive test of penile arterial inflow [13]. He used a photometer to quantify the absorption of light by the pigment oxyhemoglobin in the glans penis. An occlusion cuff at the base of the penis was

U. Jonas et al. (Eds.) Erectile Dysfunction
© Springer-Verlag Berlin Heidelberg 1991

slowly loosened and the pressure at which oxyhemoglobin became measurable in the glans indicated the systolic penile blood pressure. Efforts to clinically simplify measurements of penile blood flow were advanced by Abelson [1] who, in 1975, used the Doppler stethoscope to measure penile blood pressure in the flaccid penis and compared this value with systolic brachial pressures to yield the penile-brachial index (maximal systolic penile pressure/systolic brachial artery pressure, PBI). Michal [18] and Goldstein [14] supplemented the PBI test with a dynamic component of lower extremity and pelvic musculature exercises with measurements taken before and after. A decrease in the ratio of >0.15 was indicative of pelvic steal or significant penile inflow disease. Although inexpensive, noninvasive, and readily performed, the PBI has both experimental and conceptual flaws which have limited its use: penile pressure cuff fit is not uniform, the continuous wave Doppler receives a mixture of signals which cannot anatomically separate central cavernous from dorsal or bulbospongiosal arteries, and measurements are made in the flaccid penis when the arteries are constricted. A recent review comparing the PBI to penile pharmacoangiography found PBIs from normal patients overlapped with those from impotent patients. These investigators concluded that pressures obtained from the dorsal artery predominated, led to an overestimation of systolic penile pressure, and poorly reflected the integrity of the central cavernous arteries [24].

Arteriography remains the gold standard of vascular investigations. Adequate penile angiography requires pharmacologically induced erection, as the vessels of the flaccid shaft are not only in a low flow state but are also contracted and tortuous. High osmolality contrast agents are painful and require intravenous sedative anesthesia. Many centers routinely use epidural or spinal anesthesia, which has the additional benefit of reducing vasospasm [3, 6]. Although providing the best anatomical information about the origin of the common penile arteries, these data have been difficult to correlate with functional hemodynamic effects in the end organ. Penile angiographic imaging is improved with intracavernous agents or a combination of intracavernous and intravascular vasodilators. A very important technical question has yet to be resolved: should selective internal pudendal angiography or nonselective angiography be performed? The common penile artery may arise from the terminus of the internal pudendal or from an accessory pudendal [3, 7]. The level at which vascular investigation is begun impacts on the duration of the study, the patient's exposure to X-rays, and the volume of contrast agent. Deviations from paired penile supply (two dorsal and two cavernous arteries) have been documented in 50% of normally potent male volunteers in one penile angiography study; unilateral absence or hypoplasia of a dorsal artery has been shown in up to 30% of normally potent volunteers in the series of Bahren et al. [3].

Variation in intrapenile arterial anatomy appears to be the rule rather than the exception: with unilateral or bilateral origin of the cavernous arteries, distal shaft communications between the dorsal and central cavernous arteries, and rare but none the less documented anastomoses between the urethral and cavernous arteries [12]. The clinical problem becomes how to correlate abnormalities or variations in penile arterial anatomy with functional impairment. For the patient there remains the discomfort of the intra-arterial contrast, the exposure to ionizing radiation, the risk of minor or severe dye reaction, and the potential for temporary endothelial dysfunction following intracavernous ionic contrast agents [5]. The importance of penile angiography cannot be minimized, especially with ongoing development in interventional tools of transluminal angioplasty. However, as a screening test it is overly invasive and nonspecific of hemodynamic impairment.

Duplex Penile Sonography

In 1984, Lue et al. [16] introduced the technique of high resolution sonography and quantitative Doppler spectrum analysis (PBFS) to evaluate vasculogenic impotence. As described above, the introduction of papaverine and phentolamine revolutionized the diagnosis and management of impotence. Clearly an excellent clinical response to intracavernous vasoactive agents in a neurologically normal patient confirms the diagnosis of psychogenic impotence. All too often the clinical response to the first intracavernous agent is suboptimal. The Doppler PBFS provides an objective evaluation of a suboptimal response to vasoactive agent [22].

Duplex scanning is the combination of real-time ultrasound imaging and pulsed Doppler. The real-time image is used to evaluate thickness of the tunica albuginea, echotexture of the corporal erectile tissues, cross-sectional area of corporal bodies, cavernous arterial inner diameters, thickness of arterial wall, and pulsations. These parameters are recorded before and after intracavernous injection. The real-time image is used to visually select a penile vessel for flow velocity measurement.

We have principally used two scanners since 1984: Diasonics DRF/400V and Acuson 128 (software version 7.1, Acuson, Mountainview, Cal, USA). The former machine performs real-time small parts imaging at a frequency of 10 MHz and pulsed range-gated Doppler blood flow analysis at 4.5 MHz [16]. The latter machine has a 5-MHz, linear-array, electronically focused transducer with an offset Doppler [9]. This machine superimposes Doppler flow information on the real-time image, with different flow velocities encoded by using a color scale (color flow Doppler ultrasound).

A brief description of the physics of Doppler ultrasound is warranted, as consistently performed measurements are essential for comparing information from different investigators using a variety of machines. Flow velocity (v) is determined by: Doppler shift (Df), frequency emitted by the ultrasound probe (fe), velocity of sound (C) in the medium (penile tissue, blood), and the cosine of the angle between the probe and the vessel [10].

$$v = \frac{Df \cdot C}{2fe \cdot \cos \gamma}$$

The principal source of error is failure to standardize the Doppler angle [17]. In the blood-distended shaft, the cavernous arteries straighten, and flow in the central cavernous arteries is parallel to the vessel wall (Fig. 1a,b). The optimal angle of insonation is between 45° and 60°. Velocity should not be calculated when this angle is greater than 60°. For a complete review of the physical principles governing Doppler ultrasound, the reader is directed to the work of Merrit [17] and Frosberg [10].

Ultrasound examination begins with evaluation of the flaccid shaft. Transverse views of the base of the penis are made with the scanning hand resting

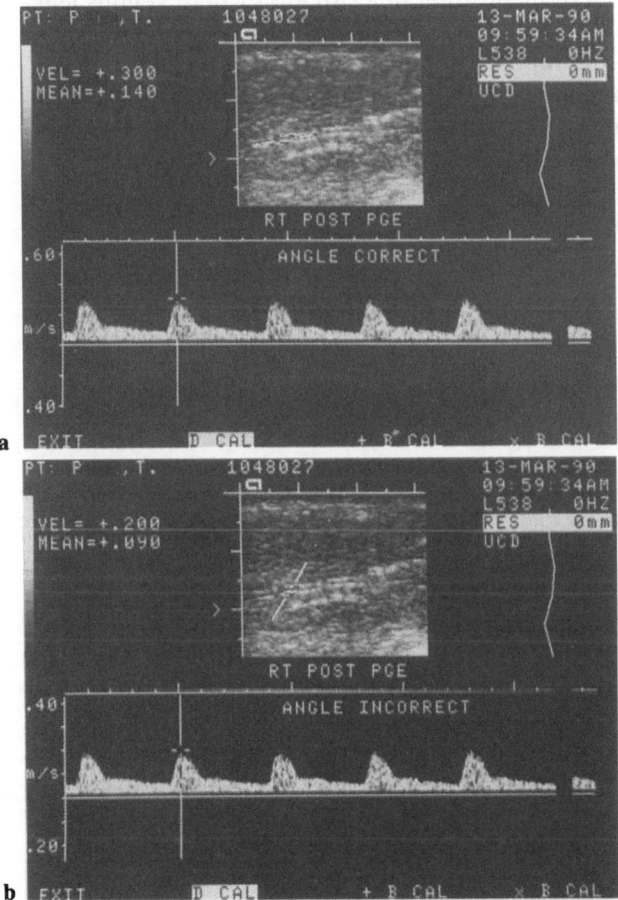

Fig. 1a,b. Longitudinal real-time views of central cavernous artery with Doppler spectral analysis. Estimation of peak systolic flow velocity depends on correct determination of the vessel angle in relation to the incident Doppler signal

gently on the patient's pubis with the other hand elevating the shaft from the glans to maintain a 90° angle with transducer. Cursors are placed to determine inner diameter of cavernous arteries and cross-sectional areas of corporal bodies. Measurement of corporal body area becomes important when comparing several interventions on a single patient at different times: evaluating a diminished response to home intracavernous injection, comparing various vasoactive agents, and comparing results from injection therapy with results of vacuum suction therapy [9]. The corporal bodies can now be scanned from base to tip to demonstrate that echotexture is homogenous, as a local fibrotic process should be relatively hyperechoic in comparison. A rubber band tourniquet is placed about the base of the penis prior to intracavernous injection with a 27 or 30 gauge needle. The band does not necessarily need to be used in patients on home therapy. For screening intracavernous shots, it allows full corporal dispersal of medication in a situation where venous leakage might otherwise eliminate the drug rapidly from the shaft. The rubber band is removed at 2 min, and repeat transverse imaging performed at 5 min. In the anxious patient or patient with compromised inflow, dispersal of medication may be delayed, and this will be visually evident by hyperechoic microbubbles at the site of injection (Fig. 2). The bubbles and medication can be promptly redistributed across both corpora by milking blood from the base to the tip of penile shaft twice. Blood-distended sinusoids are relatively hypoechoic. Hyperechoic thickening of the tunica is easily visualized against this background (Fig. 3).

Flow velocities are assessed from the longitudinal plane, 90° from the course of the deep dorsal vein. Timing is important, as arterial diameter and peak systolic velocity will maximize before full erection. Rising intracavernous

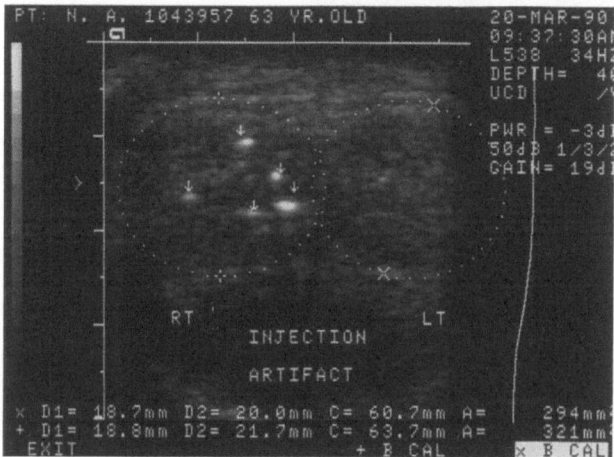

Fig. 2. Transverse view of right corpus cavernosum with echogenic microbubbles immediately following injection of PGE1

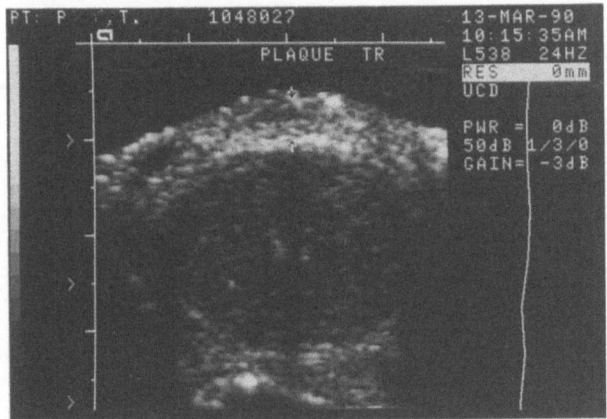

Fig. 3. Transverse view of thick Peyronie's plaque, displacing branch of deep dorsal vein to the right

pressure will decrease inflow during full erection (phase 4) or rigid erection (phase 5), as described in the animal model by Aboseif et al. [2]. Clinically, this has been demonstrated in healthy young volunteers receiving papaverine/ phentolamine [23]. Systolic velocity flow curves will peak, and diastolic flow curves will disappear before maximal intracorporal pressure is reached. In a group of seven volunteers, Schwartz et al. [23] found systolic penile occlusion pressure to range from 70 to 134 mm Hg, varying directly with the subject's own resting brachial systolic pressure. We make initial flow velocity assessment 5 min after injection; delay in response is typically evident in heavy smokers. A comfortable, warm, secure setting is essential to reduce anxiety and thus minimize sympathetic tone. Directing the patient's attention to the ultrasound screen is sufficiently distracting and often rewarding for the patient. We have found that a period of privacy and self-stimulation will enhance the penile response in more than 70% of patients. When the history is suspicious for venous leakage, this maneuver can be coupled with placement of a rubber band or a constricting ring in an attempt to isolate distal shaft, deep dorsal, and circumflex vein leakage. The duplex ultrasound study is repeated shortly after self-stimulation to reassess the systolic and diastolic flow.

An adequate response requires a >0.07-cm postinjection arterial diameter, and >25 cm/s peak systolic velocity bilaterally [19]. Benson and Vickers [4] concluded that peak systolic velocity following papaverine was the best measure of arterial adequacy. They confirm that a peak systolic velocity below 25 cm/s indicates severe arterial insufficiency; some patients with flow velocities below 25 and 30 cm/s can be treated by intracavernous therapy. Additionally, they describe marked asymmetry of flow in the paired cavernous arteries in patients with arterial insufficiency.

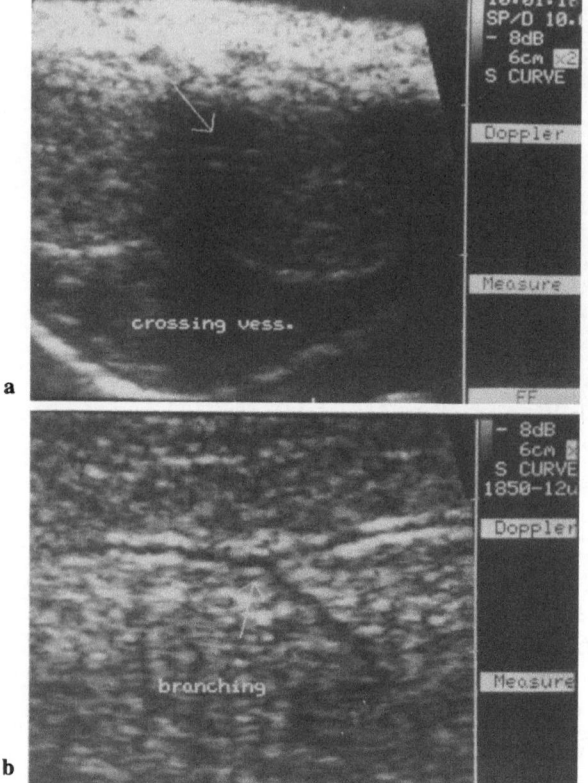

Fig. 4. Transverse (**a**) and longitudinal (**b**) views of transeptal branch of cavernous artery

    The existence of septal perforating vessels is well known from histologic studies. In our earlier examinations, we detected crossing vessels in only 14% of patients (Fig. 4a,b). With color Doppler ultrasound, a lower threshold for detecting flow is possible and superimposition of color on the real-time image has increased the detection of crossing vessels to more than 50%. Peak systolic flow prior to intracavernous injection has been detected in one or both cavernous arteries at the base of the shaft in 54% of patients. Flow in both cavernous arteries has been measured in 32% of patients with a mean of 15 cm/s. Detection of flow before injection is highly dependent on the patient's level of sympathetic tone and its predictive value uncertain. Similarly an anastomosis between the dorsal artery and central cavernous artery was noted in seven of ten cadaver specimens by Breza et al. [7]. With recent improvements in both hardware and software for Doppler PBFS, we have begun to search for such anastomoses and have noted them in only 8% of patients.

    Clinically, the suspicion of venous leakage is raised when the patient has an excellent arterial response to injected vasodilator, >30 cm/s peak systolic velocity, yet a high diastolic flow after self-stimulation. A high diastolic flow

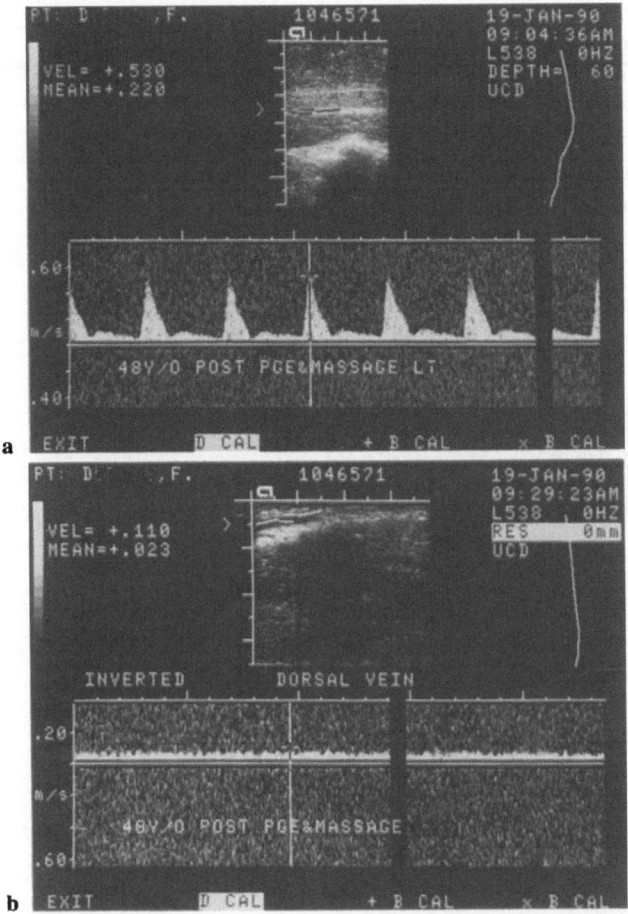

Fig. 5. a Forty-eight-year-old patient with transient rigidity following 15 µg of PGE1 and self-stimulation. Arterial peak systolic inflow is 53 cm/s. Diastolic flows are maintained at >5 cm/s. **b** Persistent venous flow through deep dorsal vein

indicates low intracavernous pressure and is highly suggestive of venous leakage at this stage. This is accompanied by inadequate or transient rigidity after self-stimulation [30].

Quam et al. [21] found end diastolic flows ranging between 0 and 24 cm/s after intracavernous papaverine (Fig. 5a,b). Among their patients, all with peak systolic velocities >25 cm/s, venous leakage on cavernosometry was predicted with a sensitivity of 90% and specificity of 56% when end diastolic flow was >5 cm/s. The authors performed dynamic infusion cavernosometry and cavernosography following papaverine injection, with an abnormal maintenance infusion rate of >30 ml of saline/min being an indicator of venous incompetence. It is unclear whether the final Doppler PBFS measurements were made after privacy and self-stimulation and what the mean peak systolic velocity was among this group.

Although the machines are currently expensive, Doppler PBFS is the most reliable means of assessing penile arterial inflows before and after intra-cavernous vasoactive agents. With attention to peak systolic velocities and end diastolic velocities, patients can appropriately be selected to undergo cavernosometry and cavernosography. Preliminary evidence for both non-selective and selective pelvic arteriography indicates excellent correlation with Doppler PBFS [15, 20]. Quam et al. [21] noted that all their patients with abnormal arteriography had peak systolic flows <25 cm/s. Others describe a more than 90% correlation between duplex sonography and selective

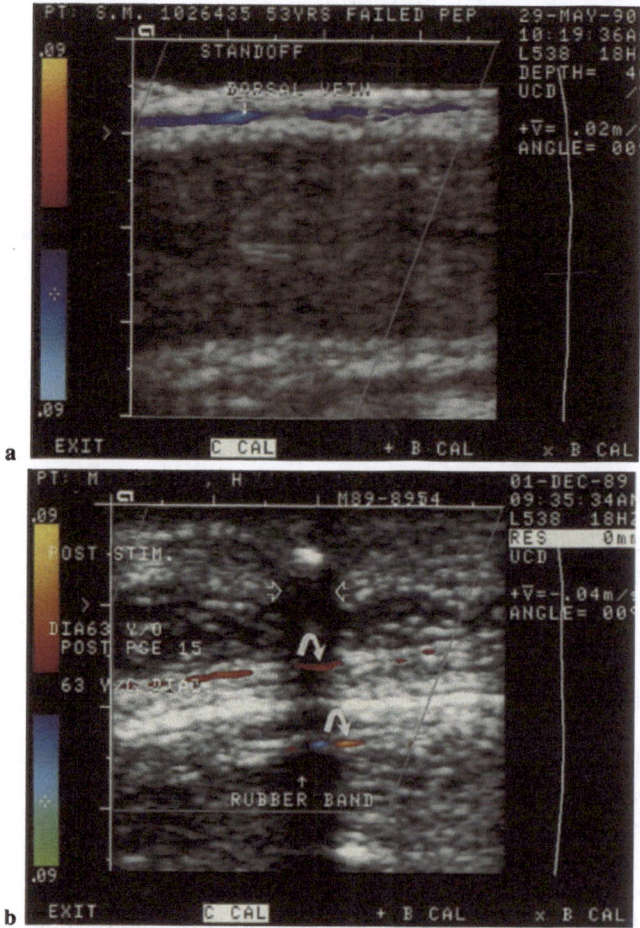

Fig. 6. a Color Doppler PBFS with real-time color flow. **b** Sixty-three-year-old diabetic following 15 μg of PGE1; rubber band obstructs deep dorsal vein flow but not the flow of the cavernous arteries

internal iliac penile pharmacoangiography [11, 19]. Doppler PBFS appears to have good correlation with nocturnal penile tumescence [25], although the parameters of peak flow velocity following a standard dosage of intra-cavernous agents have yet to be correlated with number of nocturnal erectile events or quality of events.

Color Doppler Penile Blood Flow Study

The new technology of color Doppler will increase the information obtained from PBFS. Real-time color images can: detect arterial flow in the flaccid shaft, reveal anastomoses between dorsal and cavernous arteries, crossing branches between the paired cavernous arteries, and detect venous out flow (Fig. 6a,b). For the physician learning to perform PBFS studies, color Doppler rapidly localizes the cavernous arteries and facilitates angle correction. With color Doppler PBFS, the physician may eventually perform a complete vascular examination without exposing the patient to radiation or contrast agents. Color Doppler casts a new and informative light on the gray-scale images of ultrasound.

References

1. Abelson D (1975) Diagnostic value of the penile pulse and blood pressure: a Doppler study of impotence in diabetics. J Urol 113:636
2. Aboseif SR, Lue TF (1988) Hemodynamics of penile erection. Urol Clin North Am 15:1
3. Bahren W, Gall H, Scherb W, Stief C, Thon W (1988) Arterial anatomy and arteriographic diagnosis of arteriogenic impotence. Cardiovasc Intervent Radiol 11:195
4. Benson CB and Vickers MA (1989) Sexual impotence caused by vascular disease: diagnosis with duplex sonography. AJR 153:1149
5. Bookstein JJ (1990) Letter to the Editor. AJR 286
6. Bookstein JJ, Lange EV (1987) Penile magnification pharmacoarteriography: details of intrapenile arterial anatomy. AJR 148:883
7. Breza J, Aboseif S, Orvis B, Lue TF, Tanagho EA (1989) Detailed anatomy of penile neurovascular structures: surgical significance. J Urol 141:437
8. Brindley GS (1983) Cavernosal alpha-blockade: a new technique for investigating and treating erectile impotence. Br J Psychiatry 143:332
9. Broderick GA, McGahan JP, Stone AR, deVere White RW (1990) The hemodynamics of vacuum constriction erections: assessment by color Doppler ultrasound. J Urol
10. Forsberg L, Olsson AM (1988) Doppler studies of the penile circulation. Urol Radiol 10:129
11. Gall H, Bahren W, Scherb W, Stief C, Thon W (1988) Diagnostic accuracy of Doppler ultrasound technique of the penile arteries in correlation to selective arteriography. Cardiovasc Intervent Radiol 11:225
12. Garibyan H, Lue TF (1990) Anastomotic network between the dorsal and cavernous arteries in the penis. J Urol 143:221A (Abstract 89)
13. Gaskell P (1971) The importance of penile blood pressure in cases of impotence. Can Med Assoc J 105:104

14. Goldstein I, Siroky MB, North RI et al (1982) Vasculogenic impotence: role of the pelvic steal test. J Urol 128:300
15. Krysiewicz S, Mellinger BC (1989) The role of imaging in the diagnostic evaluation of impotence. AJR 153:1133
16. Lue TF, Hricak H, Marich KW, Tanagho EA (1985) Vasculogenic impotence evaluated by high-resolution ultrasonography and pulsed Doppler spectrum analysis. Radiology 155:777
17. Merritt CR (1987) Doppler color flow imaging. J Clin Ultrasound 15:591
18. Michal V, Kramer R, Pospichal J (1978) External iliac "steal syndrome". J Cardiovasc Surg 19:355
19. Mueller SC, Lue TF (1988) Evaluation of vasculogenic impotence. Urol Clin North Am 15:65
20. Paushter, DM (1989) Role of duplex sonography in the evaluation of sexual impotence. AJR 153:1161
21. Quam JP, King BF, James EM, Brakke DM, Ilstrup DM, Parulkar BG, Hattery RR (1989) Duplex and color Doppler sonographic evaluation of vasculogenic impotence. AJR 153:1141
22. Robinson LQ, Woodcock JP, Stephenson RP (1989) Duplex scanning in suspected vasculogenic impotence: a worthwhile exercise? Br J Urol 63: 432
23. Schwartz AN, Wang KY, Mack LA, Lowe M, Berger RE, Cyr DR, Feldman M (1989) Evaluation of normal erectile function with color Doppler sonography. AJR 153:1155
24. Schwartz AN, Lowe MA, Ireton R, Berger RE, Richardson MI, Graney DO (1990) A comparison of penile brachial index and angiography: evaluation of corpora cavernosa arterial inflow. J Urol 143:510
25. Shabisgh R, Fishman IJ, Shottland Y, Karacan I, Dunn JK (1990) Comparison of penile duplex ultrasonography with nocturnal penile tumescence monitoring for the evaluation of erectile impotence. J Urol 143:924
26. Tanagho EA, Lue TF, McClure RD (1988) Functional evaluation of penile arteries with papaverine. In: Kist (ed) Contemporary management of impotence and infertility. Williams & Wilkins, Baltimore, chap 5, pp 57–69
27. Virag R (1982) Intracavernous injection of papaverine for erection failure: Letter to the Editor. Lancet 2:938
28. Virag R, Bouilly P, Frydman D (1985) Is impotence an arterial disorder? A study of arterial risk factors in 440 impotent men. Lancet 1:181
29. Virag R, Frydman D, Legman M, Virag H (1984) Intracavernous injection of papaverine as a diagnostic and therapeutic method in erectile failures. Angiology 35:79
30. Wesper E, Delcour C, Rondeux C, Struyven J, Schulman CC (1987) The erectile angle: objective criterion to evaluate the papaverine test in impotence. J Urol 138:1171

Pharmacoarteriography in Chronic Erectile Dysfunction

W. Bähren, H. Gall, W. Scherb, G. Holzki, and C. Sparwasser

Owing to the complex nature and often multifactorial genesis of chronic erectile dysfunction, diagnosis and management require a comprehensive testing program. Noninvasive morphologic and functional assessment of the penile arterial supply followed by selective bilateral pharmacoarteriography of pudendal and penile arteries is necessary to define the extent and vascular nature of pathomorphologic change, especially prior to invasive therapeutic procedures. A valid indication must exist after careful evaluation of preceeding multidisciplinary investigations.

Limitations of pharmacoarteriography are that only morphologic interpretation of number, origin, diameter, and obstruction of pudendal and penile vessels is possible. Functional aspects and quantification of normal or impaired inflow can only be estimated and are dependent on a variety of parameters not evaluated during arteriography. Arteriography alone is inadequate because more than 50% of patients reveal more than one pathophysiologic factor (e.g., arterial, venous/cavernous, neurogenic, hormonal, psychogenic) as the cause of erectile failure [3, 6].

Technical aspects regarding catheterization, projection, amount and flow-rate of contrast medium, first described by Ginestie and Romieu [9], are still valid today. Further refinements of the technique such as intracavernous application of vasoactive substances, epidural anesthesia and intra-arterial digital subtraction arteriography have led to a marked improvement in the quality of visualization of distal vessels [3, 6, 20, 27, 31]. Pharmacoarteriography is the diagnostic goldstandard in arteriogenic impotence, but only when arteriographic quality is excellent. Otherwise angiography can be misleading, resulting in both false positive and false negative diagnoses [45].

Technique of Pharmacoarteriography

General Aspects

A detailed explanation of the possible consequences of the planned diagnostic procedure, including side effects and complications, is mandatory, as is the patient's informed consent.

U. Jonas et al. (Eds.) Erectile Dysfunction
© Springer-Verlag Berlin Heidelberg 1991

With this procedure, the region to be investigated extends from the infrarenal aorta to the terminal branching of penile vessels. It is important to demonstrate the major pelvic vessels in order to detect pathology. It is additionally necessary to show the inferior epigastric artery preoperatively and determine any possible arterial contribution via the external pudendal artery and the accessory internal pudendal artery. Selective arteriography of the internal pudendal artery has to be bilateral because of numerous anatomical variations [5].

Though Ginestie and Romieu [9] performed arteriography during general anesthesia, comparative studies have shown that penile arteries could be better illustrated under epidural anesthesia and using vasoactive substances [3]. After establishing criteria of quality (Table 1), 126 bilateral selective arteriograms were judged and correlated with the type of anesthesia and the pharmacologic stimulation applied. Image quality after intracavernous (i.c.) injection of vasoactive substances and epidural anesthesia was markedly superior to that performed under local anesthesia alone [5]. Intra-arterial digital subtraction arteriography (i.a. DSA) shows good results when combined with i.c. injection of vasoactive substances, although there is a distinct

Table 1. Criteria for assessing quality of pharmacoarteriography

Range	Visible structures	With vasoactive drugs		Without vasoactive drugs	
		(n)	(%)	(n)	(%)
1	Int. pudendal artery Penile arteries with terminal branching Helicine arteries Shunt arteries	94	64.4	12	10.7
2	Int. pudendal artery Penile arteries Helicine arteries with low contrast Shunt arteries with low contrast	40	27.4	54	48.2
3	Int. pudendal artery Main stem of penile arteries	12	8.2	36	32.2
4	Int. pudendal artery Main stem of penile arteries – low contrast	0	0	4	3.6
5	Int. pudendal artery – low contrast No penile arteries	0	0	6[a]	5.3
	Total	146	100	112	100

n = 258 selective arteriograms of internal pudendal arteries in 126 patients.
[a] Were repeated with vasoactive substances.

loss of spatial resolution when compared with conventional arteriography; this is partially compensated by improved contrast of the penile arteries.

Due to dilution and the use of less contrast medium during i.a. DSA, the reaction is less painful and there are fewer vascular spasms, so that some authors believe epidural anesthesia is unnecessary [20]. To clarify this question we performed i.a. DSA without epidural anesthesia in nine patients and with epidural anesthesia in seven patients (Fig. 1). The comparison of the angiograms according to our rating scale in Table 1 revealed a mean value of 2.44 for the group without epidural anesthesia and superior quality with a mean of 1.57 for the group with epidural anesthesia. When the pharmacoarteriography is performed under local anesthesia, selective probing of the internal pudendal arteries is mandatory in order to obtain images of high quality.

In general, there is a loss of quality from the intra-arterial application of vasoactive substances except for those cases where superselective catheterization of internal pudendal artery is performed. Moreover the advantage of penile arterial stretching in the tumescent phase is lost, thus limiting the assessment of peripheral arteriosclerotic lesions.

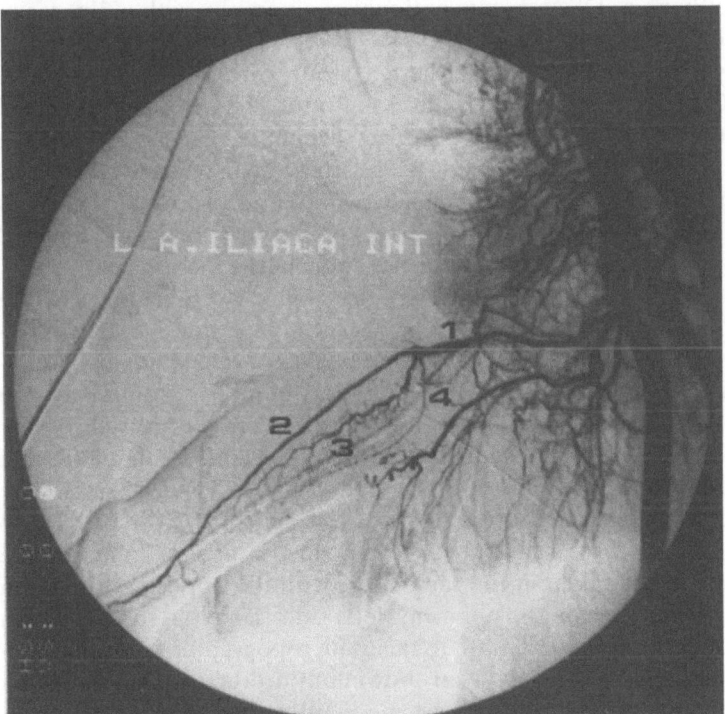

Fig. 1. Selective left pharmacoarteriography with epidural anesthesia – intra-arterial digital subtraction angiography. *1*, Penile artery; *2*, dorsal artery; *3*, cavernosal artery with helicine arteries; *4*, bulbar artery

To provide diagnostic arteriograms of pudendal and penile vessels, i.c. injection of vasoactive substances is mandatory (Table 1). Functional testing of vasomotor erectile capacity by i.c. application of a vasoactive drug combination has proven valuable in differentiating between nonvascular causes, pathologically diminished inflow, and pathologically increased outflow [10, 20]. For functional testing we administer a mixture of papaverine (15 mg/ml) and phentolamine (0.5 mg/ml) by i.c. injection and define in a stepwise and standardized manner the dosage required for complete erection. Doses range from 0.25 ml to 3 ml; normal subjects achieve a complete erection after administration of 0.5 ml [4]. To take full advantage of invasive arteriography, an i.c. injection of vasoactive substances in a dosage leading to penile tumescence is necessary.

Technical Aspects of Pharmacoarteriography

In the Seldinger technique the right femoral artery is punctured and a 5 F catheter introduction set is placed into the femoral artery. Using a 5 F pigtail catheter, arteriography of the pelvic arteries in anterior-posterior view is performed by either i.a. DSA or conventional angiography with a film series for up to 8 seconds postinjection (p.i.).

After completion of the pelvic series, a guide wire (Radiofocus guide wire, Terumo Corporation, Tokyo) is placed into the left external or internal iliac artery via the pigtail catheter in crossover technique. The pigtail catheter is replaced by a visceral catheter (C 2), and the left hypogastric artery is selectively catheterized. By using the DSA technique, a short series shows the branching pattern of the hypogastric artery. After identifying the internal pudendal artery, selective probing of this vessel is performed.

The patient is placed in a 20° left posterior oblique projection, and the penis is placed and fixed on the right thigh. After i.c. injection of papaverine-phentolamine, tumescence of the penis appears (dosage depends on preangiographic testing and varies from 0.5 to 3 ml) and 40 ml of contrast medium is injected at a flow rate of 4 ml/s. It is important not to induce full rigidity because of the resultant induced reduction of cavernosal artery diameter and flow. Filming takes place at 2, 4, 6, 8, 10, 11, 12, 14, 17 and 20 s p.i. The visceral catheter is then replaced by a Simmonds catheter (SIM I or II) to selectively catheterize the ipsilateral right hypogastric artery. Films of the right arterial system are taken in the same way, with the opposite projection and placement of the penis on the opposite (left) side. To avoid superposition by contrast medium in the bladder and to facilitate topographic determination of the urethra, it is useful to insert an indwelling urethral catheter. When i.a. DSA is used, the amount of contrast medium can be reduced to 25 ml. Injection by machine with a flow rate of 3 ml/s and a series of 20 s is employed.

Incorrect projection, patient malposition, and wrong penile position lead to vascular superimposition, which impairs identification and interpretation

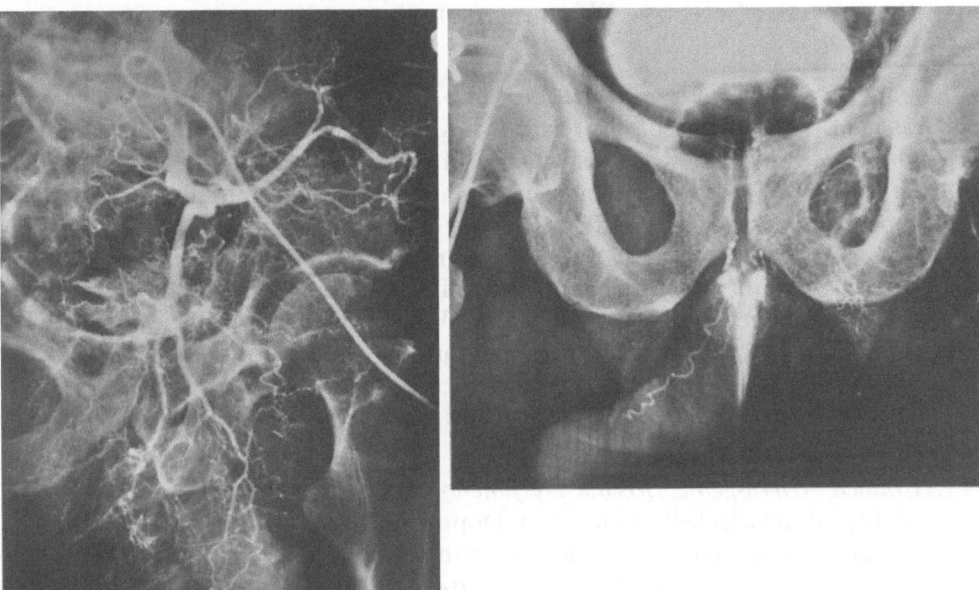

Fig. 2a,b. Technical problems. **a** Wrong projection – the contralateral side is elevated and the penis is not placed upon the opposite thigh. Pudendal and penile arteries are superposed and cannot be judged. **b** Anterior-posterior view and no application of vaso-active substances. No penile stretching. Arteries at the base of the penis cannot be evaluated

of penile arteries (Fig. 2). At a flow rate of more than 5 ml/s, marked reflux into the common iliac artery occurs. The reduced amount of contrast medium is no longer sufficient to demonstrate terminal penile arteries in the late phase with good contrast. Performance of arteriography without i.c. injection of papaverine-phentolamine leads to insufficient dilatation of pudendal and penile vessels and leads to the risk of false positive results. Additionally, the arteries appear tortuous when the penis is flaccid, making it difficult to detect arteriosclerotic stenoses (Fig. 2). Penile arteries can be missed if shorter series of exposure is used. Under normal conditions they are demonstrated after 10–12 s increasing to 20 s p.i. when pathologically disturbed.

In case of penile blood supply via an accessory internal pudendal artery deriving from other branches of the hypogastric artery, superselective probing of this branch should be attempted. The application of vasoactive substances in a dose that leads to complete erection with full rigidity is followed by poor visualization of cavernosal arteries. This correlates with the findings of Lue et al. [22] showing a late decrease in cavernosal artery flow after full erection induced by i.c. papaverine.

Indications for Selective Pharmacoarteriography

Therapeutically relevant information can be expected if the penile Doppler ultrasound and pharmacologic testing with vasoactive substances suggest a hemodynamically significant disturbance of arterial inflow [4]. If pathologic results are shown by neurologic examination and neurophysiologic tests [bulbocavernosus reflex (BCR) latency measurements; somato-sensory-evoked potential of pudendal nerve; electromyogram (EMG)], the patient most likely will not benefit from operative revascularization procedures. For this reason, a neurophysiologic evaluation should rule out neurologic damage prior to angiography, and still more important, prior to operative arterial bypass.

We perform selective bilateral pharmacoarteriography when noninvasive examinations suggest:

1. *Isolated Arteriogenic Erectile Dysfunction.* This is to determine the possibility of revascularization when Doppler ultrasound and testing with vasoactive substances demonstrate pathologic inflow (Fig. 3). Arteriography is also indicated when percutaneous transluminal angioplasty (PTA) is planned in pelvic arteries. Obstruction of pelvic vessels can be treated by PTA without injury to the neural structures that control the erectile function [7, 44, 45]. Positive effects on penile hemodynamics can be expected if there is no additional distal occlusion or stenosis in pudendal or penile arteries, especially at the level of the urogenital diaphragm.

2. *Primary Erectile Dysfunction.* Arterial malformation alone or combined with additional causes can be observed in over 60% of patients with

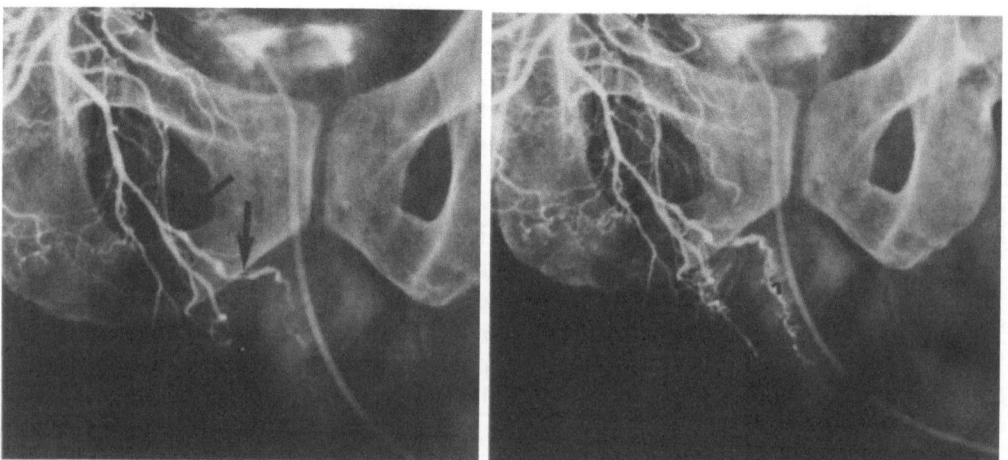

Fig. 3. a Severe stenoses of terminal internal pudendal artery and penile artery (→).
b Obstruction of dorsal penile artery. Cavernosal artery (*1*)

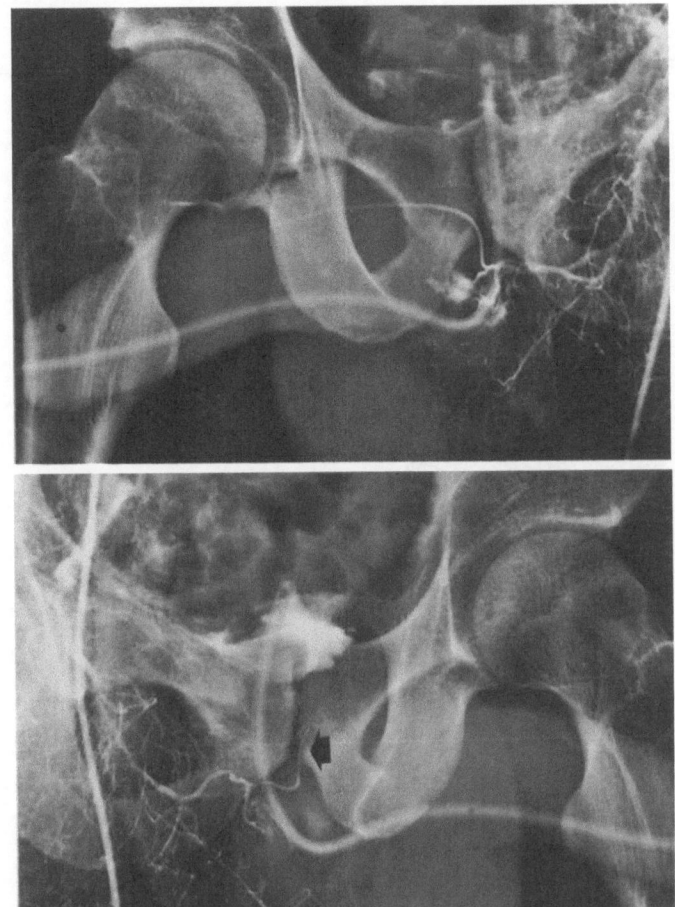

Fig. 4a,b. Vascular erectile dysfunction in a 27-year-old patient with primary erectile dysfunction. There is complex arterial malformation. **a** Two very short proximal cavernosal arteries arise from the left internal pudendal artery, indicating unilateral hypoplastic cavernosal supply. **b** Hypoplasia of the right dorsal artery. No filling of the cavernosal artery (→)

primary erectile dysfunction [3] (Fig. 4). Even if there is no chance for promising operative procedures, the positive confirmation of the organic nature gives tremendous psychologic relief to these young patients. Moreover, it prevents unnecessary, costly, and unsuccessful psychotherapy.

3. *Posttraumatic Erectile Dysfunction.* Arterial revascularization shows good results in posttraumatic erectile dysfunction if there is no complicating nerve injury present [10]. Preoperative angiography and neurophysiologic examination are mandatory. Since much pelvic trauma occurs in traffic

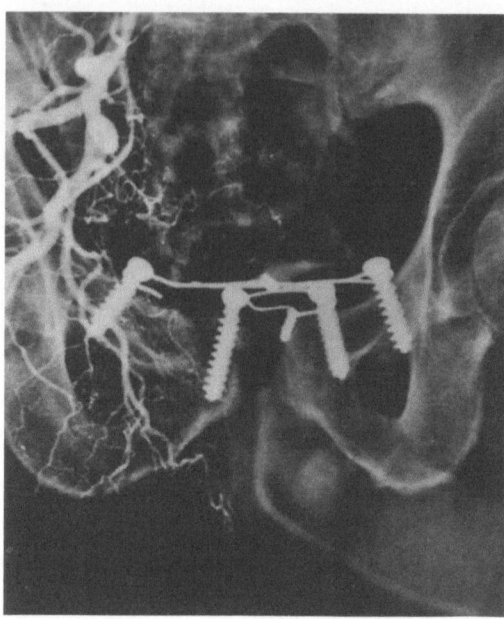

Fig. 5. A 45-year-old patient with posttraumatic erectile dysfunction after symphysical rupture. Occlusion of the penile artery at the level of urogenital diaphragm. No opacification of cavernosal and dorsal artery

accidents, it is often necessary for insurance or legal purposes to demonstrate the vascular and/or neurogenic etiology of erectile dysfunction (Fig. 5).

Side Effects, Complications, and Contraindications

Severe stenosis or occlusion of major pelvic vessels, especially involving the origin of the internal pudendal artery (IPA), generally represents a contraindication for selective catheterization unless PTA or thromboendarterectomy of the internal iliac artery seems promising. In these rare cases, selective arteriography should be performed carefully to demonstrate patent distal pudendal arteries.

In 194 arteriographic procedures, we encountered mild allergic reactions with urticaria, nausea, and vomiting in three patients. In one patient, a local hematoma occurred in the punctured inguinal region; surgical intervention was not required. In more than 50% of the patients that were investigated under local anesthesia, a painful sensation of heat in the perineal, gluteal, and genital area occurred, lasting for half a minute after selective injection of contrast medium. After intracavernous application of papaverine-phentolamine, no local side effects such as hematoma, infection, or fibrosis were observed. In all the patients who were investigated under epidural anesthesia (n = 151), continuous monitoring of vital functions showed no significant deviation of systolic or diastolic pressure after i.c. injection of 0.5–1.5 ml of papaverine-phentolamine mixture.

Normal Anatomy and Variations

The IPA is the major artery of the erectile organ. As a terminal branch of the internal iliac artery, it runs in a curve with an anterior superior concavity in the intrapelvic section at the dorsolateral pelvic wall, remote from the viscera. The IPA enters the lesser pelvis through the small sciatic notch and accompanies the internal pudendal nerve. In its posterior perineal section the IPA enters the ischiorectal fossa where it runs along the inferior insertions of the internal obturator muscle in Alcock's canal [19, 33]. At the dorsal part of the urogenital diaphragm it gives rise to the superficial perineal artery, which goes forward in the ischiobulbous triangle to end at the base of the genitals [16, 33]. Beyond the origin of the superficial perineal artery, the IPA is known as the penile artery. In its anterior perineal section, the penile artery sends inferior branches – the bulbar artery, the bulbo urethral artery, and the cavernosal artery. The cavernosal artery penetrates the middle aponeurosis and tunica albuginea of the corpus cavernosum [12]. The penile artery terminates in the dorsal penile artery, which runs outside the corpus cavernosum on the dorsum of the penis to the glans. There it divides, usually anastomosing with the contralateral dorsal artery and distal branches of the urethral artery.

The cavernosal artery is functionally of greatest significance for erectile hemodynamics [23]. There is a large individual variability in branching patterns, sites of penetration of the tunica albuginea, and communication with the other penile arteries [30] (Fig. 6). In many cases there is a short proximal retrograde branch to the crus of the corpus cavernosum. En route through the center of the cavernous bodies, the main cavernosal artery sends off numerous helicine arteries which enter the sinusoidal spaces. Additionally, several (up to 10) anastomoses between the cavernosal artery and the corpus spongiosum can be found in pharmacoangiography (called "shunt" arteries) (Fig. 6). The dorsal artery of the penis gives superficial branches to the skin as well as deep branches through the tunica albuginea. Helicine-like arteries arising from the dorsal artery cannot be observed arteriographically, although they are described anatomically [42].

Variations in the penile arterial system are common; the most frequent observations are shown in Fig. 7. Adachi [1] reported on the occurrence of accessory IPA in 10.9% of male specimens. Angiographically, this additional artery was described in 6% [16] to 9% [9] of cases. We found one or more additional supplying arteries in 10.8% of patients who did not show arterial malformation [3]. If arteriography revealed penile arterial malformation, this

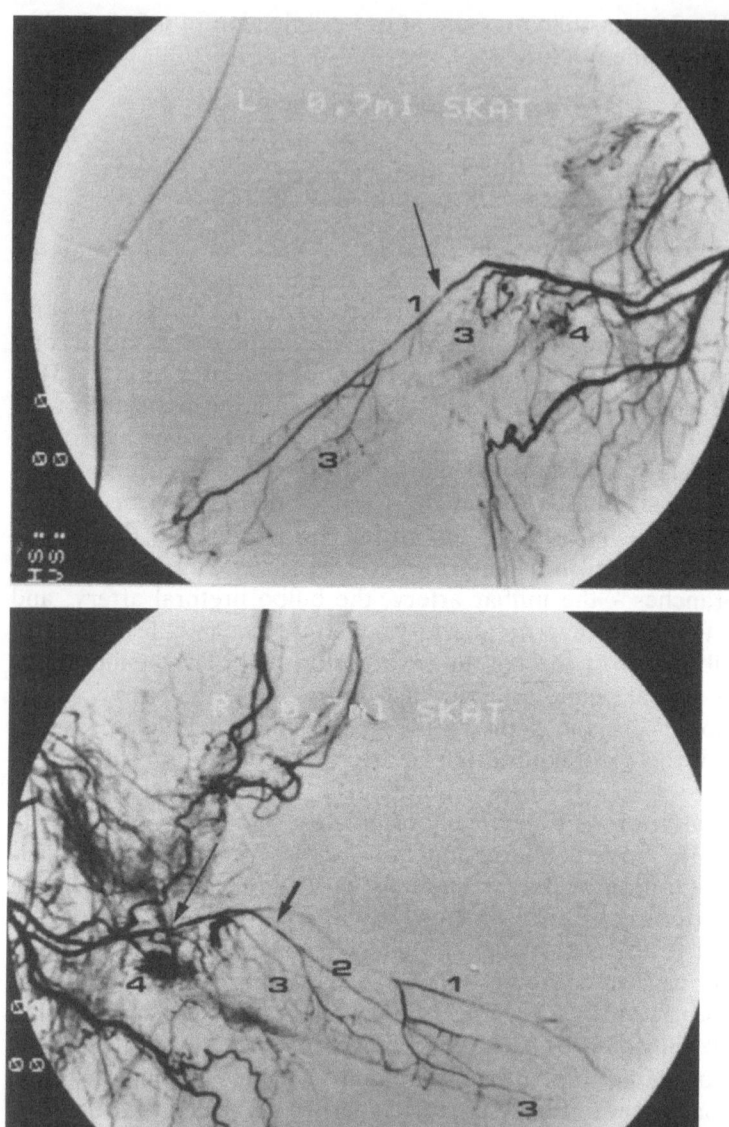

Fig. 6a,b. i.a. DSA in a 50-year-old patient with moderate arteriosclerotic lesions (→). Epidural anesthesia; multiple cavernosal arteries, partially anastomosing between both sides supply the cavernous bodies *1*, Left dorsal artery; *2*, Right dorsal artery; *3*, Cavernosal arteries with helicine and shunt arteries; *4*, Artery of the bulb

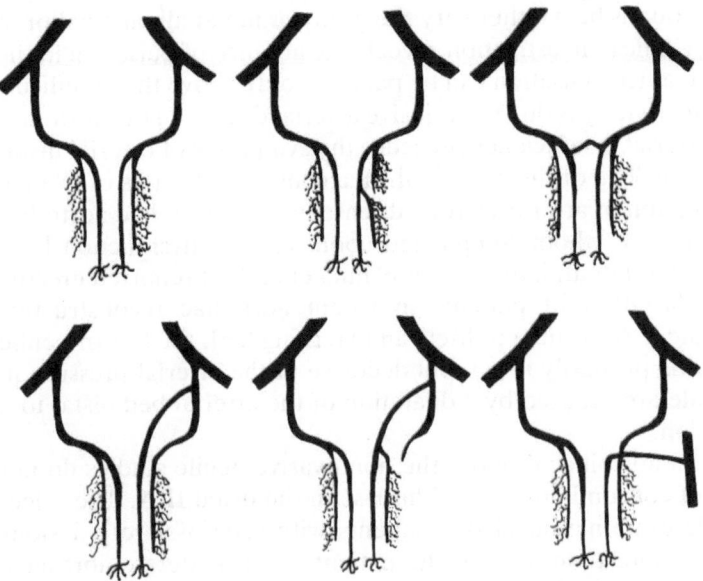

Fig. 7. Variation of penile arteries

supplementary vessel with its typical appearance and course, occurred in 45%, either unilaterally or bilaterally [3].

Patients

From February 1981 until February 1990, 194 of 625 patients with chronic erectile dysfunction underwent bilateral selective pudendal arteriography after multidisciplinary evaluation. The mean age was 39 years (19–65). Mean duration of erectile dysfunction was 2½ years. Since 1984 all arteriograms were performed after intracavernous application of vasoactive substances. A total of 48 patients were evaluated by arteriography because of primary erectile dysfunction. In 17 patients, arteriography was applied in post-traumatic erectile dysfunction.

Occlusive Arterial Disease in Aorta and Iliac Arteries

In 1923, Leriche described a syndrome related to thrombotic obliteration of the aortic bifurcation [21]. In this syndrome patients are, as a rule, young adults who complain of the following symptoms: inability to keep a stable erection; fatigue of both lower limbs; global atrophy of both lower limbs; no trophic changes; wounds heal either very sluggishly or not at all; and pallor of the legs and feet. Clinical investigation reveals the absence of pulsation in the legs or groins. The aortic pulsation can be palpated only above the umbilicus. When loss of penile rigidity is due to occlusive arterial disease in the aortoiliac area, the penile arterial insufficiency precedes the symptoms of arterial insufficiency of the legs in 30% of the cases [26]. In a consecutive series of 98 men admitted for evaluation of arteriosclerotic disease in the leg, 70 had aortoiliac occlusions, 39 (58%) of whom complained about erectile dysfunction [26]. Nath et al. [34], Queral et al. [36], and De Palma et al. [35] reported erectile dysfunction in 71%–81% of patients in whom aortoiliac reconstructive surgery was indicated. According to Metz and Herning [26], the loss of penile rigidity could be due primarily to a rapid decrease of the arterial pressure in the pudendal-penile area caused by a dilatation of the arterial bed distal to a stenosis or occlusion.

In patients with aortoiliac disease, the noninvasive penile studies do not allow evaluation of concomitant arterial disease in the distal IPA. The selective arteriographic examination of our patients with arteriosclerotic lesions demonstrated that more than 60% of the patients with moderate aortoiliac lesions (stenoses) also had occlusion and hemodynamically significant stenoses distally in the internal pudendal and penile arteries [3].

In patients who develop impotence following aortoiliac reconstructive vascular surgery [18, 25, 26, 30, 36, 39] several possible causes exist which are difficult to distinguish: preexisting distal arteriosclerosis; inadequate central restoration of blood flow; surgical interference with the autonomic nervous system; and concomitant venogenic impotence.

Some authors [41, 50] conclude that surgical intervention tends to further impair erectile function, but Sabri and Cotton [38] and Michal et al. [28] reported significant improvement in prospective studies. They especially were interested in preservation of the integrity of the hypogastric plexus by increased use of thromboendarterectomy of the internal iliac arteries.

A special constellation of occlusive arteriosclerosis of the aortoiliac vessels can cause a syndrome consisting of inability to maintain the erection after initiation of strenuous coital movements. The syndrome is thought to be due to a redistribution of a limited blood flow in favor of the activated muscles and is therefore named the "pelvic steal syndrome" (PSS) or "external iliac steal syndrome" [11, 25, 29, 46] analogous to the subclavian steal syndrome.

Arteriosclerosis of Internal Pudendal Arteries and Penile Vessels

The changes in morphology and structure of pudendal-penile arteries correspond to arteriosclerotic alterations in other vascular regions [37]. The dramatic circulatory event of penile erection requires sufficient elasticity and compliance of supplying arteries, as well as cavernosal structures [23]. If

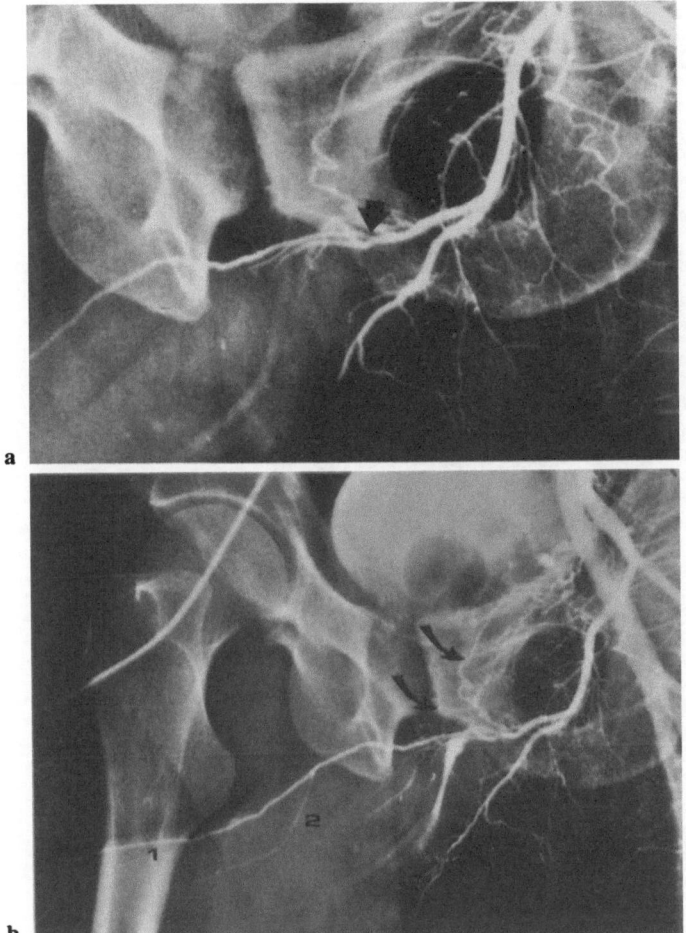

Fig. 8. a A 39-year-old patient with severe stenosis of the penile artery (→). **b** Distal cavernosal artery (2) derives from the dorsal artery (1), which has reduced inflow. Beginning collateral circulation (→)

arteriosclerosis reduces cavernosal arterialization, collateral connections are adequate to maintain organ viability. The functional increase in arterial inflow, however, becomes insufficient to produce intracavernosal pressure adequate for full erection (38) and progressive erectile dysfunction develops.

It has been shown that coincidental risk factors increase the rate of organic erectile dysfunction up to 90% [47]. Virag [47] concluded that 10% of the men between 40 and 60 years can expect to suffer from erectile dysfunction. At least 60% of these men will experience erectile dysfunction of organic nature with vascular causes in ⅔ of them [47]. The studies that include selective arteriography in the diagnostic workup of impotent patients

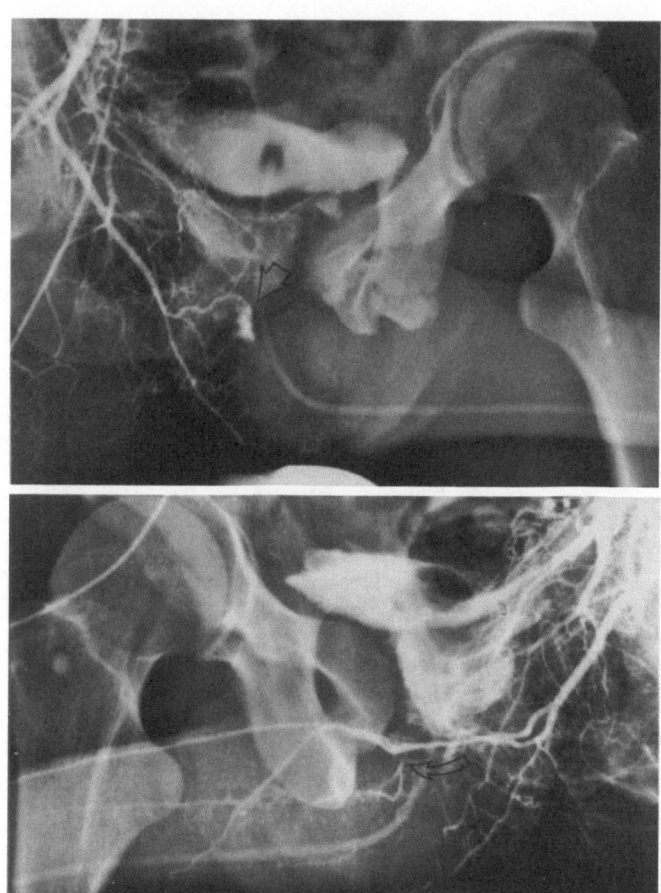

Fig. 9a,b. A 22-year-old patient with posttraumatic erectile dysfunction after fracture of the anterior pelvic girdle and urethral rupture. **a** Except for the artery of the bulb (→), there is no opacification of penile arteries on the right side. **b** Note obstruction of the proximal cavernosal artery at the level of the urogenital diaphragm (→). There is unilateral cavernosal supply. Retrograde filling is via an anastomosis from the dorsal artery

[13, 17, 31] revealed a vascular etiology in up to 85.5% [31]. The arteriographic appearance of obstructed peripheral arteries in erectile dysfunction is rather uniform [13, 31]. Stenoses and occlusions are most frequently situated bilaterally at the terminal part of the IPA at the level of the urogenital diaphragm (Fig. 8). In these cases the artery of the bulb can usually still be visualized because of its further proximal branching, whereas the dorsal and cavernosal arteries are often completely obstructed. Only poor collateralization can be found in these cases. Segmental stenoses alone or in combination with obstruction and partly effective collateralization can be observed in the IPA before and during its course in Alcock's canal. Isolated stenosis at its origin from the ischiopudendal trunk can also occur. Bookstein et al. [6] also found remarkable symmetry in occlusive disease of the internal pudendal and penile arteries. The hemodynamic significance of demonstrated stenosis can often be judged angiographically by the presence of collateral circulation [6].

Posttraumatic Erectile Dysfunction

Due to their proximate location, the penile nerves and arteries are frequently injured in association with injury to the urethra or urogenital diaphragm. Noniatrogenic injuries are caused by blunt or perforating trauma to the external genitalia. Characteristic fractures that result in injury to the lower urinary tract are single or multiple fractures of the ischiopubic ramus and the symphysis. About 5% – 10% of pelvic fractures are accompanied by injuries to the lower urinary tract [14, 40].

Injury to the urethra and the accompanying nerves and vessels is caused by a shearing mechanism. Because of the extremely mobile fragments of the fractured pelvic girdle and the puboprostatic ligaments, the energy of the trauma is transmitted to the anatomical structures attached to the urogenital diaphragm (Fig. 9) [32]. In an analysis of 16 patients with documented noniatrogenic posttraumatic impotence, Lurie et al. showed that posttraumatic arterial occlusion most frequently involves the internal pudendal artery, followed in frequency by the cavernosal and dorsal arteries. According to Lurie, the primary site of injury and obstruction is usually where the penile arteries course through the urogenital diaphragm. Internal iliac artery occlusion was seen only after pelvic fracture [24] (Fig. 10).

The multidisciplinary evaluation of our 17 patients showed that the vascular lesions – occurring alone or in combination with neurogenic damage – should be given primary consideration in the pathogenesis of posttraumatic erectile dysfunction (Fig. 11). The most frequent vascular posttraumatic changes were observed in the distal IPA at the level of the urogenital diaphragm. This is even more important because, due to the development and improvement in vascular surgery in the last 5 years [15, 48], revascularization can be offered to all those patients who do not show an additional neurogenic etiology.

Penile Arterial Malformation

Bilateral selective pudendal arteriography was performed to prove a pathological Doppler finding in 48 of 70 patients with primary erectile dysfunction. Fifteen patients revealed a normal penile arterial anatomy or anatomical variation like a unilateral cavernosal supply not considered hemodynamically

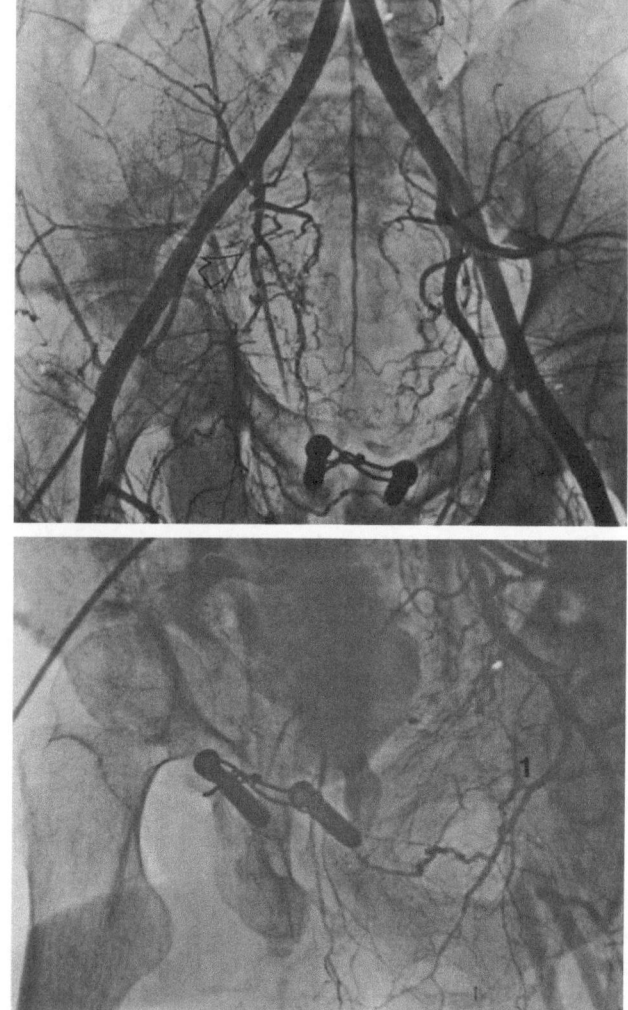

Fig. 10. a Posttraumatic arterial damage at the internal iliac artery and its mainstems after pelvic fracture. **b** Additional occlusion of pudendal vessels at the level of urogenital diaphragm after symphysial rupture and fracture of the anterior pelvic girdle. *1*, Left internal pudendal artery

relevant in young men without arterisclerotic risk factors (Figs. 12 and 13). Bilateral hypoplasia or aplasia of at least two penile arteries was found in 12 patients. Nineteen patients showed complex arterial anomalies with a mixture of unilateral supply of dorsal and/or cavernosal artery in combination with aplasia or severe hypoplasia regularly involving both axes (Figs. 4 and 14). The arteriographic findings showed that arterial maldevelopment has to be severe and bilateral in order to cause primary erectile dysfunction on a pure

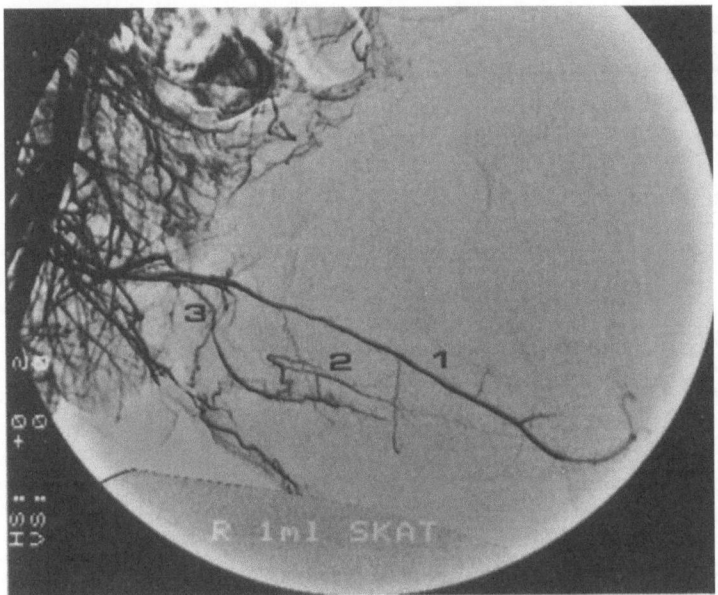

Fig. 11. Posttraumatic erectile dysfunction after blunt direct penile trauma (straddle trauma) in a 25 year old patient. *1*, Dorsal artery. *2*, Cavernosal artery with interruption of flow from penile artery. *3*, Collateral circulation via a mighty urethral artery

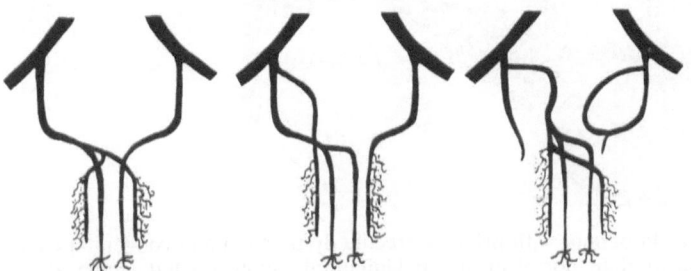

Fig. 12. Unilateral cavernosal or penile supply

arterial basis. Hypoplasia or aplasia of one dorsal artery is of no significance to erectile function in young men. As reported by Zorgniotti et al. [52], primary erectile dysfunction can be associated with pudendal arteriovenous malformation. It seems to be a rare cause of erectile failure and was found in two of our patients with primary erectile failure (Fig. 15).

Current arteriographic reports primarily describe arteriosclerotic lesions as a cause of vascular erectile dysfunction [9, 13, 17, 27, 31, 43, 51]. Aplasia and hypoplasia of penile arteries were reported by Ginestie and Romieu [9]

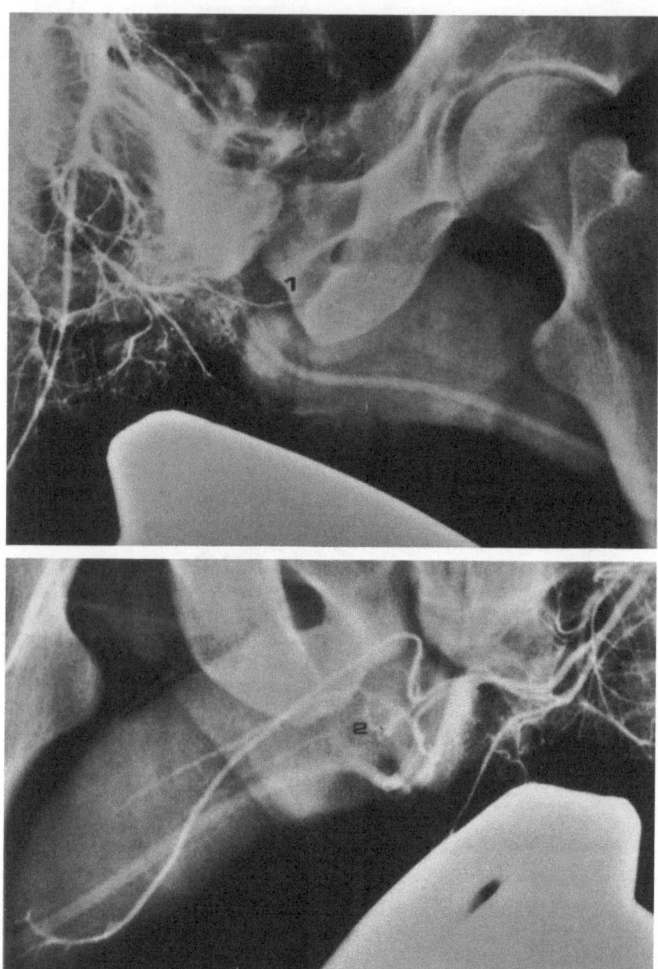

Fig. 13a,b. A 21-year-old patient with primary erectile dysfunction and congenital curvature. **a** *1*, Hypoplasia of right dorsal artery. **b** Unilateral supply via left penile artery; atypical circular vessel at the base of the penis (*2*). Only moderate disturbance of arterial supply can be assumed. Additionally the patient showed venous and neurogenic factors

as a cause for primary erectile dysfunction. Michal, one of the first to attain a modern diagnosis of erectile dysfunction and a pioneer in revascularization surgery, described the occurrence of aplasia or hypoplasia of the cavernosal artery and correlated it with "constitutional" impotence [31].

The basic problem in the assessment of abnormal penile arterialization is to find a correlation between the number, caliber, and wall structure of the penile arterial system and the extent of the associated functional impairment.

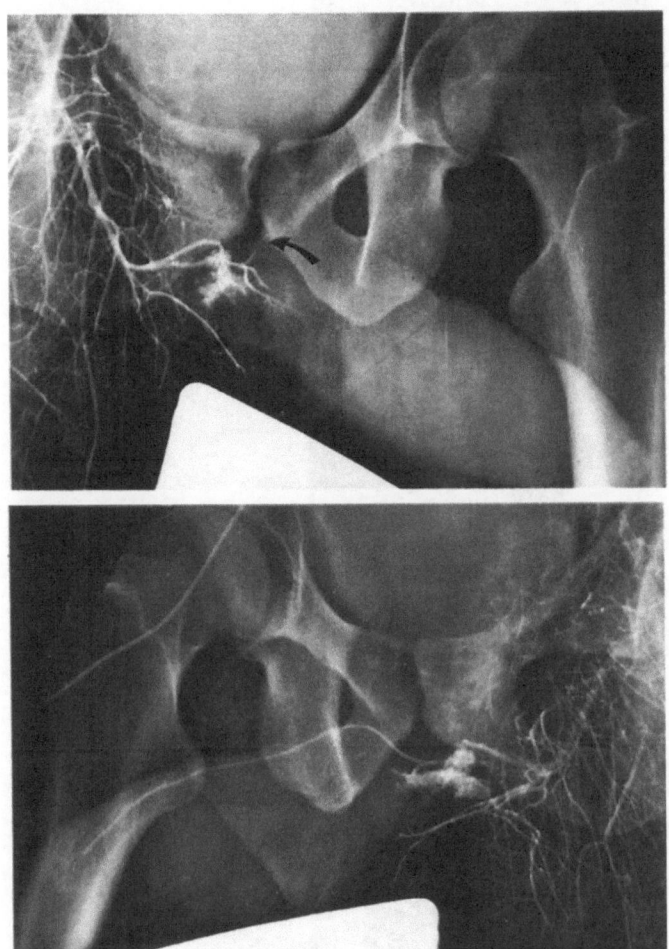

Fig. 14a,b. A 24-year-old patient with primary erectile dysfunction. Severe hypoplasia of right dorsal artery (→) and both cavernosal arteries

Our conclusions about the impact of arterial malformation, derived from the study of a group of patients with primary erectile dysfunction due to isolated arterial genesis and a control group of normally potent young men (n = 30) investigated by detailed Doppler examination [3], are as follows: Deviations from the paired penile supply (two dorsal arteries and two cavernosal arteries) frequently occur. Only 50% of the normally potent showed an anatomically normal arterial pattern. Unilateral hypoplasia or aplasia of a dorsal artery was demonstrated in 30% of the volunteers. Unilateral hypoplasia of both penile arteries does not lead to primary erectile dysfunction. Depending on the extent of hypoplasia, age and risk factors of arteriosclerosis,

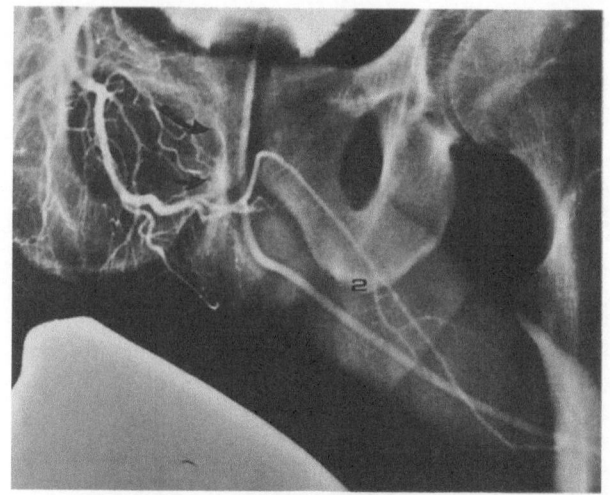

a

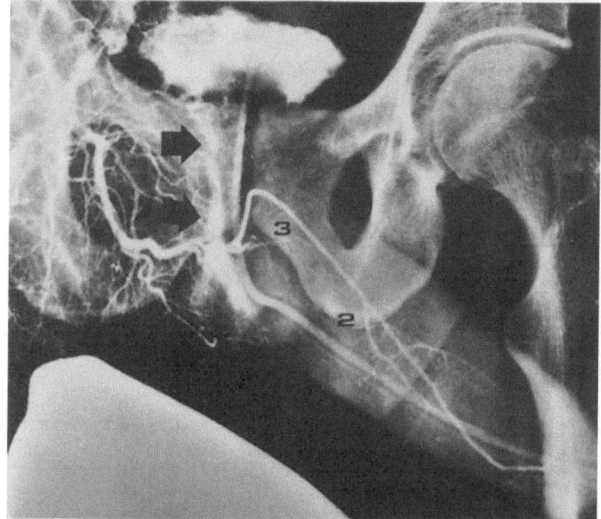

b

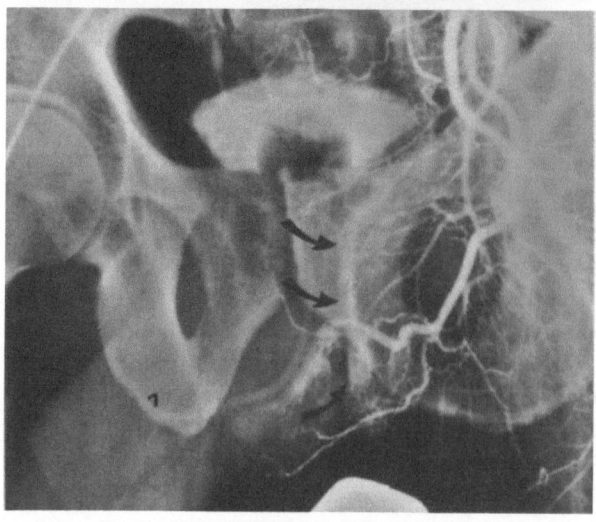

c

Fig. 15a–c. A 35-year-old patient with incomplete primary erectile dysfunction. **a** Selective right, arterial phase: Opacification of an AV fistula at the penile base (→). Distal cavernosal artery (2) with branching derived from the dorsal artery. **b** Selective right, late phase: Strong opacification of AV fistula (→). 2 Unilateral supply of distal cavernosal bodies; 3, dorsal penile artery. **c** Selective left: Early opacification of AV malformation (→). No cavernosal arteries filled. 1, Hypoplasia of dorsal artery

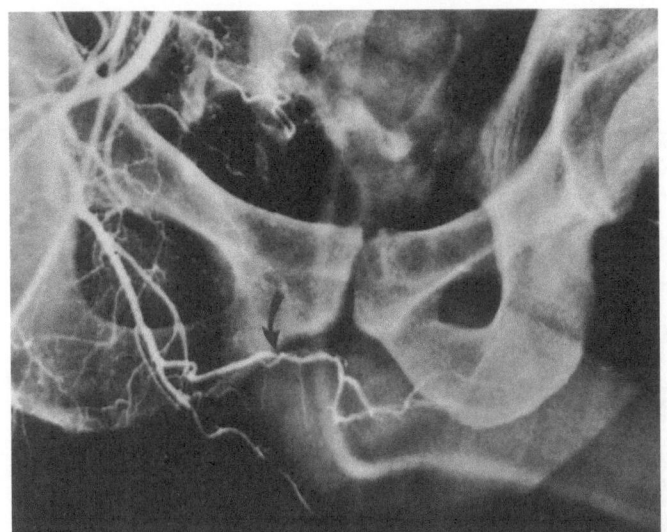

a

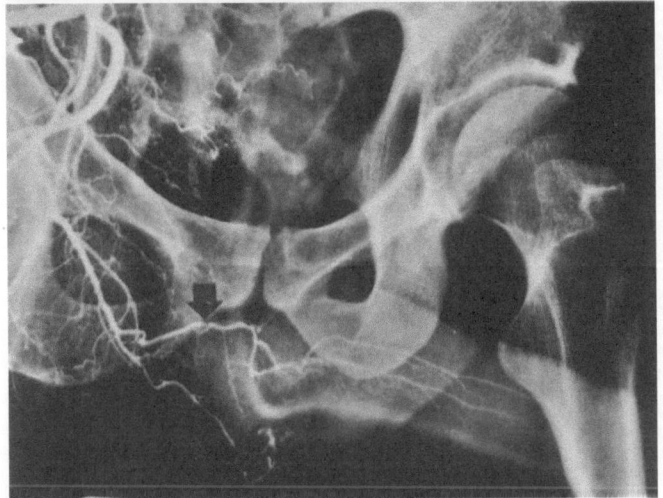

b

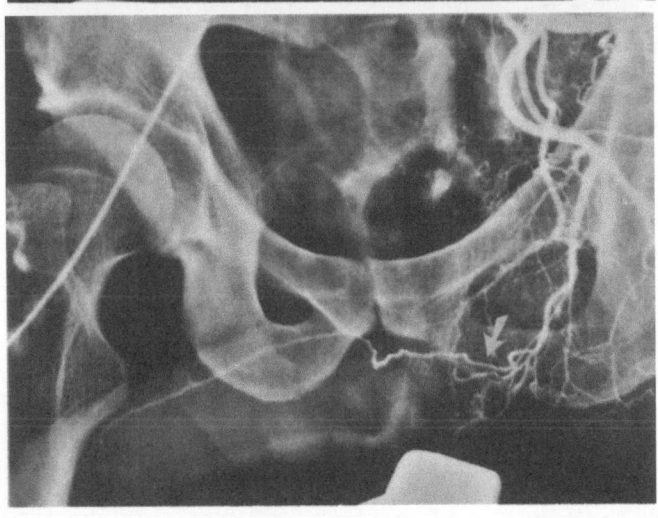

c

Fig. 16a–c. A 42-year-old patient with increasing loss of rigidity for 3 years. Selective pharmaco-arteriography in epidural anesthesia shows a combination of unilateral supply of cavernous bodies and arteriosclerosis. **a,b** Right side – stenosis of penile artery (*arrow*). Unilateral cavernosal supply. Severe hypoplasia of dorsal artery. **c** Left side – minor stenosis in the distal part of internal pudendal artery (→)

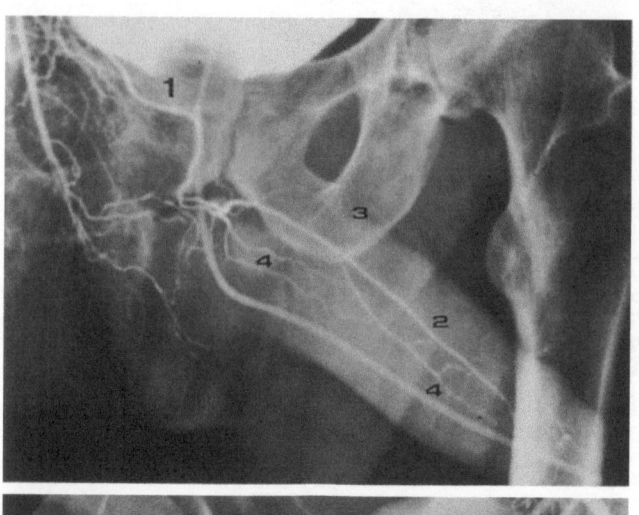

a

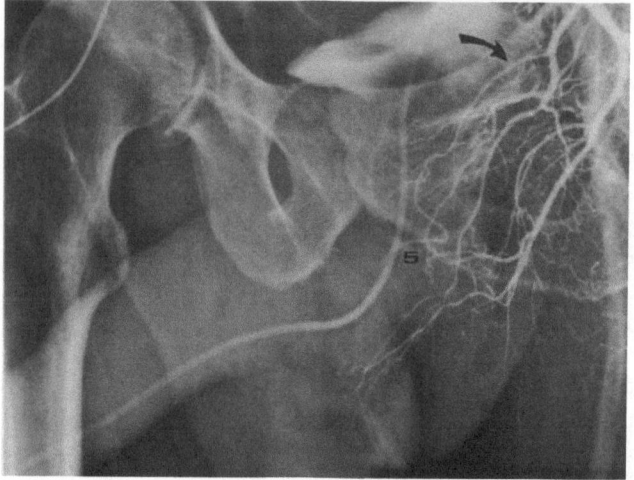

b

Fig. 17a,b. A 41-year-old patient with gradually developing erectile dysfunction over 2 years. **a** Right side – Complete penile arterialization via right accessory internal pudendal artery (*1*). *2*, Right dorsal artery; *3*, left hypoplastic dorsal artery; and *4*, proximal and distal cavernosal arteries. **b** Left side. *5*, Small artery of the bulb in early arterial phase. No other penile vessels are to be seen. Small accessory internal pudendal artery coming from obtuator artery (→)

hypoplasia can be a cause of secondary failure. Bilateral aplasia or hypoplasia or complex anomalies involving the cavernosal arteries represent the essential condition for primary erectile dysfunction.

Unilateral supply of the dorsal arteries can be defined as a variant of normal; unilateral supply of the cavernosal arteries or the whole penile arterial bed does not cause primary erectile dysfunction, but may predispose to secondary erectile dysfunction (Fig. 16). The onset of erectile dysfunction is influenced by age and risk factors of arteriosclerosis. Penile arterial anomalies are often combined with pathologic outflow conditions. It remains to be determined whether lack of cavernosal compliance, insufficient inflow, or pathologic drainage is responsible for the venous insufficiency.

With aging, all the arteries show typical changes, e.g., a large increase of nonelastic fibrous tissue and diminished elastic content [2]. This leads to a reduction in arterial compliance with increasing age. Thus in cases of unilateral cavernosal supply, the loss of 50% inflow by the absence of a pudendal artery can be compensated by the contralateral side for many years (Fig. 17). This vasomotor erectile reserve becomes progressively reduced with increasing age, and more importantly, when risk factors of arteriosclerosis are present.

References

1. Adachi B (1927) Das Arteriensystem der Japaner, Bd II. Supp ad Acta scholae medicinalis unversitatis imperialis Kyoto 9:95–125
2. Ahmed MM (1967) Age and sex differences in the structure of the tunica media of the human aorta. Acta Anat 66:45–53
3. Bähren W (1985) Erektile Dysfunktion: Selektive arteriographische Diagnostik und Therapie unter Anwendung vasoaktiver Substanzen. Habilitationsschrift Ulm, S 126–130
4. Bähren W, Stief CG, Scherb W, Gall H, Gallwitz A, Altwein JE (1986) Rationelle Diagnostik der erektilen Dysfunktion unter Anwendung eines pharmakologischen Testes. Akt Urologie 4:177–180
5. Bähren, W, Gall H, Scherb W, Stief C, Thon W (1988) Arterial anatomy and arteriographic diagnosis of arteriogenic impotence. Cardiovasc Intervent Radiol 11:195–210
6. Bookstein JJ, Valji K, Parsons L, Kessler W (1987) Pharmacoarteriography in the evaluation of impotence. J Urol 137:333–337
7. Castaneda-Zuniga WR, Smith A, Kaye K, Rusnak B, Herrera M, Miller R, Amplatz K, Weens C, Ketchum D (1982) Transluminal angioplasty for treatment of vasculogenic impotence. AJR 139:371–373
8. Forster A (1903) Beiträge zur Anatomie der äußeren männlichen Geschlechtsorgane des Menschen. Z Morphol Anthropol 6:435–501
9. Ginestie JF, Romieu A (1976) L'exploration radiologique de l'impuissance. Malonie, Paris, pp 2–24
10. Goldstein I (1986) Revascularization procedures. Semin Urol IV(4): 252–258
11. Goldstein I, Siroky MB, Nath RL, McMillan TN, Menzoian JV, Krane RJ (1982) Vasculogenic impotence: Role of the pelvic steal test. J Urol 128:300–306
12. Gray H (1973) Gray's anatomy of the human body. Lea & Febinger, Philadelphia, p 648
13. Gray R, Keresteci A, St. Louis E, Grosman H, Jewett M, Rankin J, Provan J (1982) Investigation of impotence by internal pudendal angiography: Experience with 73 cases. Radiology 144:773–780
14. Hartmann K (1955) Blasen- und Harnröhrenverletzungen bei Beckenbrüchen. Langenbecks Arch Klin Chir 282:943–949
15. Hauri D (1984) Vascular reconstruction. Read at Symposium: Controversy in the Diagnosis and Treatment of Erectile Impotence, Nov 30–Dec 1, 1984, Leiden, The Netherlands

16. Huguet JF, Clerissi J, Juhan C (1981) Radiologic anatomy of pudendal artery. Eur J Radiol 1:278–284
17. Juhan CM, Huguet JF, Clerissi JA, Courjaret P (1980) Classification of internal pudendal artery lesions in one-hundred cases. In: Zorgniotti AW, Rossi G (eds) Vasculogenic impotence. Thomas, Springfield, pp 153–169
18. Kholoussy AM, Gain T, Matsumoto T (1981) Impotence after aorto-iliac surgery: Current concepts. Angiology 32 (9):589–594
19. Langer C (1862) Über das Gefäßsystem der männlichen Schwellorgane. Sitzungsber Akad Wiss Wien Math Naturwiss Kl 46:120–129
20. Leipner N, Porst H, Köster O, Nadstawek J (1986) DSA und konventionelle Angiographie im Vergleich bei der angiographischen Diagnostik der Impotentia coeundi. Fortschr Röntgenstr 144 (5):515–522
21. Leriche R (1923) Des oblitérations artérielles hautes comme cause d'une insuffisance circulatoire des membres inférieurs. Bull Soc Chirurgie 49:1404–1406
22. Lue T, Tanagho EA (1985) Diagnostische Abklärung der erektilen Impotenz. Akt Urol 16:244–249
23. Lue TF, Jünemann KP, Fournier GR, Tanagho EA (1986) Mechanism of penile erection. ISIR (ed) Proc 2nd World Meeting on Impotence (Abstract 1.1) Prag
24. Luric AL, Bookstein J, Kessler W (1988) Angiography of posttraumatic impotence. Cardiovasc Intervent Radiol 11:232–236
25. May AG, Weese JA de Rob CG (1969) Changes in sexual function following operation on the abdominal aorta. Surgery 65(1):41–47
26. Metz P, Herning M (1984) Impotence and aorto-iliac disease with special reference to the pelvic steal syndrome. Int Angiol 3:259–262
27. Michal V, Pospichal J (1978) Phalloarteriography in the diagnosis of erectile impotence. World J Surg 2:239–248
28. Michal V, Kramar R, Bartak V (1974) Femoro-pudendal bypass in the treatment of sexual impotence. J Cardiovasc Surg 15:356–359
29. Michal V, Kramar R, Pospichal J (1978) External iliac "steal syndrome". J Cardiovasc Surg 19:355–357
30. Michal V, Kramar R, Highal L, First P (1980) Aortoiliac occlusive disease. In: Zorgniotti AW, Rossi G (eds) Vasulogenic impotence. Thomas, Springfield, pp 185–215
31. Michal V, Kovac J, Belan A (1984) Arterial lesions in impotence: Phalloarteriography. Int Angiol 3:247–254
32. Mitchell JP (1968) Injuries to the urethra. Br J Urol 4:649–654
33. Müller J (1935) Entdeckung der bei der Erektion wirksamen Arterien. Arch Anat 202–213
34. Nath RL, Menzoian JO, Kaplan KH, McMillian TN, Siroky MB, Krane RJ (1981) The mutlidisciplinary approach to vasculogenic impotence. Surgery 89 (1):124–133
35. Palma RG de Levine SB, Feldman S (1978) Preservation of erectile function after aorto-iliac reconstruction. Arch Surg 113:958–962
36. Queral LA, Whithehouse WM, Flinn WR, Zarins CK, Bergan JJ, Yao JS (1979) Pelvic hemodynamics after aortoiliac reconstruction. Surgery 86 (6):799–808
37. Rotter W, Schürmann R (1950) Die Blutgefäße des menschlichen Penis. Virchows Arch 318:352–393
38. Sabri S, Cotton C (1971) Sexual function following aorto-iliac reconstruction. Lancet 2:1218–1219
39. Schweiger H, Zirngibl H, Raithel D (1984) Potenzstörungen vor und nach Beckenarterienrekonstruktion: Objektivierung durch Messung des Penisarteriendrucks. Chirurg 55:95–99
40. Sigel A, Chlepas S (1981) Verletzungen der Harnröhre. In: Lutzeyer W (Hrsg) Traumatologie des Urogenitaltraktes. Springer, Berlin Heidelberg New York, S 131–199
41. Spiro M, Cotton CT (1970) Aorto-iliac thrombendarterectomy. Br J Surg 57:161–168
42. Stieve H (1930) Männliche Genitalorgane. In: Möllendorf W (Hrsg) Handbuch der mikroskopischen Anatomie des Menschen, Bd VII/2. Springer, Berlin

43. Struyven J, Gregoir W, Giannakopoulos X, Wauters E (1979) Selective pudendal arteriography. Eur Urol 5:233–242
44. Unnik JG van, Marsman IW (1984) Impotence due to the external iliac steal syndrome treated by percutaneous transluminal angioplasty. J Urol 131:544–545
45. Valji K, Bookstein J (1988) Transluminal angioplasty in the treatment of arteriogenic impotence. Cardiovasc Intervent Radiol 11:245–252
46. Virag R (1981) Pelvic steal syndrome. Vasa 9:304–307
47. Virag R (1984) Impotence: A new field in angiology. Int Angiol 3:217–220
48. Virag R (1984) The treatment of angiogenic impotence. Int Angiol 3:275–280
49. Wagner G, Green R (1981) Impotence. Plenum Press, New York London, pp 62–72
50. Watt JK, Gillespie G, Pollack JG (1974) Arterial surgery in intermittent claudication. Br Med J 1:23–27
51. Zorgniotti AW, Padula G, Shaw WW (1983) Selective arteriography for vascular impotence. World J Urol 1:213–217
52. Zorgniotti AW, Shaw WW, Padula G, Rossi G (1984) Impotence associated with pudendal arteriovenous malformation. J Urol 132:128–131

Evaluation of the Cavernous Occlusive System

C.G. Stief

Introduction

Recent experimental studies show that the smooth muscle of the cavernous tissue plays a key role in the hemodynamics of penile erection [5, 8]. A fully rigid erection requires, in addition to cavernous relaxation, a large reduction in the cavernous outflow [2], which is brought about both by the passive compression of venous cushions between the cavernous sinusoids and the tunica albuginea [2], and the squeezing of the obliquely running venae perforantes within the tunica albuginea [7]. Therefore, excessive cavernous outflow can be caused by incomplete cavernosal relaxation, e.g., by cavernous fibrosis due to diabetes, or by disturbances of the squeezing mechanism within the tunica albuginea, or by both.

In 1852, Kölliker was the first to describe the phenomenon of artificial erection by direct perfusion of the cavernous bodies [6]. He observed that the flow needed to maintain an erection could be reduced as soon as full rigidity was reached. He concluded that this phenomenon was due to a reduction in the cavernous outflow caused by the squeezing of the venae perforantes within the tunica albuginea.

To evaluate the cavernous outflow in impotent patients, Wagner and Virag introduced dynamic cavernosography [1, 13], allowing quantification of venous leakage by maintenance flow and qualification using X-rays after contrast medium perfusion. Virag proposed that the opacification should be performed during artificial erection to occlude the physiologically open venous channels and thereby to identify abnormal cavernous drainage.

Recent experimental studies have shown dynamic cavernosometry and cavernosography during saline perfusion alone to be unphysiological [10, 11]. Only after cavernous smooth muscle relaxation induced by intracavernous injection of vasoactive drugs cavernosometry and cavernosography can evaluate the cavernous occlusive system in a physiological way.

Anatomy

The superficial dorsal veins which primarily drain the glans and the penile skin drain into the pudendal plexus and/or the saphenous vein(s). They are

U. Jonas et al. (Eds.) Erectile Dysfunction
© Springer-Verlag Berlin Heidelberg 1991

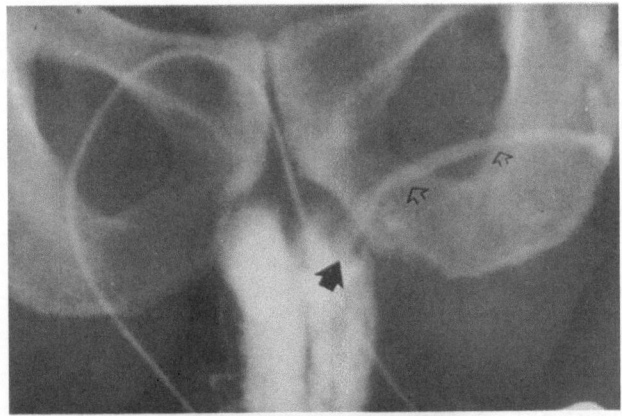

a

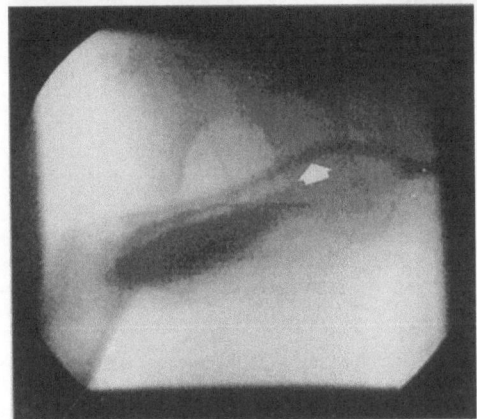

b

Fig. 1. a Abnormal cavernosal drainage via an ectopic vein (*arrows*) into the left saphenous vein. **b** Videoimage of the early filling phase shows the immediate (abnormal) efflux from the cavernous bodies via the ectopic vein (*arrow*), long before the cavernous bodies are entirely filled with contrast medium

called ectopic veins when they drain into the saphenous vein(s) (Fig. 1), and they communicate with the deep dorsal vein that drains the glans and the corpora cavernosa (Fig. 2). The deep dorsal vein drains into the periprostatic plexus and into the internal pudendal veins via communications. Additionally, the cavernous drainage runs, via the cavernous veins merging at the hilum of the penis, medially from the tip of the crura and via numerous small veins at the tip of the crura (crural veins). In the flaccid state, there are venous shunts between the corpora cavernosa and between the corpus cavernosum and the glans [3].

Indications

Cavernosometry and cavernosography are invasive diagnostic methods that require strict indications, based on the results of noninvasive and minimally invasive work-up, especially on the results of pharmacotesting [12], Doppler

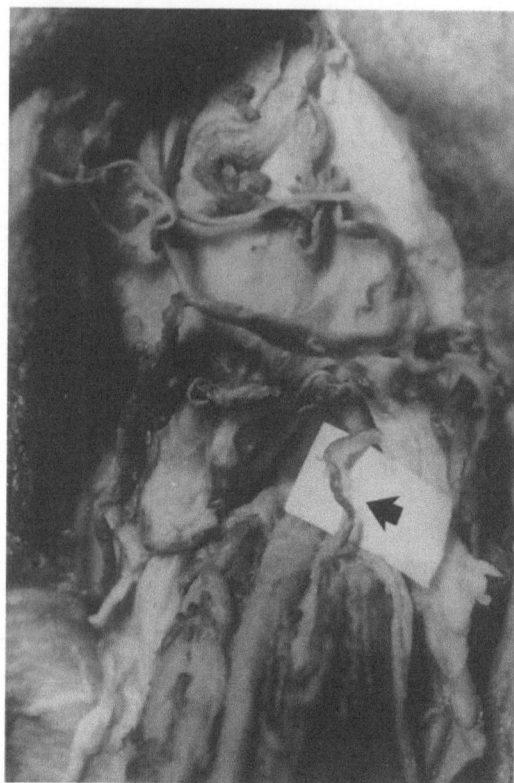

Fig. 2. Anatomical dissection showing connection of the superficial dorsal and deep dorsal penile venous drainage (*arrow*)

sonography [4] and SPACE (*s*ingle *p*otential *a*nalysis of *c*avernous *e*lectric activity). We see two major groups of patients: (a) good candidates for venous procedures with a good chance for spontaneous erections after the procedure (normal results in Doppler sonography, full erection after administration of 15 mg papaverine and 0.5 mg phentolamine or more, normal SPACE), and (b) candidates for venous procedures that refuse prosthetic surgery and who must presumably rely on autoinjection therapy even after successful venous surgery (abnormal results in Doppler sonography, poor response to pharmacotesting, abnormal SPACE).

Method

Under sterile conditions, the proximal left cavernous body is punctured with a 19G cannula and connected to a perfusion pump. The proximal right cavernous body is then punctured with a 26G needle and connected to a Stattham transducer for continuous intracavernous pressure recording (Fig.

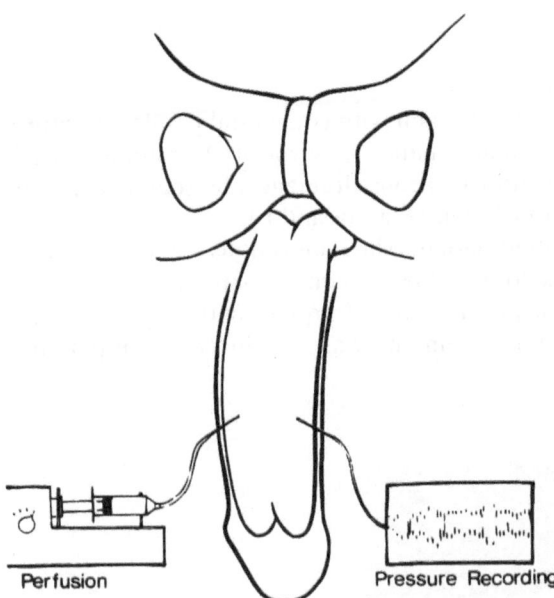

Fig. 3. Needle placement for cavernosometry and cavernosography

3). To induce cavernous smooth muscle relaxation, 30 mg papaverine and 1 mg phentolamine are injected intracavernously via the left butterfly cannula. After 5 min and subsequent cavernous relaxation, cavernosometry is performed by perfusing the penis with saline at a flow rate of 200 ml/min. The temperature of the saline is 37°C to avoid cavernous smooth muscle contraction with subsequently false positive results due to cold saline. As soon as full rigidity is reached (corresponding to an intracavernous pressure of about 80 mm Hg), the minimum flow to maintain a full erection is determined ("maintenance flow"). If full rigidity cannot be achieved within 120 s (corresponding to 400 ml saline), measurement of the maintenance flow is abandoned to prevent circulatory side effects, and opacification is done in the semirigid state. The maintenance flow is the quantitative measure of cavernous venous outflow (diagnosis of venous leakage).

Cavernosography is then performed. Artificial erection is maintained by perfusing with undiluted nonionic contrast medium (Solutrast[R]). For exact localization of the abnormal cavernous venous draining system, X-rays are taken in the anteroposterior and in oblique (30°) positions. Cavernosography visualizes the anatomy of the venous leakage. Because of possible endothelial alterations of the sinusoids, the penis is then perfused with 30–50 ml of saline to wash out the hyperoncotic contrast medium. To prevent hematomas, the cannulas are removed and the puncture sites are compressed manually for at least 5 min.

Results

As a control group, eight young potent men with congenital penile curvature underwent cavernosometry. The maintenance flow was 4–14 ml/min (mean 7 ml/min). In cavernosography, no cavernous drainage was seen except for the opacification of the deep dorsal vein (Fig. 4a and b).

In about a third of the impotent patients showing venous leakage, a single abnormal drainage system was found, the remaining patients presented a combination of different systems [9]. The most frequent pathologic drainage was found to run via the deep dorsal vein and was seen in 27.4% of patients

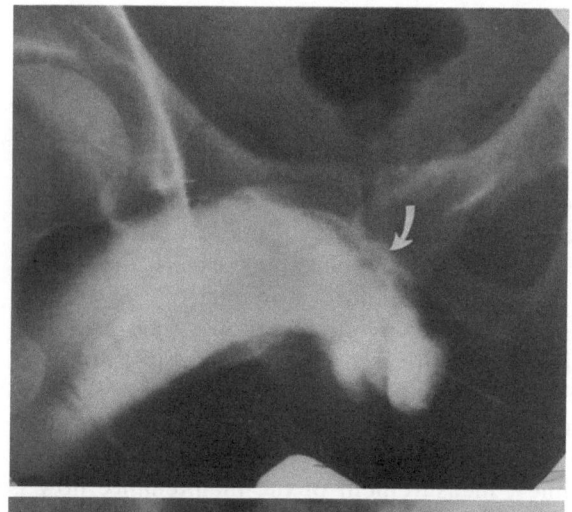

a

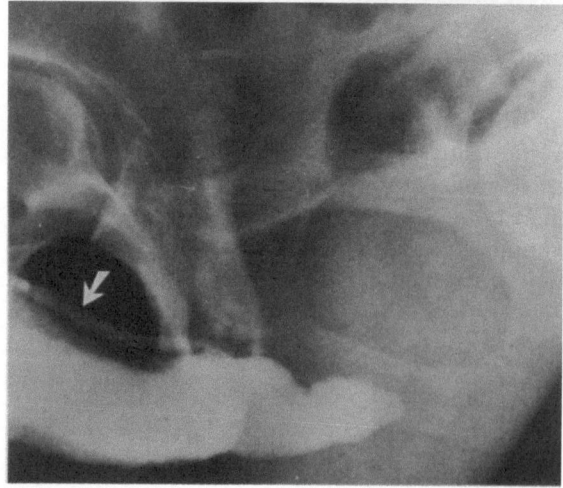

b

Fig. 4a,b. Cavernosography of a normal potent man with congenital penile curvature from an anteroposterior (**a**) and an oblique (**b**) position. Beside slight opacification of the deep dorsal vein (*arrows*), no cavernous drainage is seen

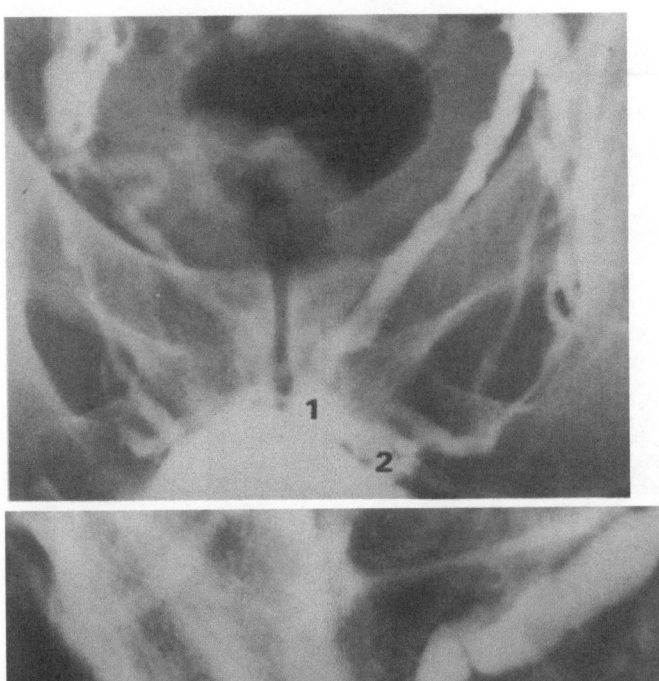

Fig. 5a,b. Abnormal cavernous drainage via the deep dorsal vein (*1*), cavernous veins (*2*) and crural veins (*arrow*), visualized by cavernosography in an anteroposterior (**a**) and (**b**) plane. The latter oblique projection proves the abnormal drainage to be via the cavernous veins (*2*)

with secondary impotence and in 15.6% with primary impotence. The combination of deep dorsal and cavernous vein drainage was found in 24.8% of patients with secondary impotence and 25% of patients with primary impotence (Fig. 5a and b) and deep dorsal and ectopic vein drainage occurred in 18.6% and 18.7%, respectively. There were no significant differences between the maintenance flows corresponding to the type of pathologic drainages, except in the case of drainage via ectopic veins. There was also no

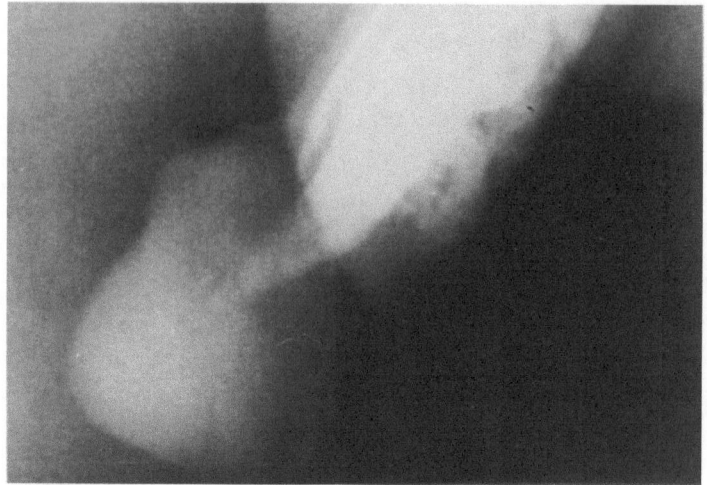

a

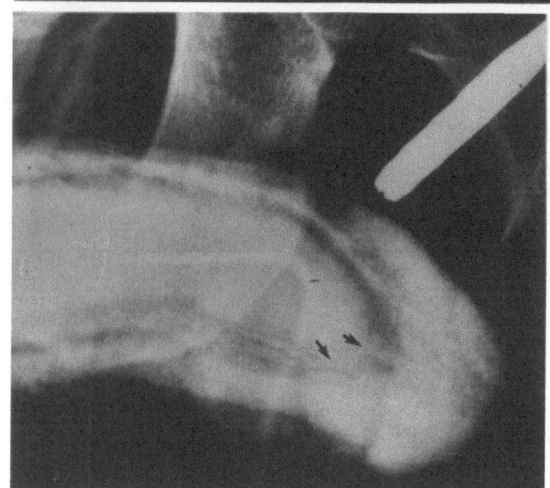

b

Fig. 6. a No opacification of the glans in a normally potent patient. **b** Corporoglandular fistula (*arrows*) with opacification of the glans. **c** Retrograde filling of the glans via the deep dorsal vein after deep dorsal vein ligation (*1*, before contrast medium filling; *2–4*, after contrast medium perfusion)

significant difference between pharmacotesting results for different types of drainage.

The deep dorsal vein (or veins) was involved in the anomalous drainage in 81.3% of patients with primary impotence and in 92% of patients with secondary impotence. The ectopic vein (or veins) was involved in the anomalous drainage in 59.4% of patients with primary impotence and 45.1% of patients with secondary impotence, the cavernous vein (or veins) in 34.4% and 43.3% of the patient groups, respectively. A cavernosoglandular shunt (Fig. 6) was found in 18.8% of patients with primary impotence and 7.0% of patients with secondary impotence. In 28% of the patients with cavernous vein drainage, crural vein drainage was also visualized (Fig. 5b).

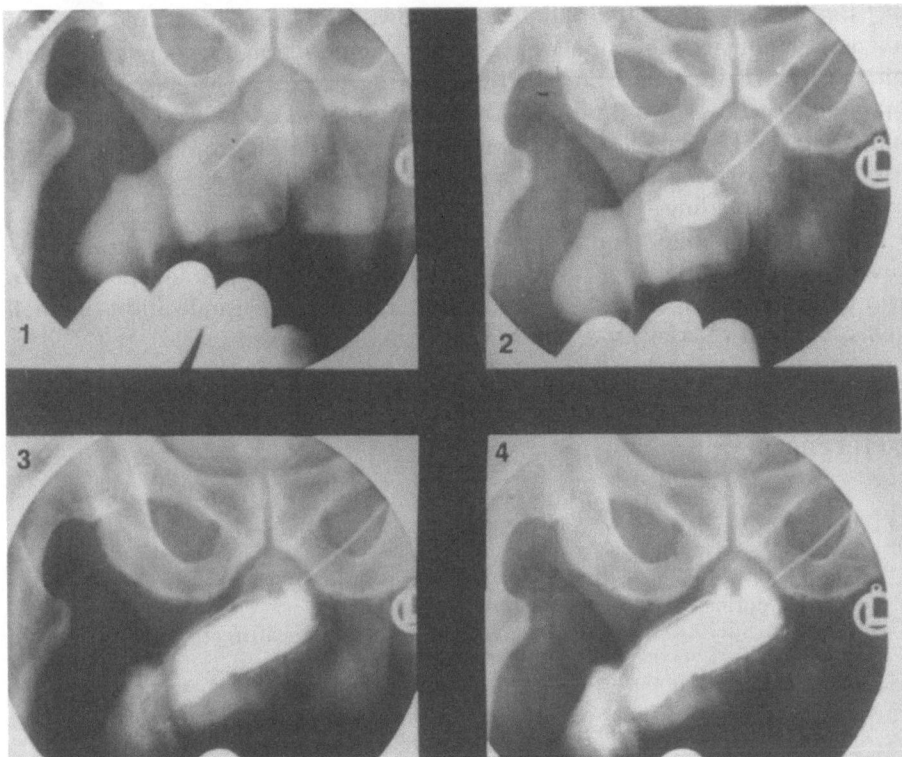

c

Side Effects

Ecchymosis (<5 mm) occurred in 27% of the patients, mainly at the site of the 19G needle. We saw three important subcutaneous edemas of the penile shaft. Two occurred during saline perfusion by displacement of the needle out of the corpora. They rapidly resorbed without any further treatment. One occurred during contrast medium perfusion and was followed by continuous penile shaft swelling caused by the hyperoncotic contrast medium. This edema was also resorbed without further therapy within 2 days.

Conclusion

Cavernosometry and cavernosography should be done only after cavernous smooth muscle relaxation induced by intracavernous injection of vasoactive drugs.

Beside measuring the maintenance flow, Virag also measured the flow needed to induce an erection [13]. Because the induction flow depends mainly on the size of the penis and on the cavernous drainage (measured by the maintenance flow), we think that the determination of the induction flow is unnecessary. The maintenance flow seems to be the appropriate parameter for diagnosis of venous leakage. This clinical assumption was substantiated by experimental findings [10].

Successful penile venous surgery depends on precise localization of the cavernous venous leakage. Therefore, cavernosography should be done in two planes (anteroposterior and oblique). For proper visualization of small veins, dilution of contrast medium should be abandoned.

References

1. Ebbehoj J, Wagner G (1979) Insufficient penile erection due to abnormal drainage of cavernous bodies. Urology 13:507
2. Fournier GR, Jünemann KP, Lue TF, Tanagho EA (1987) Mechanisms of venous occlusion during canine penile erection. J Urol 137:163
3. Gilbert P, Stief CG (1987) Spongiosolysis: A new surgical treatment of impotence caused by distal venous leakage. J Urol 138:784
4. Jevtich MJ (1980) Importance of penile arterial pulse sound examination in impotence. J Urol 124:820
5. Jünemann KP, Lue TF, Fournier GR, Tanagho EA (1986) Hemodynamics of papaverin- and phentolamin-induced erections. J Urol 136:158
6. Kölliker A (1852) Das anatomische und physiologische Verhalten der cavernösen Körper der Sexualorgane. Verh Phys-Med Ges Würzburg 2:118
7. Lierse W (1982) Blood vessels and nerves of the human penis. Urol Int 37:145
8. Lue TF, Takamura T, Umraya M., Schmidt RA, Tanagho EA (1984) Hemodynamics of canine corpora cavernosa during erection. Urology 24:347
9. Stief CG, Wetterauer U (1989) Quantitative and qualitative analysis of dynamic cavernosographies in erectile dysfunction due to venous leakage. Urology 34:252
10. Stief CG, Diederichs W, Benard F, Bosch R, Lue TF, Tanagho EA (1988) The diagnosis of venogenic impotence: dynamic or pharmacologic cavernosometry? J Urol 140:1561
11. Stief CG, Benard F, Diederichs W, Bosch R, Lue TF, Tanagho ET (1988) The rationale for pharmacologic cavernosography. J Urol 140:1564
12. Stief CG, Bähren W, Gall H, Scherb W (1988) Functional evaluation of penile hemodynamics. J Urol 139:734
13. Virag R, Legman M, Zwang G, Dermange H (1979) L'utilisation de l'erection passive dans l'exploration de l'impuissance d'origine vasculaire. Contraception Fertilite Sexualite 7:707

Monitoring of Penile Tumescence and Rigidity

W.F. Thon

Erectile dysfunction is defined as the inability to obtain and/or sustain an erection adequate for vaginal penetration and satisfactory completion of sexual intercourse. Differential diagnosis of the two main causes of erectile dysfunction – organic and psychogenic impotence – is often impossible during a routine examination. Psychological exploration fails to discriminate between organic and psychogenic impotence [18]. Men with suspected psychogenic erectile dysfunction have neither more nor fewer pathological deviations on the Minnesota Multiphasic Personality Inventory (MMPI), California Psychological Inventory (CPI), or Derogatis Sexual Functioning Inventory (DSFI) than do those with objective organic disorders [20, 25].

The development of effective treatment alternatives for impotence has increased the importance of distinguishing between psychogenic and organic erectile dysfunction. Psychogenic impotence is frequently successfully reversed by sexual behavior modification techniques such as systematic desensitization and assertive training [24]. Arterial disorders are successfully treated by intracavernous pharmacotherapy [13, 27, 31], angioplasty [2], or revascularization procedures [22].

In 1970, Karacan [16] suggested the use of nocturnal penile tumescence (NPT) monitoring as a clinical tool for the diagnosis of erectile dysfunction. The changes in penile circumference are measured by two thin mercury filled silicone tubing loops which are positioned around the penis – one just behind the corona and one at the base. NPT is a naturally occurring sleep-related phenomenon with four to five erections nightly during REM sleep lasting approximately 25–35 min. Total tumescence time declines with increasing age. Patients with psychogenic impotence and a normal NPT have an intact erectile mechanism and thus a potential for normal erectile capacity.

Patients with organic etiology have absent or abnormal NPT monitoring measurements. Abnormal NPT monitoring measurements during the first night of testing are known to be of limited diagnostic value due to the influence of the patient's unfamiliarity with the testing situation [5] and to some extent due to occult sleep disorders [23, 29]. In about 20%, of patients, abnormal NPT is noted without any identifiable organic etiology. In 17%, of the patients with normal NPT monitoring, rigidity is inadequate for vaginal penetration [29].

U. Jonas et al. (Eds.) Erectile Dysfunction
© Springer-Verlag Berlin Heidelberg 1991

The source of the NPT monitoring error is the phenomenon of significant penile expansion without sufficient rigidity for vaginal penetration. There is only limited data concerning the measurement of penile expansion and intracavernous pressure during erection. The increase in circumference only correlates well with intracavernous pressure to a certain extent [12]. Metz and Wagner [21] recorded maximal penile circumference at an intracavernous pressure below the pressure required for full rigidity.

Desai et al. [7] conducted tests on a flexible tubular model and demonstrated a linear relationship between force and pressure ($r = 0.99$) and between radial and axial rigidity ($r = 0.99$). They also noted interindividual variation in intracavernosal pressure and rigidity measured at the moment the penis became erect and at an angle of 90° or more from the horizontal. Wespes et al. [30] described a simple method to evaluate rigidity by measuring the angle between the penis and the legs with the patient in the standing position. Patients with normal rigidity on palpation had an angle greater than 110°.

In 1985 Bradley et al. [4] first described a device for the continuous and simultaneous measurement of penile rigidity and circumferential expansion of the penis (RigiScan, Dacomed, Minneapolis, MN; (Fig. 1). RigiScan monitors the penile circumference every 15 s with two wire loops. When the penis increases 1 cm in circumference the loops gently tighten around the penis every 30s with a linear force of 10 ounces in order to record the cross sectional response to radial compression which is recorded as 0%–100% rigidity. Nocturnal RigiScan monitoring of penile tumescence and rigidity (Fig. 2) during at least two consecutive nights has proven to be a reliable and objective test [15]. Still there is a discrepancy between NPT status and performance in a sexual situation. Desai et al. [7] observed a significantly higher degree of sustained rigidity achieved during visual sexual stimulation than during nocturnal sleep erections. A positive penile response to visual erotic stimuli proves that the neurogenic pathways involved in the sexual response are functionally intact.

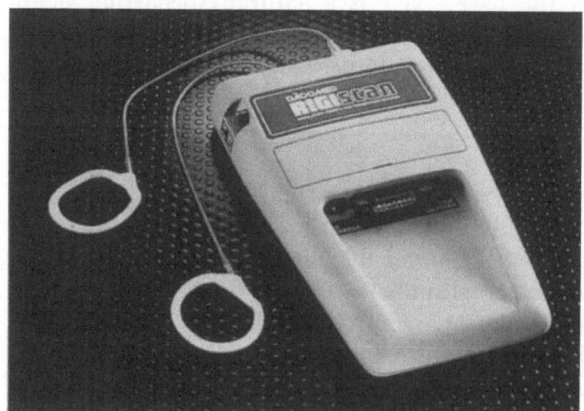

Fig. 1. RigiScan device (Dacomed Corp., Minneapolis, MN) for continuous monitoring of penile tumescence and rigidity. Loops are applied to penile base and shaft

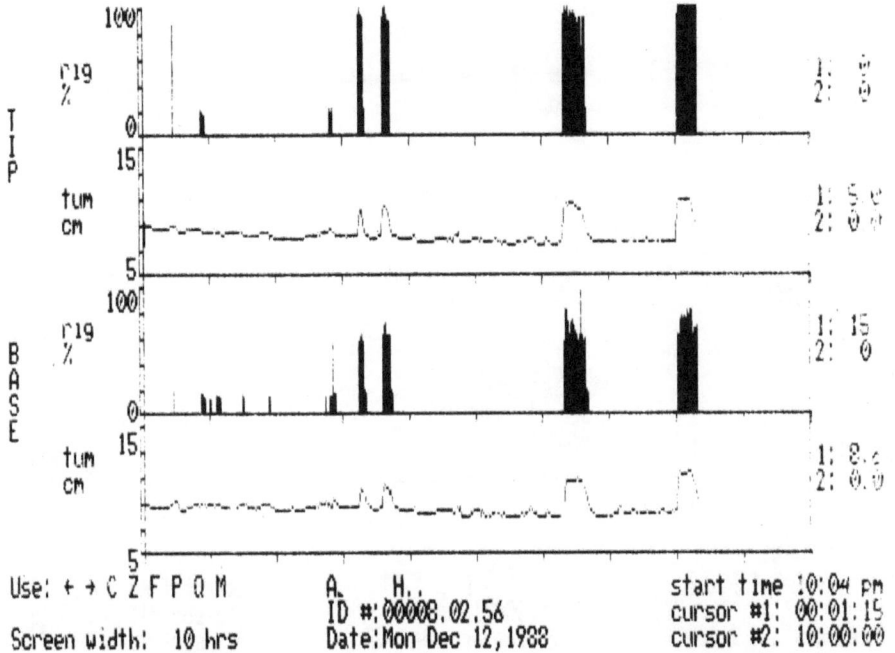

Fig. 2. Nocturnal RigiScan of normal pattern of erections as seen in a 34-year-old man with psychogenic erectile dysfunction. *Tip* represents tumescence (*tum*) and rigidity (*rig*) of distal penis; *Base* represents tumescence and rigidity of proximal penis. RigiScan documents four normal erections with normal rigidity

For routine evaluation of patients complaining of erectile dysfunction, it is advisable to examine them first with RigiScan real-time monitoring during visual sexual stimulation (Fig. 3) in combination with intracavernous pharmacotesting [11]. Patients who reported having erectile dysfunction, but who had a good response to visual erotic stimulation (VES) can be easily classified as psychogenically impotent. Patients with no response to VES, but with a good response to VES after pharmacotesting probably have an organic etiology. In patients who have no response even after the injection of a maximum dose of a vasoactive drug (20 µg Prostaglandin E1), there is a relatively high suspicion of venous insufficiency.

Other than RigiScan, only a few commercially available devices exist for monitoring penile tumescence and rigidity: Surgitek ART-1000 (Surgitek Med. Eng. Corp., Racine, WI), PERIN [7], and RIGIDMETRE [28]. None of these devices is able to predict accurately the success of vaginal penetration because the result also depends partly upon partner acceptance. The selection of our rigidity criteria was based upon results obtained during intracavernous injection tests, in which we found that 70% rigidity would be fully sufficient for vaginal intromission. No standards of objective measurements have yet been established for penile rigidity which can be directly related to vaginal

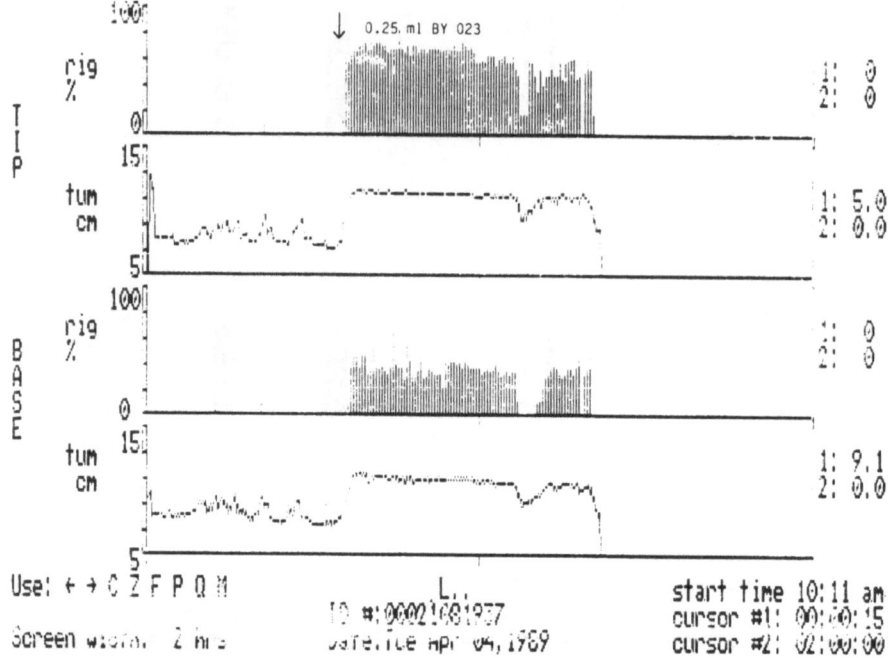

Fig. 3. RigiScan real-time monitoring during visual sexual stimulation in a 42-year-old man with arteriogenic erectile impotence shows no rigidity during visual sexual stimulation alone but 65% rigidity on proximal penis and 45% rigidity on distal penis after intracavernous injection of 3.75 mg papaverine and 0.125 mg phentolamine (0.25 ml test solution BY 023, TOSSE, Hamburg, FRG)

penetration. Bradley et al. [4] demonstrated that circumferential rigidity is linearly related to the buckling force. Prior studies by Karacan et al. [17] have shown that intromission is possible when buckling pressure is more than 100 mm Hg and is unlikely to be accomplished if penile buckling force is less than 100 mm Hg.

Increase in circumference as well as rigidity can also be measured semi-quantitatively with simple devices like the JONAS Erectiometer [14] (ESKA; Fig. 4) or the Snap-Gauge band [9] (Dacomed Corp., Minneapolis, MN; Fig. 5). The JONAS Erectiometer consists of a calibrated band with a sliding collar fastened to one end. The collar has a slot of predetermined size which requires a force of approximately 250 grams (yellow collar) or 450 grams (green collar) in order to pull the band through the slot. Circumference changes can be monitored during sleep or during VES with a good correlation to maximum rigidity as monitored by RigiScan (personal observation). Slob et al. [26] recently proved the usefulness of the erectiometer in conjunction with VES while examining male patients complaining of erectile dysfunction. The Snap-Gauge band consists of a three-film layer mounted on a Velcro fastener. The plastic sheets are arranged parallel to one another and are

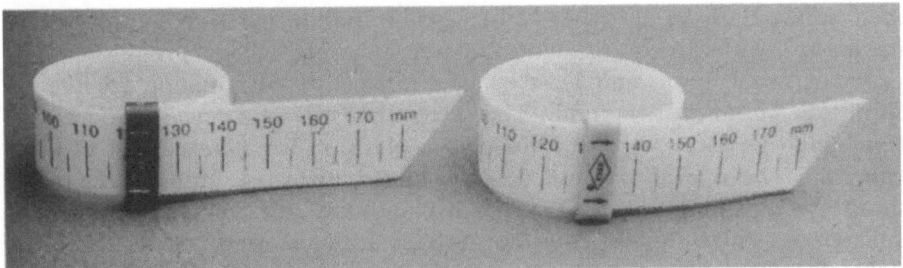

Fig. 4. JONAS Erectiometer (ESKA, Geisenheim, FRG). Calibrated band with a sliding collar fastened to one end. The sliding collar correlates to the force (250 g, yellow; 450 g, green) necessary to pull the band through the slot

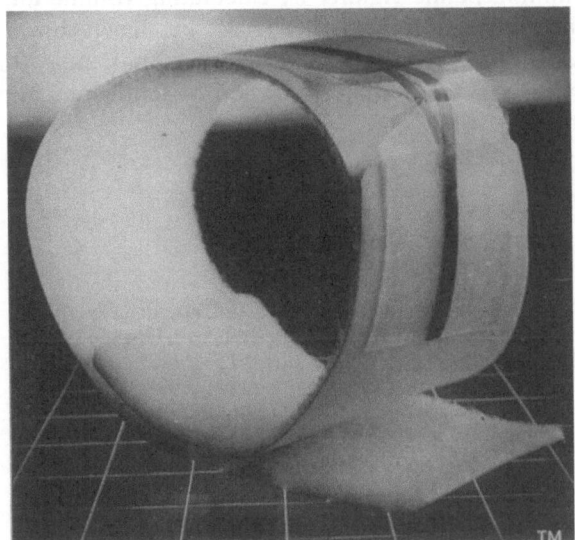

Fig. 5. Snap-Gauge (Dacomed Corp., Minneapolis, MN) with Velcro fasteners and three film layers, which rupture at different force constants (blue stripe, 10 ounces; red stripe, 15 ounces; clear film, 20 ounces)

designed to rupture at different force constants: the blue stripe at 10 ounces, the red stripe at 15 ounces, and the clear film at 20 ounces. Snap-Gauge and JONAS Erectiometer only measure maximum rigidity. The application of these devices for measuring NPT and their use in conjunction with erotic sexual stimulation are simple screening procedures for men with erectile dysfunction. Abnormal results attained with these semiquantitative devices have to be precisely evaluated by RigiScan monitoring.

Condra et al. [6] and Ellis et al. [10] reported discrepancies between Snap-Gauge and NPT monitoring. Allen and Brendler [1] even questioned the diagnostic accuracy of the Snap-Gauge test while comparing Snap-Gauge and NPT monitoring.

To avoid psychogenic disturbances during evaluation, noncontact methods of recording penile configuration changes are regarded as the most ideal tools. Earls et al. [8] described penile monitoring with a camera connected to a video recorder. We evaluated a system called "Priapus", which provides an accurate and least invasive means of determining erectile response to visual erotic stimuli. The system consists of a sensory and operations unit. The sensory unit consists of a platform for a stereo pair of CCD cameras. The operations unit consists of a Unix workstation, a Sun 386i desktop microcomputer with graphic display printer, and an image processing subsystem. Video signals from the cameras are converted into digital image data. The system is capable of making detailed measurements of circumference including penile shape, length, volume, curvature, and erection angle. The system allows objective determinations of penile configuration in patients complaining of penile deviation during erection. The system's accuracy in indirectly determining penile rigidity by calculating volume and angle changes per s has to be determined in further trials. Further technical developments will help assist the urologist in his evaluation of patients with erectile dysfunction and help to discriminate between psychogenic and organic causes of impotence.

References

1. Allen R, Brendler CB (1990) Snap-Gauge compared to a full nocturnal penile tumescence study for evaluation of patients with erectile impotence. J Urol 143:51–54
2. Becker GJ, Rowe DM, Holden RW, Dalsing MC, Bendick PJ (1986) Percutaneous transluminal angioplasty for vasculogenic impotence. Indiana Med 79(3):256–262
3. Bradley WE (1987) New techniques in evaluation of impotence. Urology 29(4): 383–388
4. Bradley WE, Timm GW, Gallagher JM, Johnson BK (1985) New method for continuous measurement of nocturnal penile tumescence and rigidity. Urology 26:4–9
5. Brooks ME (1983) Validity of monitoring nocturnal penile tumescence for a single night. Urol Res 11:187–189
6. Condra M, Fenemore J, Reid K, Phillips P, Morales A, Owen J, Surridge DH (1987) Screening assessment of penile tumescence and rigidity. Clinical test of Snap-Gauge. Urology 29:254
7. Desai KM, Floyd TJ, Follet DH, Peake DR, Gingell JC (1988) Development of a penile rigidity indicator and new concepts in the quantification of rigidity. Br J Urol 61:254–260
8. Earls C, Marshall WL, Marshall PG, Morales A, Surridge DH (1983) Penile elongation: a method for the screening of impotence. J Urol 130:90–92
9. Ek A, Bradley WE, Krane RJ (1983) Snap-Gauge-band: new concept in measuring penile rigidity. Urology 21:63–67
10. Ellis D, Doghramji K, Bagley DH (1988) Snap-Gauge band versus penile rigidity in impotence assessment. J Urol 140:61
11. Giesbers AAGM, Bruins JL, Kramer AEJL, Jonas U (1987) New methods in the diagnosis of impotence: RigiScan penile tumescence and rigidity monitoring and diagnostic papaverine hydrochloride injection. World J Urol 5:173–176
12. Godec CJ, Cass AS (1981) Quantification of erection. J Urol 126:345–347
13. Ishii N, Watanabe H, Irisawa C, Kikuchi Y, Kubota Y, Kawamura S, Suzuki H, Chiba R, Tokiwa M, Shirai M (1989) Intracavernous injection of prostaglandin E1 for the treatment of erectile impotence. J Urol 141(2):323–325

14. Jonas U (1982) Erectiometer: Ein einfacher und sicherer Test in der Diagnostik der erektilen Impotenz. Akt Urol 13:324–327
15. Kaneko S, Bradley WE (1986) Evaluation of erectile dysfunction with continuous monitoring of penile rigidity. J Urol 136:1062–1069
16. Karacan J (1970) Clinical value of nocturnal REM erection in the differential diagnosis of sexual impotence. Med Aspects Hum Sex 4:27–34
17. Karacan J, Aslan C, Hirshkowitz M (1983) Erectile mechanisms in man. Science 220:1080–1082
18. Levenson H, Olkin R., Herzoff N, deLancy M (1986), MMPI evaluation of erectile dysfunction: failure of organic vs. psychogenic decision rules. J Clin Psychol 42: 752–754
19. Marshall P, Morales A, Surridge D (1981) Unreliability of nocturnal penile tumescence recording and MMPJ profiles in assessment of impotence. Urology 17:136–139
20. Martin LM, Rodgers DA, Montague DK (1983) Psychometric differentiation of biogenic and psychogenic impotence. Arch Sex Behav 12:475–485
21. Metz P, Wagner G (1981) Penile circumference and erection. Urology 18:268–270
22. Michal V, Kramar R, Pospichal J, Ruzbarsky V, Simana J, Blazkova J, Lachman M, Hejhal L (1980) Vascular surgery in the treatment of impotence; its present possibilities and prospects. Czech Med 3(3):213–217
23. Pressman MR, DiPhilippo MA, Kendrick JI, Conroy K, Fry JM (1986), Problems in the interpretation of nocturnal penile tumescence studies: disruption of sleep by occult sleep disorders. J Urol 136:595–598
24. Schilling E, Loth NA (1980) Psychisch bedingte Potenzstörungen, psychologische Diagnose und psychotherapeutische Behandlungsmöglichkeiten. Fortschr Med 98: 1748–1751
25. Seagraves RT, Schönberg HW, Zarins CK, Knopf J, Camic P (1981) Discrimination of organic versus psychological impotence with the DSFI: a failure to replicate. J Sex Marital Ther 7:230–238
26. Slob AK, Blom JHM, van der Werft Ten Bosch JJ (1990) Erection problems in medical practice: differential diagnosis with relatively simple method. J Urol 143:46–50
27. Virag R (1982) Intracavernous injection of papaverine for erectile failure. Letter to the Editor. Lancet 2:938
28. Virag R, Virag H, Lajuie J (1985) A new device for measuring penile rigidity. Urology 25:80–81
29. Wein AJ, Fishkin R, Carpiniello VL, Mallory TR (1981) Expansion without significant rigidity during nocturnal penile tumescence testing: a potential source of misinterpretation. J Urol 126:343–344
30. Wespes E, Delcour C, Rondeux C, Stryven J, Schulman CC (1987) The erectile angle: objective criterion to evaluate the papaverine test in impotence. J Urol 138(5): 1171–1173
31. Zorgniotti AW, Lefleur RS (1985) Auto-injection of the corpus cavernosum with a vasoactive drug combination for vasculogenic impotence. J Urol 133:39–41

Neurophysiological Evaluation of Erectile Dysfunction

W.H. Scherb

Introduction

Diagnosing the neurogenic causes underlying erectile dysfunction represents a special challenge within the framework of a complete multidisciplinary evaluation of impotency. Neurogenic disturbances that result in erectile dysfunction can be caused by lesions in the autonomic nervous system or within somatic nerve fibers. Only indirect evaluation of the autonomic nervous system is clinically possible. Lesions ascribed to the somatic nervous system can be easily measured and recorded using routine diagnostic methods [1–7, 9, 14, 15]. Measurement of the latency times of the bulbocavernous reflex (BCR) and somatosensory evoked potentials (SSEP) after stimulation of the dorsal penile nerve are proven clinical neurological tests, which are performed routinely [7, 16]. Recording of the bulbocavernous reflex after cortical magnetic stimulation [8], sleep polygraphy and late somatosensory evoked potentials (LSSEP) of the dorsal penile nerve are further methods used in the diagnosis of central nervous system disturbances responsible for erectile dysfunction [10].

Neurogenic Causes of Erectile Dysfunction

A complete and uncomplicated approach toward the neurological evaluation or erectile dysfunction has not been defined. Classification according to anatomical or diagnostic criteria is possible, with further division into patients with definite neurological diseases and those diagnosed using only certain neurophysiological tests. The clinical symptoms usually do not allow an unequivocal classification into the anatomical or diagnostic group. The numerous neurogenic causes of erectile dysfunction are easily classified when they are arranged according to their anatomical lesions (Table 1). Anatomical lesions in the mechanism of erection can be located either in the central nervous system or in the peripheral nervous system. Central nervous system lesions can be further subdivided into cerebral, supranuclear, or spinal lesions. The peripheral nervous system lesions are either radicular, nuclear, or neural [11].

U. Jonas et al. (Eds.) Erectile Dysfunction
© Springer-Verlag Berlin Heidelberg 1991

Table 1. Classification of neurogenic causes of erectile dysfunction

Etiology	Localization			Examples
– Space occupying – Vascular – Traumatic/iatrogenic – Systemic disease – Metabolic – Toxic	Central	Cerebral		Stroke Parkinson disease Temporal lobe epilepsy Myotonic dystrophy
		Spinal		Multiple sclerosis Spinal cord transection
	Peripheral	Nuclear		Conus-cauda lesion Meningomyelocele
		Radicular		Polyradiculitis Intervertebral disc prolaps
		Neural		Polyneuropathy Nerve damage

Table 2. Systematic neurophysiological procedures to be used in differential diagnosis of erectile dysfunction in order of increasing complexity and amount of time

5. EEG and Topographic brain mapping (TBM)
  4. Somatosensory evoked potentials (SSEP)
    3. Reflex measurements
      2. Electromyography
        1. Hard objective signs

Neurophysiological Procedures in the Differential Diagnosis of Erectile Dysfunction

The numerous causes of erectile dysfunction make a precise and objective evaluation of the underlying causes imperative. A careful evaluation of patient history concerning erection, ejaculation, and bladder function is important. The presenting symptoms often provide valuable information concerning innervation of the urogenital tract. Differential diagnosis of erectile dysfunction is still quite difficult because it can be the result of autonomic, reflexogenic, or psychogenic disorders. A psychological cause of erectile dysfunction is often diagnosed hastily due to a lack of objective neurogenic causes for the erectile dysfunction.

The development of new neurophysiological diagnostic methods in the differential diagnosis of erectile dysfunction offers the patient noninvasive and reproducible diagnostic evaluations (Table 2). These new diagnostic methods give the physician indications of the location of neurogenic lesions.

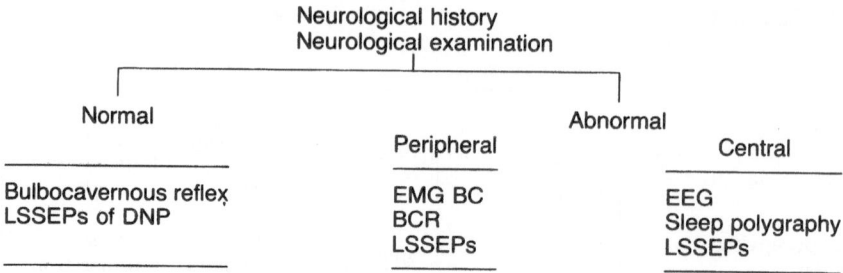

Fig. 1. Differential diagnosis of neurogenic causes of erectile dysfunction. *DNP*, dorsal nerve of penis; *BC*, bulbocavernous muscle

Clinical neurophysiology together with adequate technical expertise and experience can deliver critical information in the differential diagnosis of erectile dysfunction. Figure 1 outlines the type of neurophysiological diagnostic methods that should be employed after the patient's neurological status has been determined.

BCR Latency Measurements

Method

BCR latency is measured with the patient lying in the supine position. Both the dorsal penile nerve and the pudendal nerve are stimulated with a ring electrode placed around the penis. The anode is placed proximal to the corona glandis and the cathode is placed 3 cm proximally from the anode. Square wave impulses with a duration of 0.2 ms are applied in intervals of 40–60 via a direct current (DC) stimulator. The stimulus intensity is two to three times the predetermined invidual stimulus threshold. The average stimulus threshold lies between 5 and 15 mA. Concentric needle electrodes that have been placed in the right and left bulbocavernous muscles are used to record the stimulus response.

The signals are recorded with a sensitivity of 50 mV/cm amplified over a range from 200 Hz to 3 Hz − 3 dB. At least four successive stimulus responses are recorded and evaluated. The latency period for each stimulus response is measured from the beginning of the stimulus to that of the response. The stimulus response is measured with a cursor on the oscilloscope screen (Fig. 2a–c). The following parameters can be determined:

1. The minimum latency of each side
2. The maximum latency of each side
3. The mean latency of each side
4. The distribution of the latencies on each side
5. The minimum difference between both sides
6. The maximum difference between both sides

Somatosensory Evoked Potentials

The same electrode configuration is used for SSEP measurements as described above for the BCR measurements. The stimulus intensity lies between two and three times the predetermined individual stimulus threshold; the stimulus frequency is 3/s. SSEPs are recorded from the scalp using either self-adhesive electrodes or subcutaneous platinum irridium needle electrodes. The active electrode is placed 2 cm dorsal from the C and the reference electrode is placed at the FP. The signals are recorded with a sensitivity of 20 mV/cm amplified over a range from 2 Hz to 3 Hz − 3 dB. The signals are recorded twice electronically and analyzed 200 ms after the stimulus (Fig. 2d).

Differential Diagnosis of Neurogenic Causes of Erectile Dysfunction

Patient history and physical examination are two valuable instruments used in postulating a presumptive diagnosis for the neurogenic cause of erectile dysfunction. Objective neurophysiological diagnostic methods must be used in order to identify the damaged nerve or central nervous system structure. Clinical neurophysiology can help identify and classify the neurogenic causes of erectile dysfunction. Even with a normal patient history and physical examination, a pathological BCR can be the only indication for disturbances in the segmental reflex involving the dorsal penile nerve and pudendal nerve (S2-S4). At the present time it is not known how often a "normal erection" occurs even though a pathological BCR was observed. It is also not known how often a pure autonomic lesion can result in erectile dysfunction even though the BCR latency was normal. Evidence of disturbances occurring in the S2-S4 segments can be substantiated by a pathological electrogram (Fig. 3). Usually, routine measurement of the BCR latency can be achieved by using self-adhesive surface electrodes with or without averaging. Needle electrodes should be used when one of the following is observed or presumed: abnormal patient history, abnormal physical examination, and evidence of peripheral nerve damage. If needle electrodes are used, then a simultaneous EMG of the bulbocavernous muscle can be recorded.

Transcranial Magnetic Stimulation

Transcranial magnetic stimulation (TMS) is a complementary method used to examine the central motor pathways leading to the striated muscles of the urogenital system [8]. We examined 20 control patients and 24 patients with neurogenic causes of erectile dysfunction. The examinations were per-

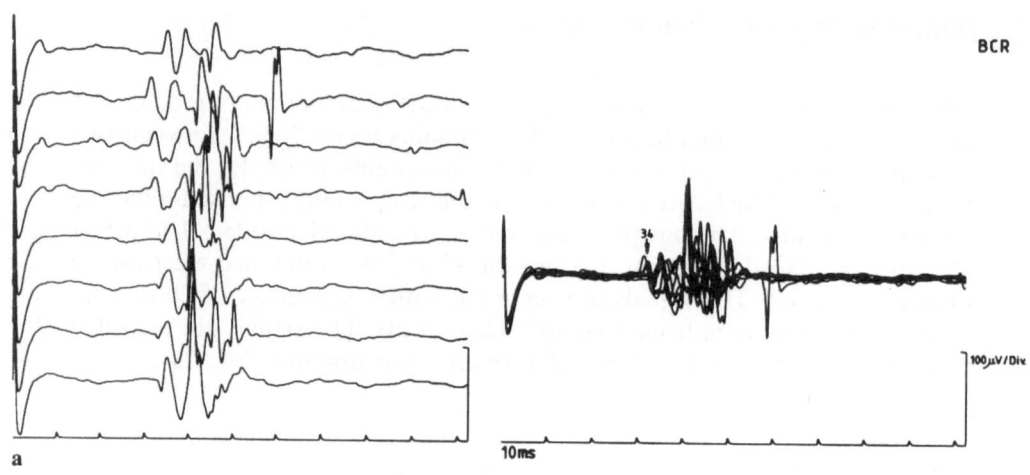

BCR

100 µV/Div

10ms

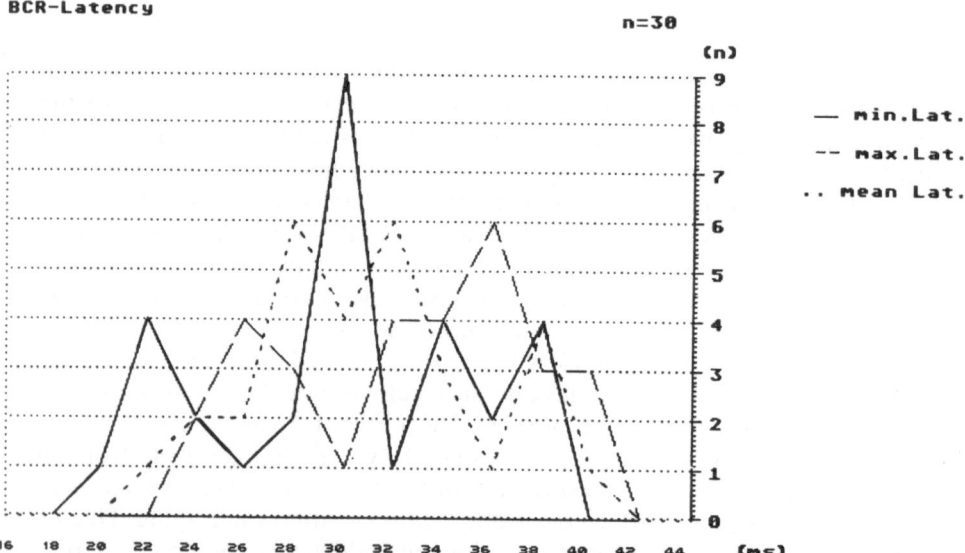

BCR-Latency   n=30

— min.Lat.
-- max.Lat.
.. mean Lat.

b **Fig. 2. a** *Left*, eight consecutive recordings with a needle electrode; control patient. *Right*, The same recordings superimposed upon one another. **b** Statistical distribution of the minimum, maximum, and mean latencies for 30 control patients. Mean min., 30 ms Standard Deviation 5.5 ms; Mean max., 34 ms Standard Deviation 5.1 ms. **c** BCR latency averaged over 32 sweeps; control patient. Latency right (*R*) 30 ms; Latency Left (*L*) 32 ms. **d** Cortical recording over Cz–Fpz of a normal SSEP of the pudendal nerve

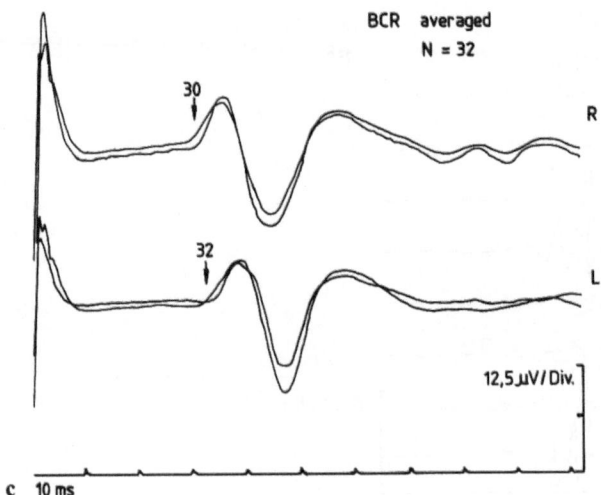

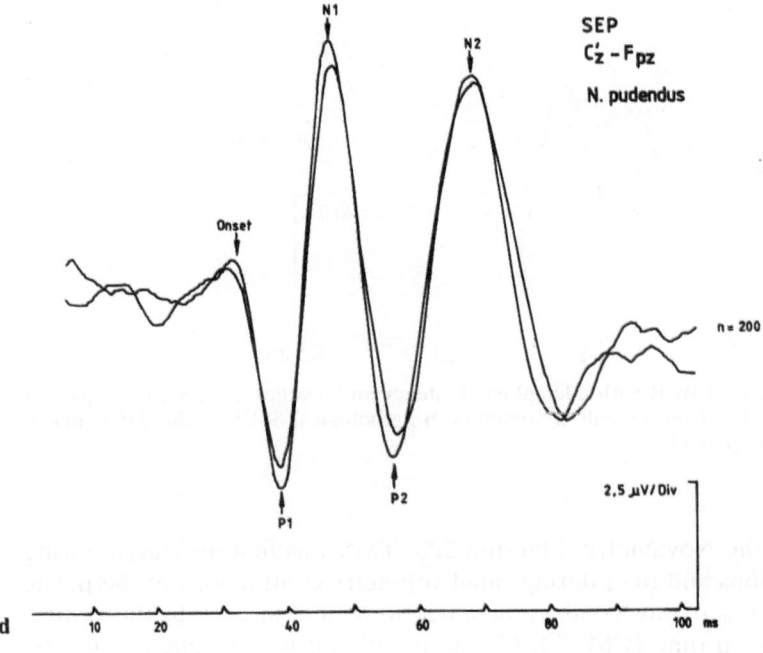

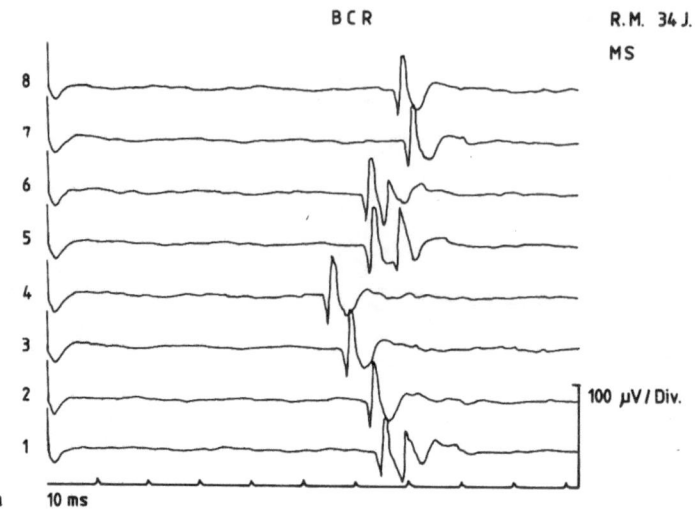

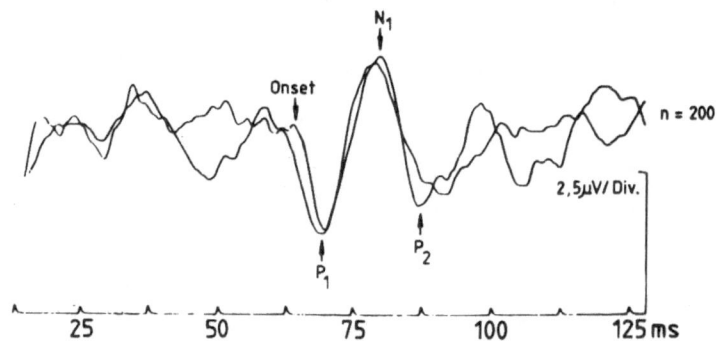

Fig. 3. a Pathological BCR with a lengthened latency and a wider dispersion in a patient with multiple sclerosis and erectile dysfunction. **b** Pathological SSEP of the dorsal penile nerve in the same patient

formed using the Novametrix Magstim 200. TMS was first measured during resting conditions and then during small voluntary contractions of the pelvic muscles. Three separate conduction times were measured: (1) the central motor conduction time (CMCT); (2) the peripheral motor conduction time (PMCT); and (3) the difference between CMCT and PMCT.

Prolonged central motor latencies are found in patients with hemiplegia, multiple sclerosis, and amyotrophic lateral sclerosis. Prolonged peripheral latencies are found in diabetics, alcoholics, and in some patients posttraumatically or postoperatively. Pathological central sensory latencies as well as combinations of prolonged CMCTs and SSEPs were observed in patients suffering from alcoholism, diabetus mellitus, and multiple sclerosis.

Table 3. Typical sacral root latency testing, evoked potentials and transcranial magnetic stimulation in a control patient

	Mean (ms)	SD
A. Sacral Root Latency Testing		
Bulbocavernous Reflex (BCRL)	31.5	4.1
Anal Reflex (ARL)	35.4	4.5
B. Evoked Potentials		
SSEP of DNP		
Cortical:	39.8	1.7
T12:	26.7	1.6
Difference (cortical minus T12)	13.1	1.4
C. Transcranial Magnetic Stimulation		
Central Motor Conduction Time		
(CMCT)		
at rest:	28.4	2.8
contraction:	21.2	2.3
Peripheral Motor Conduction Time		
(PMCT)		
at rest:	22.1	1.7
contraction:	12.2	2.1
Difference (CMCT minus PMCT)		
at rest:	6.3	1.0
contraction:	9.0	1.1

TMS resulted in better objective examination in the section of the pyramidal tract that innervates the pelvis and also allowed for more precise localization within the tract (Table 3). Voluntary contractions lead to fasciculations which result in shortened latencies due to summation effects. TMS is painless and no side effects have been observed.

Summary

Clinical neurophysiological examinations such as BCR latency and the simultaneous recording of SSEPs of the dorsal penile nerve are standardised and reliable examinations. These diagnostic examinations are used in the evaluation of the pathways responsible for somatic penile innervation. TMS is an important supplement in the evaluation of the long motor pathways. Without the knowledge of these pathways no therapeutic measures should be undertaken. Sleep polygraphy and LSSEPs of the dorsal penile nerve are further examinations that are so far complicated and very time consuming. These two examinations yield additional information to simplify the differential diagnosis of central nervous system disturbances responsible for erectile dysfunction.

Acknowledgement. I thank Mrs. S. Rief and Mrs. E. Schenk for technical assistance, and F. Schaebsdau, MD, for translating the manuscript.

References

1. Bradley WE, Lin JTY, Johnson B (1984) Measurement of the conduction velocity of the dorsal nerve of the penis. J Urol 131:1127–1129
2. Chantraine A, Leval J de, Okelinx A (1973) Motor conduction velocity in the internal pudendal nerves. In: Desmedt JE (ed) New developments in electromyographiy and clinical neurophysiology, vol 2. Karger, Basel, pp 433–438
3. Dick HC, Bradley WE, Scott FB, Timm GW (1974) Pudendal sexual reflexes. Urology 3:376–379
4. Ertekin C, Reel F (1976) Bulbocavernosus reflex in normal men and in patients with neurogenic bladder and/or impotence. J Neurol Sci 28:1–15
5. Haldemann S, Bradley WE, Bhatia NN, Johnson BK (1982) Pudendal evoked responses. Arch Neurol 39:280–283
6. Krane, RJ, Siroky MB (1980) Studies on sacral evoked potentials. J Urol 124:872–876
7. Opsomer RJ, Guerit JM, Wese FX, van Cough PJ (1986) Pudendal cortical somatosensory evoked potentials. J Urol 135:1216–1218
8. Opsomer RJ Pesce F, van Caugh PJ, Rossini PM (1988) Motor evoked potentials: A new method to study the motor pathways to the striated muscles of the genital tract. Proceedings: Third Biennial World Meeting on Impotence, 24
9. Rushworth G (1967) Diagnostic value of the electromyographic study of reflex activity in man. Electroencephalogr Clin Neurophysiol 25:65–73
10. Scherb WH (1988) Neurophysiologische Verfahren bei der Diagnostik der erektilen Dysfunktion. In: Bähren W, Altwein JE (Hrsg) Impotenz. Thieme, Stuttgart New York, S 50–62
11. Scherb WH (1988) Aspekte neurogener Ursachen der erektilen Dysfunktion. In: Bähren W, Altwein JE (Hrsg) Impotenz. Thieme, Stuttgart New York, S 124–132
12. Scherb WH, Bähren W, Gall H Thon WF (1988) Neurophysiologic parameters in evaluation of erectile dysfunction. Acta Urol Belg 56:154–161
13. Scherb WH, Bähren W, Gall H, Stief CG, Thon WF (1988) Differentialdiagnose und Behandlung somatischer und funktioneller Formen der diabetischen erektilen Impotenz. In: Strian W, Hölzl R, Haselbeck M (Hrsg) Verhaltensmedizin und Diabetes mellitus. Springer, Berlin Heidelberg New York Tokyo, S 414–428
14. Siroky MB, Sax DS, Krane RS (1979) Sacral signal tracing: the electrophysiology of the bulbocavernosus reflex. J Urol 122:661–664
15. Tackmann W, Vogel P, Probst H (1987) Somatosensory evoked potentials after stimulation of the dorsal penile nerve: Normative data and results from 145 patients with erectile dysfunction. Eur Neurol 27:245–250
16. Tackmann W, Porst H, van Ahlen H (1988) Bulbocavernosus reflex latencies and somatosensory evoked potentials after pudendal nerve stimulation in the diagnosis of impotence. J Neurol 235:219–225

Testing the Autonomic System

J.H. Abicht

The diagnosis of autonomic neuropathy, which is considered an important cause of organic impotence [18, 46], is difficult. Symptoms of autonomic failure are not specific [37, 41, 50, 53], do not always correlate with impotence [38], and methods for the direct measurement and assessment of autonomic function in human subjects are not presently available.

Neurogenic erectile dysfunction reveals disorders of the somatic and/or autonomic parts of the sacral peripheral nervous system (PNS) [29, 35], but can also show affections of other parts in the PNS [9, 15, 44].

Apart from indirect testing of autonomic function, which is commonly evaluated by employing responses of an entire reflex arch of the autonomic nervous system (ANS), a direct recording of impulses conducted by the autonomic nerve fibers is only possible using microneurography. This method is suitable for testing the sympathetic part of the ANS in the vascular system [19, 52].

For detecting autonomic failure in patients with impotence, the assessment of ANS function has to include investigations of the genitourinary and other systems because of the evidential association of organic impotence with neurogenic bladder dysfunction [29], diminished testicular pain [7], decreased conduction velocity in the dorsal nerve of the penis [24, 45], prolongation of bulbocavernous reflex latency time [39, 44, 47], abnormal myographical pattern of the penile smooth muscle [49], abnormal warm and cool perception thresholds [21], and pathological cardiovascular (CV) responses of the ANS [42].

Several tests have been proposed for testing the integrity of sympathetic and parasympathetic nerves in humans, many of them stressing or tedious procedures (e.g., invasive testing of CV function, gastrointestinal motility and urinary bladder function, biochemical, physiological and pharmacological methods, testing skin vasomotor reflexes, plasma norepinephrine response to standing, measuring pupillary reaction, and pancreatic polypeptide response to hypoglycemia or a meal [3, 34]). For diagnosing autonomic neuropathy, it is necessary to use tests which are noninvasive, easy to perform, quantitative, sensitive, reliable, reproducible, based on adequate studies of normality, and which are able to distinguish between sympathetic and parasympathetic systems [10, 13, 17, 23].

The CV reflex tests, which fulfill these criteria, are as follows:

U. Jonas et al. (Eds.) Erectile Dysfunction
© Springer-Verlag Berlin Heidelberg 1991

1. Test of heart rate control (mainly parasympathetic)
   a) Heart rate variation (HRV) during quiet breathing
   b) HRV during deep breathing
   c) HRV in response to standing up
2. Test of blood pressure control (mainly sympathetic)
   a) Blood pressure response to standing up

   In healthy humans, heart rate changes constantly and is obviously influenced by breathing – a physiologic phenomenon called respiratory arrhythmia. In autonomic failure in man, the baroreceptors, as feedback transducers in cybernetic terms, do not produce the required responses in the effectors, e.g., the resistance and capacity vessels (mediated by sympathetic efferent constrictor fibers) and the heart (mediated by sympathetic and parasympathetic efferent fibers) [3].

   The proposed battery of CV tests can be performed easily with minimal equipment (ECG machine and an aneroid pressure gauge) within 15–20 min. Nowadays, measurement of the RR intervals (intervals between R waves in QRS waveform), calculation of the various ratios and grouping of the results can be done automatically with the help of a number of computer programs. Since autonomic function deteriorates with ageing, it is necessary to compare any defects in patients with results in control subjects of comparable age [4, 40].

   As the heart rate and blood pressure response can be affected and influenced by many external factors, all ANS tests should be performed under standardized conditions [5, 23], which are as follows:

- In the morning
- In a quiet relaxed atmosphere
- After the patient has become familiar with the procedure
- After 15 min of supine rest
- In patients who have avoided prescription and/or over-the-counter medicines for at least 8 h
- In patients who have not experienced vigorous exercise or severe emotional upset in the last 24 h
- In patients who have not experienced acute illness in the last 48 h
- Patients should not smoke or drink alcohol for at least 12 h before the test

Description of Four ANS Function Tests and Their Normal/Abnormal Values

HRV During Quiet Breathing

The patient lies quietly on a couch, has his eyes closed, and the ECG is recorded for 1 min. The HRV, expressed as the variation coefficient of the mean RR deviation, is calculated. Values less than 1.88 in the elderly (41–60 years old) and 2.52 in the young adult (18–40 years old) are considered pathological.

HRV During Deep Breathing

The patient is in a sitting position and breathes deeply at a rate of six breaths/min. The maximal average difference of minimal heart rate of inspiration and maximal heart rate of expiration during three successive breathing cycles is calculated. Values should be higher than 15 beats/min in the young adult and 9 beats/min in the elderly.

HRV in Response to Standing Up

After a period of 10 min lying quietly, the patient stands up as quickly as possible. After a phase of tachycardia a following phase of bradycardia can be observed. The ratio of the longest RR interval of the bradycardiac phase (normally around the 30th beat after standing up) and the shortest RR interval of the tachycardiac phase (normally around the 15 beat) should be greater than 1.11.

Blood Pressure Response to Standing Up

Systolic blood pressure is measured before and immediately after the orthostatic maneuver, described above. The postural systolic blood pressure fall should be less than 13 mm Hg.

Abnormality in one of the four tests should be recognized as a strong indicator of underlying autonomic neuropathy (AN); two or more abnormal tests establish the diagnosis of AN [1, 4, 17].

As we know from previous investigation of the ANS, erectile dysfunction/impotence, especially in diabetic patients, may be the earliest symptom of unmyelinated fiber neuropathy. The so-called small fiber neuropathy [51] is recognized by selective fiber damage affecting both autonomic innervation and unmyelinated and small myelinated fibers of the somatic nervous system [13, 22, 26, 27].

The detection of abnormal cold and warm perception thresholds can help to reveal small fiber neuropathy of the PNS. Several methods of testing thermal thresholds are available [6, 11, 28, 56]. We prefer the method developed by Fowler et al. [22] which showed a strong correlation between loss of warm perception and erectile dysfunction in diabetics. This supported the suggestion of Ewing et al. [16] that erectile dysfunction in diabetics may be the earliest symptom of unmyelinated fiber neuropathy.

Measurement of Cutaneous Thermal Thresholds

Cold and warm stimuli are applied through a Peltier thermode metallic element, which is kept in constant contact with the skin of the patient's hands and feet. The metallic element is connected to a thermode-controlling box, which is directed by a microcomputer using a special software program. Following a bleep from the computer, which the patient is asked to acknowledge or not (forced choice method), an ordered series of abrupt temperature changes are made. As the cold and warm stimuli are of gradually diminishing intensity, a level of perception is established and a threshold is calculated. The patient's reliability is assessed by his response to catch trials (no temperature change following the bleep), which are produced at random intervals during the test procedure. The warm threshold, in normal subjects without neuropathy, should be smaller than 1.4°C, the cool threshold 0.9°C [4]. Measuring a threshold for both warming and cooling takes between 20 and 30 min.

Concluding Remarks

The described and recommended battery of four tests for quantitative indirect measurement of autonomic reflexes can be used to detect autonomic failure and to monitor improvement or deterioration of autonomic nerve function in impotent patients, with and without therapy [8, 20].

In conclusion, the results of studies applying these tests suggest that parasympathetic and sympathetic damage due to autonomic failure is another major pathogenic factor of impotence, especially in patients with diabetes mellitus [36]. However, by testing only the CV reflexes and the somatic small fibers, normal results do not exclude autonomic failure in the sacral PNS, even if the patient has no specific sacral complaint and no clinical or neurophysiological evidence of sacral neuropathy [2].

These discrepancies occur due to the lack of neurophysiological techniques available to detect minor or subclinical structural and functional deficits of peripheral nerve function [15]. Nerve biopsy analysis (e.g., of the sural nerve) may help to reveal important underlying abnormalities in peripheral neuropathy such as axonal swelling, atrophy or demyelination [12], but this technique has limited application [48].

Furthermore, there is evidence that early nerve lesions, especially in autonomic fibers, are additionally characterized by neurotransmitter and neuropeptide depletion. A reliable histological method is required for detecting these deficits, especially in endorgans like corpus cavernosum penis (CCP), urinary bladder and skin. In some recent studies, depletion of neurotransmitters and neuropeptides (e.g., acetylcholine, vasoactive intestinal polypeptide, substance P, neuropeptide Y, calcitonin gene-related peptide, endothelium-derived relaxing factor) and other general neuronal markers (e.g., enolase, neurofilament triplet proteins and S-100) was detected by immunohistochemical techniques in CCP, urinary bladder and also skin biopsies of e.g., diabetic patients both with and without clinical or neurophysiological evidence of peripheral neuropathy [25, 31, 32, 33, 43]. Further studies using these methods are needed to find out whether these abnormalities in patients with impotence antedate clinical and neurophysiological abnormalities, correlate with symptoms and clinical findings, and whether this technique is a valuable tool for detection of peptidergic nerve fiber response to treatment.

References

1. Abicht J, Bautsch BW, Mitzkat HJ (1988) Untersuchungen zur Beurteilung von Validität und Empfindlichkeit verschiedener Funktionstests des autonomen Nervensystemes bei Typ-I- und Typ-II-Diabetikern. Akt Endokrin Stoffw 9:124
2. Alloussi S, Mast GJ, Kopper B, Ziegler M (1985) Harnblasenentleerungsstörung als Folge einer sakralen autonomen diabetischen Neuropathie. Urologe (A) 24:291–295
3. Bannister R, Mathias C (1988) Testing autonomic reflexes. In: Bannister R (ed) Autonomic failure. A textbook of clinical disorders of the autonomic nervous system, 2nd edn. Oxford University Press, New York, pp 289–308
4. Bautsch BW (1990) Untersuchungen zur Diagnostik der diabetischen autonomen Neuropathie. Standardisierung und Beurteilung der Aussagekraft von sechs kardiovaskulären Tests und eines Verfahrens zur Prüfung der Temperatursensibilität. Thesis, Medical School Hannover
5. Bennett T, Gardiner SM (1988) Cardiovascular pathophysiology in diabetes mellitus. In: Bannister R (ed) Autonomic failure. A textbook of clinical disorders of the autonomic nervous system, 2nd edn. Oxford University Press, New York, pp 654–666
6. Bertelsmann FW, Heimaans JJ, Weber EJM, van der Veen EA, Schouten JA (1985). Thermal discrimination thresholds in normal subjects and in patients with diabetic neuropathy. J Neurol Neurosurg Psychiatry 48:686–690
7. Campbell IW, Ewing DJ, Clarke BF, Duncan LJP (1974) Testicular pain sensation in diabetic autonomic neuropathy. Br Med J 2:638–639
8. Cicmir I, Kashiwagi S, Berger H, Koschinski T, Gries FA (1983) Improvement of autonomic nerve function after one year of continuous subcutaneous insulin infusion. Diabetologia 25:147
9. Clarke BF, Ewing DJ, Campbell IW (1979) Diabetic autonomic neuropathy. Diabetologia 17:195–212
10. Consensus Statement (1988) Report and Recommendations of the San Antonio Conference on Diabetic Neuropathy. Diabetes Care 9:592–597
11. Dyck PJ, Zimmerman IR, O'Brian PC, Ness A, Caskey PE, Karnes J, Buskek WC (1978) Automated systems to evaluate touch-pressure vibration anf thermal cutaneous sensation in man. Ann Neurol 4:502–510
12. Dyck PJ, Karnes J, Lais A, Lofgren EP, Stevens JC (1984) Pathological alterations of the peripheral nervous systems of humans. In: Dyck PJ, Thomas PK, Lambert EH, Runge R (eds) Peripheral neuropathy, 2nd edn. Saunders, Philadelphia, pp 760–870
13. Dyck PJ, Karnes J, O'Brien PC (1987) Diagnosis, staging and classification of diabetic neuropathy and association with other complications. In: Dyck PJ, Asbury AK, Winegrad AI, Porte E jr (eds) Diabetic neuropathy. Saunders, Philadelphia, pp 36–44
14. Dyck PJ, Buskek W, Spring E, Karnes J, Litchy WJ, O'Brian PC, Service FJ (1987)

Vibratory and cooling detection thresolds compared with other tests in diagnosing and staging diabetic neuropathy. Diabetes Care 10:432-440

15. Ewing DJ, Clarke BF (1986) Diabetic autonomic neuropathy: Present insights and future prospects. Diabetes Care 9:648-665
16. Ewing DJ, Campbell IW, Clarke BF (1980) The natural history of diabetic autonomic neuropathy. Q J Med, 193:95-108
17. Ewing DJ, Martyn CN, Young RJ, Clarke BF (1985) The value of cardiovascular autonomic function tests: 10 years experience in diabetes. Diabetes Care 8:491-498
18. Faerman I, Glocer L, Fox D, Jadinsky MN, Rapaport M (1974) Impotence and diabetes. Histological studies of the autonomic vervous fibres of the corpora cavernosa in impotent diabetic males. Diabetes 23:971-976
19. Fagius J (1985) Autonomic neurophysiology in long-term diabetes. J Clin Physiol (Suppl 5) 5:74-78
20. Fedele D, Negrin P, Cardone, C (1984) Influence of continuous subcutaneous insulin infusion (CSII) treatment on diabetic somatic and autonomic neuropathy. J Endocrinol Invest 7:623-628
21. Fowler CJ, Carroll MB, Burns D, Howe N, Robinson K (1987) A portable system for measuring cutaneous thresholds for warming and cooling. J Neurol Neurosurg Psychiatry 50:1211-1215
22. Fowler CJ, Ali Z, Kirby RS, Pryor JP (1988) The value of testing for unmyelinated fibre sensory neuropathy in diabetic impotence. Br J Urol 61:63-67
23. Genovely H, Pfeifer MA (1988) RR-variation: The autonomic test of choice in diabetes. Diabet Metab Rev 4:255-271
24. Gerstenberg TC, Bradley, WE (1983) Nerve conduction velocity measurement of dorsal nerve of penis in normal and impotent males. Urology 22:90-92
25. Gu J, Polak JM, Lazarides M et al (1984) Decrease of vasoactive intestinal polypeptide (VIP) in the penises from impotent men. Lancet 2:315-318
26. Guy RJC, Watkins PJ (1985) The relationship of autonomic and peripheral neuropathy in diabetes mellitus. J Auton Nerv Syst 14:103
27. Guy RJC, Clark CA, Malcolm PN, Watkins PJ (1985) Evaluation of thermal and vibration sensation in diabetic neuropathy. Diabetologia 28:131-137
28. Jamal GA, Hansen S, Weir AI, Ballantyne JB (1986) An improved automated method for the measurement of thermal thresholds. J Neurol Neurosurg Psychiatry 48:354-360
29. Kirby RS, Fowler CJ (1988) Bladder and sexual dysfunction in diseases affecting the autonomic nervous system. In: Bannister R (ed) Autonomic failure. A textbook of clinical disorders of the autonomic nervous system, 2nd edn. Oxford University Press, New York, pp 413-431
30. Lehmann WP, Haslbeck M, Müller J, Melmert H, Strian F (1985) Frühdiagnose der autonomen Diabetes-Neuropathie mit Hilfe der Temperatursensibilität. Dtsch Med Wochenschr 110:639-642
31. Levy DM, Karanth SS, Springall DR, Polak JM (1989) Depletion of cutaneous nerves and neuropeptides in diabetes mellitus: an immunocytochemical study. Diabetologia 32:427-433
32. Lincoln J, Crowe R, Blackley PF, Pryor JP, Lumley JS, Burnstock G (1987) Changes in vipergic, cholinergic and adrenergic innervation of human penile tissue in diabetic and non-diabetic males. J Urol 137:1053-1059
33. Lindberger M, Schröder HD, Schultzberg M, Kristensson K, Persson A, Östmann J, Link H (1989) Nerve fibre studies in skin biopsies in peripheral neuropathies. I. Immunohistochemical analysis of neuropeptides in diabetes mellitus. J Neurol Sci 93:289-296
34. Low PA (1984) Quantitation of autonomic responses. In: Dyck PJ, Thomas PK, Lambert EH, Bunge R (eds) Peripheral neuropathy, 2nd edn, vol 1. Saunders, Philadelphia, pp 1139-1165
35. Lue TF, Zeineh SJ, Schmidt RA et al. (1984) Neuroanatomy of penile erection: Its relevance to iatrogenic impotence. J Urol 131:273-280

36. McCulloch DK, Young RJ, Prescott RJ, Campbell IW, Clarke BJ (1984) The natural history of impotence in diabetic men. Diabetologia 26:437–440
37. McLeod JG (1988) Autonomic dysfunction in peripheral nerve disease. In: Bannister R (ed) Autonomic failure. A textbook of clinical disorders of the autonomic nervous system, 2nd edn. Oxford University Press, New York, pp 607–624
38. Palmer JDK, Fink S, Burger RH (1986) Diabetic secondary impotence: neuropathic factor as measured by peripheral motor nerve conduction. Urology 28:197–200
39. Parys BT, Evans CM, Parsons KF (1988) Bulbuscavernosus reflex latency in the investigation of diabetic impotence. Br J Urol 61:59–62
40. Pfeifer MA, Halter JB, Weinberg CR, Cook D, Best L, Reenan A, Porte D Jr (1983) Differential changes of autonomic nervous system function with age in man. Am J Med 75:249–258
41. Pozza G, Comi G, Librenti MC, Canal N (1987) Clinical aspects and treatment of diabetic peripheral and autonomic neuropathy. Front Diabetes 8:160–176
42. Quadri R, Veglio M, Flecchia D, Tonda L, Lorenzo F de, Chiandussi L, Fonzo D (1989) Autonomic neuropathy and sexual impotence in diabetic patients: Analysis of cardiovascular reflexes. Andrologia 21:346–352
43. Saenz de Tejada I, Goldstein I, Azadzoi K, Krane RJ, Cohen RA (1989) Impaired neurogenic and endothelium-mediated relaxation of penile smooth muscle from diabetic men with impotence. N Engl J Med 320:1025–1030
44. Sarica Y, Karacan I (1987) Bulbuscavernosus reflex to somatic and visceral nerve stimulation in normal subjects and in diabetics with erectile impotence. J Urol 138: 55–58
45. Scherb WH, Bähren W, Stief CG, Gallwitz A, Thon W, Kriebel J (1987) Neurophysiological evaluation of patients with neurogenic erectile dysfunction. Clin Neurol Neurosurg (Suppl 1) 89:88
46. Sharlip ID (1984) Clinical andrology. In: Smith DR (ed) General urology, 11th edn. Lange Medical Publications, Los Altos, CA, pp 622–626
47. Siroky MB, Sax DS, Krane RJ (1979) Sacral signal tracing: The electrophysiology of the bulbuscavernosus reflex. J Urol 122:661–664
48. Solders G (1988) Discomfort after fascicular nerve biopsy. Acta Neurol Scand 77: 503–504
49. Stief CG (1991) Diagnosis of autonomic impotence (SPACE). In: Jonas U, Thon WF, Stief CG (eds) Erectile dysfunction. Springer, Berlin Heidelberg New York Tokyo
50. Sundkvist G (1981) Autonomic nervous dysfunction in asymptomatic diabetic patient with signs of peripheral neuropathy. Diabetes Care 4:529–534
51. Thomas PK, Brown MJ (1987) Diabetic polyneuropathy. In: Dyck PJ, Thomas PK, Asbury AK, Winegrad AI, Porte D Jr (eds) Diabetic neuropathy. Saunders, Philadelphia, pp 56–65
52. Wallin BG (1988) Intraneural recordings of normal and abnormal sympathetic activity in man. In: Bannister R (ed) Autonomic failure. A textbook of clinical disorders of the autonomic nervous system, 2nd edn. Oxford University Press, New York, pp 177–196
53. Wieling W, Borst C, Lieshout, JJ van. Sprangers RLH, Karemaker JM, Brederode JFM van, Montfrans GA, Dunning AJ (1985) Assessment of methods of estimate impairment of vagal and sympathetic cardiovascular innervation of the heart in diabetic autonomic neuropathy. Neth J Med 28:383–392
54. Wrabek AJ (1985) Bulbuscavernosus reflex testing in 100 consecutive cases of erectile dysfunction. Urology 25:495–498
55. Young RJ, MacIntyre CA, Martyn CN et al (1986) Progression of subclinical polyneuropathy in young patients with type I (insulin-dependent) diabetes: associated with glycaemic control and microangiopathy (microvascular complications). Diabetologia 29:156–161
56. Ziegler D, Mayer P, Gries F (1988) Evaluation of thermal, pain and vibration sensation thresholds in newly diagnosed type I diabetic patients. J Neurol Neurosurg Psychiatry 51:1420–1424

Single Potential Analysis of Cavernous Electrical Activity: A Possible Diagnosis of Autonomic Cavernous Dysfunction and Cavernous Smooth Muscle Degeneration*

C.G. Stief

Introduction

The diagnosis of vasculogenic erectile dysfunction has been substantially refined by the introduction of the intracavernous injection of vasoactive drugs. Penile arterial inflow can be assessed rather precisely by pulsed Doppler sonography [6] and cavernous venous outflow by pharmacocavernosometry and pharmacocavernosography [7]. Standardized intracavernous injection of vasoactive drugs [10] allows a good overall evaluation of penile vascular status and of cavernous smooth muscle function.

To elucidate the status of cavernous autonomic innervation, somatosensory penile innervation was examined because of the lack of tests available for the autonomic nervous system itself. Measurement of the latency of the bulbocavernous reflex (BCRL) was the preferred test [4, 9], but recent publications cast some doubts on the relevance of this procedure for autonomic neuropathy [5].

Thomas Gerstenberg and Gorm Wagner were the first to approach this major drawback in the diagnosis of erectile dysfunction when they suggested the registration of cavernous smooth muscle activity [11]. Cavernous electrical activity was recorded during flaccidity and during visual sexual stimulation [2, 11, 12]. If the frequency of cavernous electrical activity did not reach the electrical zero line, autonomic cavernous dysfunction ("dyscoordination") was assumed. To describe the registration of cavernous electrical activity, we use a different method of data processing from that published by Gerstenberg and Wagner. Our method allows a minimally invasive, reproducible, and refined diagnosis of autonomic cavernous neuropathy and, presumably, of cavernous smooth muscle degeneration.

Patients and Methods

Since the introduction of single potential analysis of cavernous electrical activity (SPACE) into our routine diagnostic work-up, 154 consecutive patients with erectile dysfunction were evaluated multidisciplinarily in our impotence

*This work was supported by a grant of the Deutsche Forschungsgemeinschaft (Sti 96/2–1)

clinic. In all patients, minimum duration of impotence was 1 year. Our standard work-up consisted of clinical history, physical examination, sexual history and psychometry, laboratory blood tests including testosterone and prolactin, Doppler sonography of the penile arteries [3], standardized pharmacotesting [10], neurophysiological examination including BCRL, somatosensory evoked potential testing (SSEP) [9], and SPACE. When indicated [10], pharmacocavernosometry and pharmacocavernosography or phallarteriography were performed. Furthermore, 37 patients from our urological ward (e.g., with varicocele) with normal erectile function underwent SPACE. Another 61 patients with erectile dysfunction were referred from other departments or centers especially for SPACE evaluation.

Of these patients, 27 had insulin-dependent diabetes (14 of them for more than 20 years), 11 had primary erectile dysfunction, seven chronic renal failure and one multiple sclerosis. Three patients had cystoprostatectomy, four radical prostatectomy, three abdominoperineal extirpation of the rectum and six a complete traumatic lesion of the spinal cord above T11. Two patients had posttraumatic impotence, eight underwent spinal cord surgery for prolapse and two hemipelvectomy. Three had undergone anterior extirpation of the rectum, two had a neurologically proven polyneuropathy, one a severe hypothyroidism and one a cauda equina syndrome after meningoencephalitis.

The patients were extensively informed about the procedure and possible risks and gave written consent. Both the procedure and indications for its application were approved by the university ethical committee.

A coaxial needle electrode (Dantec 9013 L) was inserted laterally into the cavernous body. The electrode was pushed forward into the proximal cavernous body until the tip of the electrode was located in the center of the cavernous body. The potentials were processed by different electrophysiological units (Wiest Space; Dantec Neuromatic 2000, Tektronix AM 502, HSE electrophysiological preamplifiers). The signals were displayed continuously on a monitor screen (Dantec 2000 and Tektronix) and simultaneously recorded (Wiest Space; Dantec 21 F 02 Rec; after modifications with the intrinsic recorder of the Neuromatic Graphtec thermowriter); paper speed was 5 mm/s. The cut off frequencies were 2–2000 Hz for the first 71 patients, then set at 0.5–500 Hz. The upper cut off frequency of the Neuromatic thermowriter was 10 Hz. Amplification was mostly at 50 μV/unit.

For an exact description of the potentials, they were analyzed for (1) first depolarization (plus or minus), (2) amplitude, (3) length, (4) polyphasity (crossing the baseline).

Examination. Because all patients with normal erectile function showed abnormal potentials up to 15 min after introduction of the needle electrode, SPACE evaluation was started 20 min after needle electrode introduction. After 25 min registration of cavernous electric activity during flaccidity, audiovisual sexual stimulation (AVSS) was used for another 25 min with the examiner leaving the room. At the end of AVSS, the examiner evaluated the erectile response by inspection, palpation, and questioning. Then recording was continued for another 10 min. Usually, the needle electrode was inserted into the left cavernous body. To evaluate if the cavernous electric activity in patients with normal erectile function is synchronous in different areas of the penis (and, therefore, cavernous electric activity represents autonomic innervation), two needles were inserted into each cavernous body in more than 50 patients.

Definitions. As in classical electromyography, *negative* depolarizations were defined to be in the up direction, *positive* depolarizations to be in the down direction in relation to the baseline. *Spikes* are extremely short-lasting depolarizations. *Bursts* are groups of spikes (Fig. 1). Due to the instrument delay of the Dantec recorder, spikes and bursts could only be documented at a paper speed of 0.5 cm/s or more. *Whips* are potentials with a very fast first phase of depolarization and a slower concave shaped repolarization phase (Fig. 2).

Results

The electrical activity of the cavernous smooth muscles could not be registered in one impotent patient and two patients with normal erectile function.

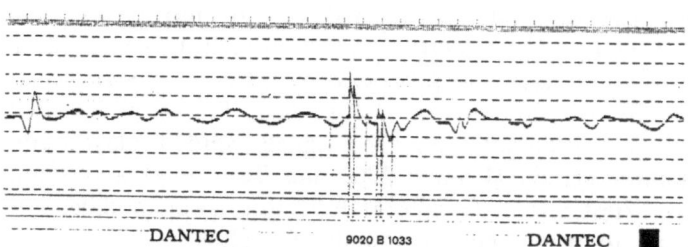

Fig. 1. Bursts in a 33-year-old patient with complete spinal cord injury at the level of T9. 1 horizontal unit corresponds to 1 s, 1 vertical unit to 50 µV

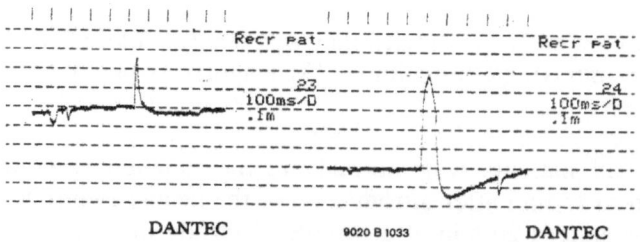

Fig. 2. Whips were the most frequent abnormal findings in patients with defined neurological lesions. 1 horizontal unit corresponds to 1 s, 1 vertical unit to 100 µV

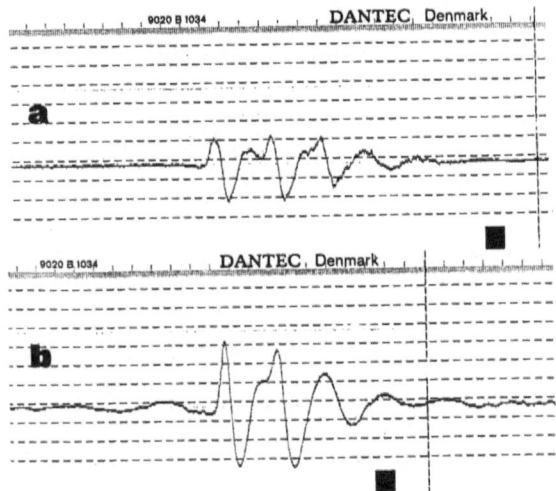

Fig. 3a,b. The Effect of changing the cut off frequencies from 2 to 2000 Hz (**a**) and from to 0.5 to 500 Hz (**b**) 1 horizontal unit corresponds to 1 s, 1 vertical unit to 50 μV

When we changed the lower cut off frequency to 0.5 Hz in the second normal patient (overall number of patients 71), potentials were easily recorded. Starting with this patient, we therefore chose 0.5 Hz as the lower cut off frequency. Lowering of the cut off frequency from 2 to 0.5 Hz resulted in an increase in amplitude of about 150% (Fig. 3). In many patients, low frequency depolarizations at the end of the potentials could be seen at 0.5 Hz that were not visible at 2 Hz. In these patients, potential length and polyphasity were consecutively changed, too.

In 34 of 36 *normal* patients with recorded activity, the potentials were similar. The potentials started with a positive depolarization or with a short-lasting negative, followed by a positive depolarization. At cut off frequencies of 2–2000 Hz, the length of the potentials was 3–12 s (mean 9.5 s; SD 0.3), the amplitude was 60–250 μV (mean 153 μV; SD 31), polyphasity was 5–11 (mean 8.5; SD 0.3). At cut off frequencies of 0.5–500 Hz, the length was 8–18 s (mean 12.8 s, SD 2.8), the amplitude 250–750 μV (mean 444 μV; SD 109) and the polyphasity 8–22 (mean 13.8; SD 3.3). The shape of the potentials was very uniform for the same individual (Fig. 4), although the frequency varied considerably, depending on the degree of relaxation of the patient. Spikes were seen at a frequency of about 0.4/min; both positive and negative spikes were recorded. The mean amplitude was 70 μV. There were many patients without any spikes in the recording. We did not record bursts or whips in this group. Simultaneous recording of cavernous electrical activity in both cavernous bodies showed synchronization of the potentials (Fig. 5).

To evaluate a possible influence of stress on the cavernous electrical activity, SPACE was done about 1 h before surgery in two normal patients. In both patients, wavelike electrical activity with no specific potentials was recorded (Fig. 6).

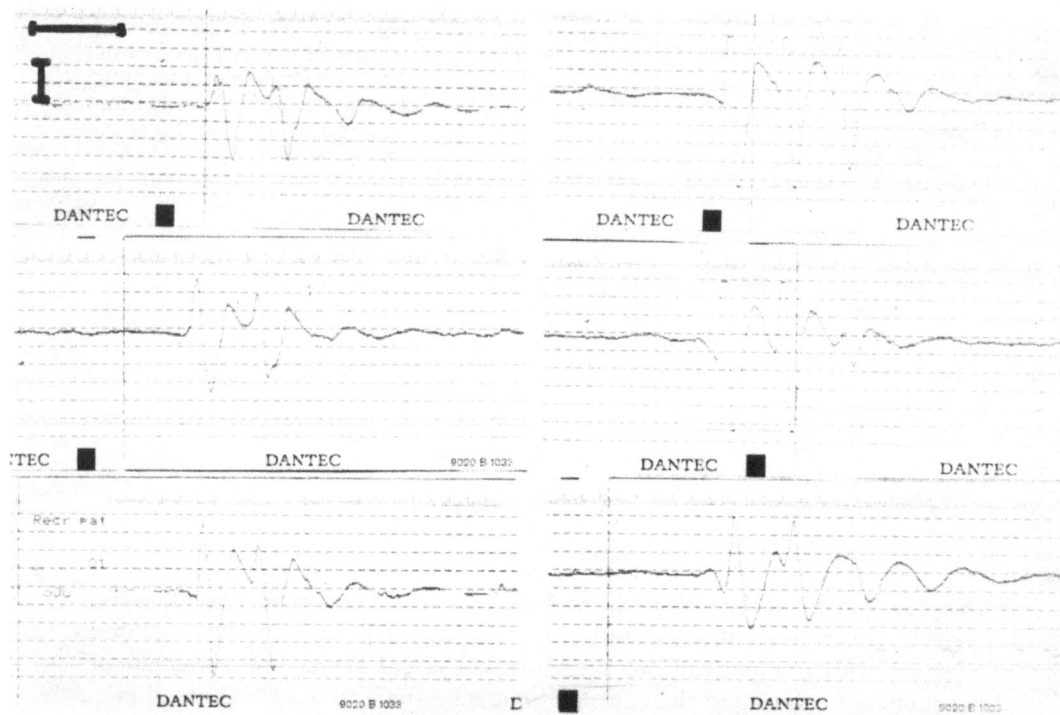

Fig. 4. Potentials recorded in a normal patient were similar to each other

All normal patients consented to AVSS. In all, 23 of 37 patients had a full or almost full erection during AVSS, 14 of 37 had only (partial) tumescence. Comparing the potentials during flaccidity and tumescence or erection, a uniform change could be observed. With increasing tumescence and rigidity, an increase in the frequency of the potentials with a simultaneous decrease in amplitude and polyphasity was seen (Fig. 7). During full erection, potentials were recorded in all patients. In contrast to this, no potentials (electrical silence) were recorded after intracavernous injection of papaverine and phentolamine or prostaglandin E1 (PGE1).

In patients with a *lesion of the upper motorneuron* (traumatic spinal cord injury above T11), potentials lasting from 28 to over 2 min were recorded (Fig. 8). The amplitude of the potentials and the time between passages of the base line were comparable to the potentials recorded in normal patients. Whips were numerous, bursts were less frequently recorded.

In the patients with a *lesion of the lower motoneuron* (e.g., after cysto-prostatectomy), two different types of potentials were recorded. On the one hand, short potentials with a significantly increased amplitude, on the other, short potentials with a significantly reduced amplitude (Fig. 9). Short whips were seen frequently.

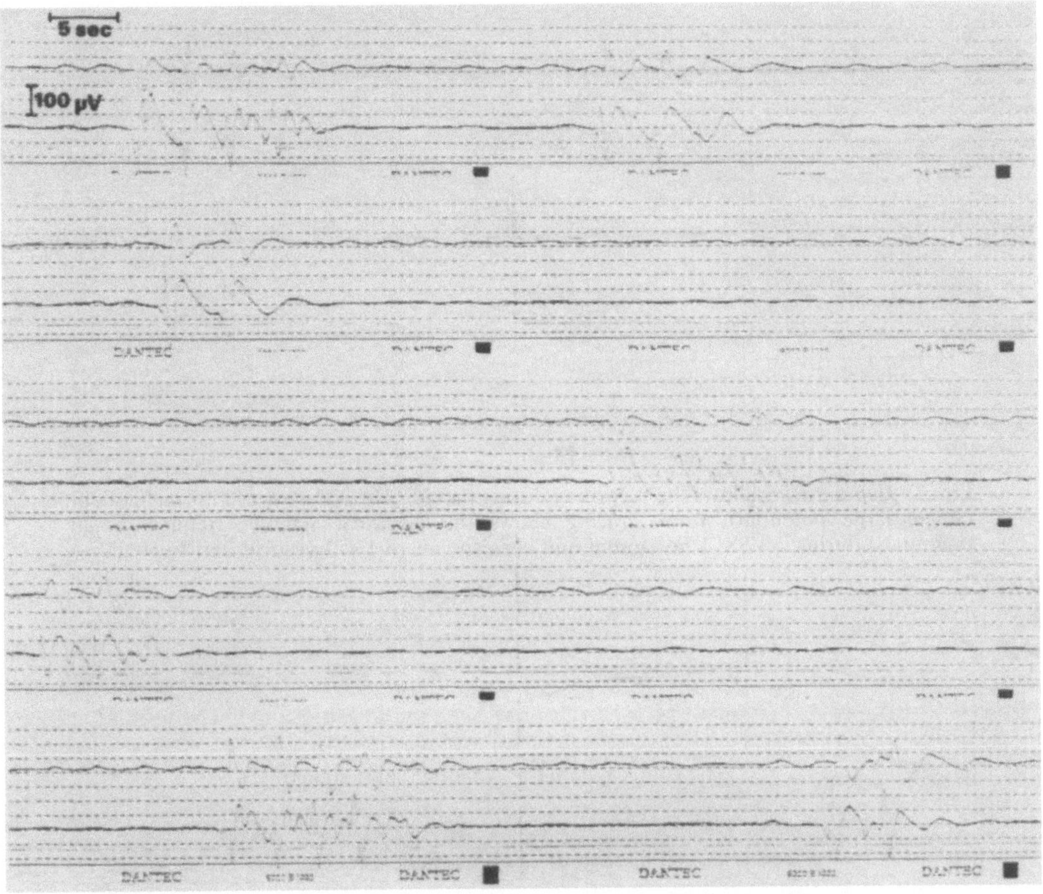

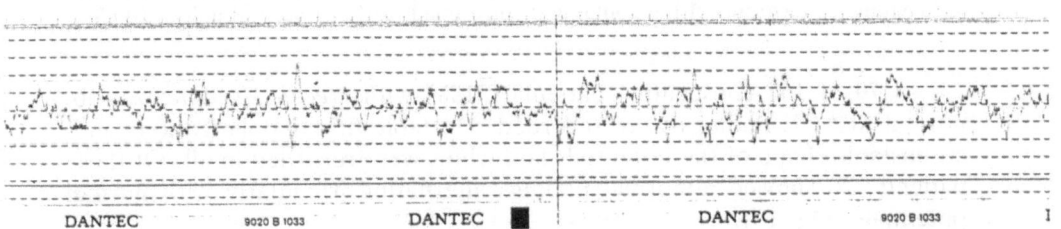

Fig. 5. Simultaneous continuous recording of cavernous electric activity in both cavernous bodies showed synchronized cavernous electrical activity

Fig. 6. Recording of a 29-year-old patient with varicocele 1 h prior to surgery. 1 horizontal unit corresponds to 1 s, 1 vertical unit to 50 μV

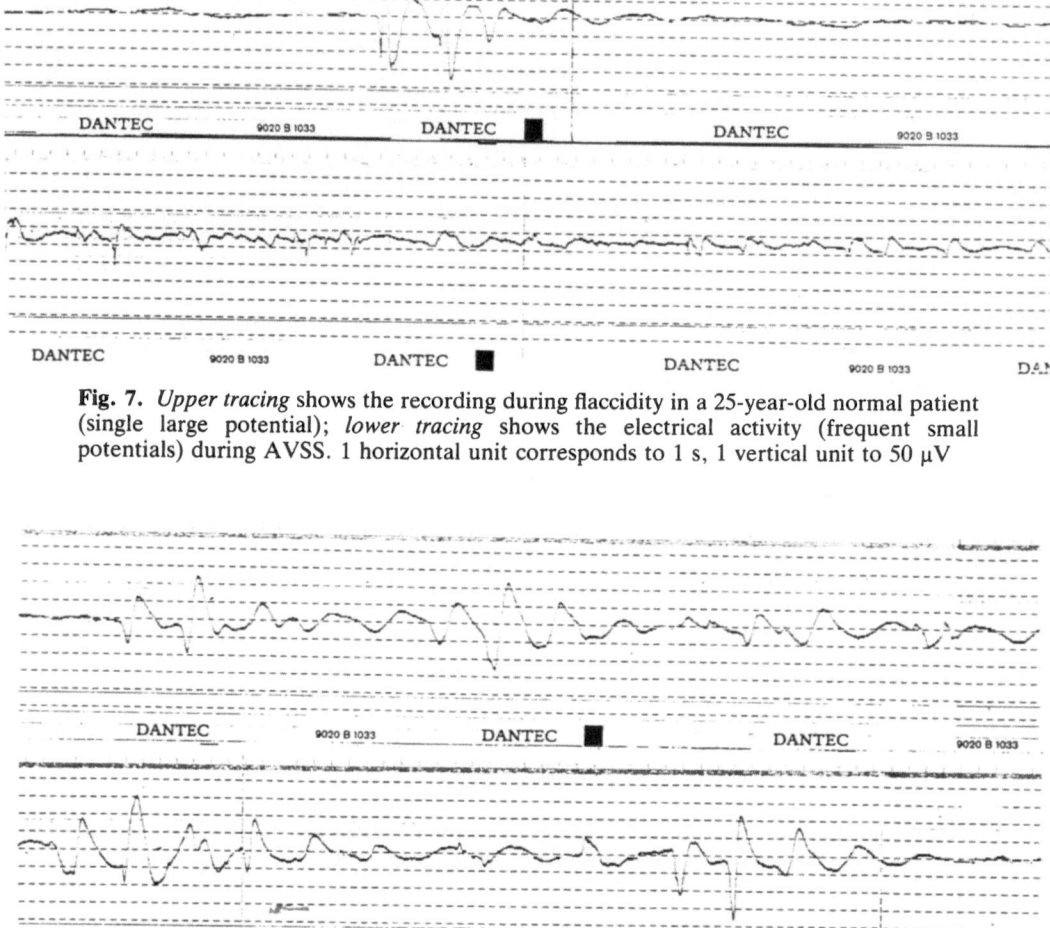

Fig. 7. *Upper tracing* shows the recording during flaccidity in a 25-year-old normal patient (single large potential); *lower tracing* shows the electrical activity (frequent small potentials) during AVSS. 1 horizontal unit corresponds to 1 s, 1 vertical unit to 50 μV

Fig. 8. Potentials of long duration, which are pathophysiognomic for upper motor neuron lesions, recorded in a 33-year-old patient (see also Fig. 1). *Upper* and *lower* lines comprise one continuous recording. 1 horizontal unit corresponds to 1 s, 1 vertical unit to 50 μV

In 79 of 154 consecutive patients (51%) with *erectile dysfunction*, abnormal SPACE findings were recorded. Unstable first depolarizations and, an unstable shape of the potentials and whips were recorded in all. Of these patients, 26 showed abnormal findings alternating irregularly with normal potentials (Fig. 10).

During AVSS, 11 of 29 patients with *psychogenic impotence* showed an increased frequency with otherwise unchanged potentials.

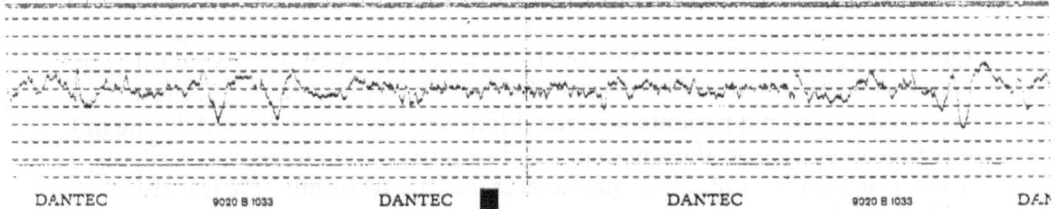

Fig. 9. Recording of a 51-year-old patient who had undergone abdominoperineal extirpation of the rectum 4 years previously. 1 horizontal unit corresponds to 1 s, 1 vertical unit
to 50 μV

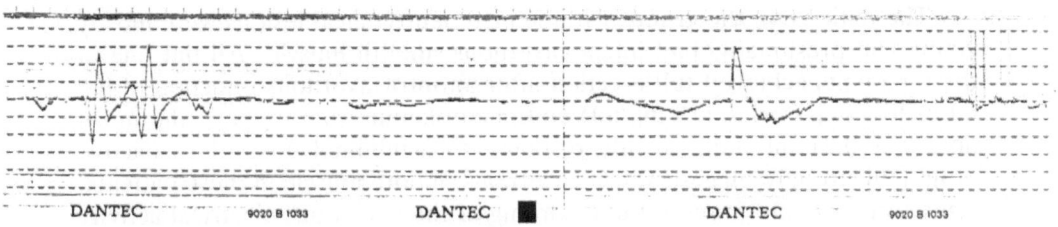

Fig. 10. 33-year-old patient who had had insulin-dependent diabetes for 18 years; normal
potentials as well as whips and bursts were seen. 1 horizontal unit corresponds to 1 s, 1
vertical unit to 50 μV

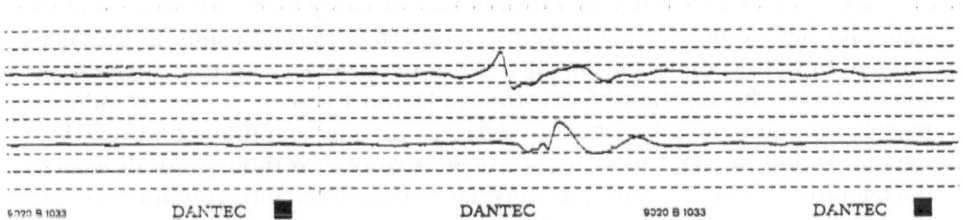

Fig. 11. Recordings in a 32-year-old patient who had had insulin-dependent diabetes for 21
years shows potentials of low amplitude and slow depolarizations (electrodes in both
cavernous bodies). 1 horizontal unit corresponds to 1 s, 1 vertical unit to 50 μV

In 11 of 14 patients with insulin-dependent *diabetes mellitus* (duration
over 20 years), multidisciplinary examination showed signs highly suggestive
of cavernous smooth muscle degeneration [8]. On palpation, the penis felt
much smaller in all these patients than in other patients. All patients had
only a poor response to the intracavernous injection of vasoactive drugs and
showed extensive venous leakage in cavernosometry and cavernosography.
In SPACE, these patients showed desynchronized potentials of low amplitude, irregular shape and slow depolarization (Fig. 11). In one patient with
erectile dysfunction, the recordings coult not be interpreted due to wavelike
baseline activity.

Discussion

Our findings show that the electrical potentials of cavernous smooth muscle activity can be recorded. The reproducible recordings, the similarity of the potentials in normal patients, and the different responses recorded during full erection to AVSS on the one hand and to intracavernous injection of vaso-active drugs on the other strongly suggest that the recordings are not artifacts. Different types of autonomic lesions may be differentiated by SPACE.

Although the etiology of potentials seems to be well correlated to the neurological status, the etiology of spikes and bursts remains unclear. Further studies must establish whether these recordings were artifacts (e.g., due to apparatus close to the examination room) or physiological events.

The patients in the groups with defined neurological lesions were mostly young and presumably had intact cavernous smooth muscle. All but one of these patients achieved full erection after an intracavernous injection of 0.5 ml or less papaverine (15 mg/ml) and phentolamine (0.5 mg/ml); the mean dose was 0.31 ml. Full erectile response to a minimal dose of vasoactive drugs [10] strongly suggests intact cavernous smooth muscle in these patients. Therefore, the alteration in the recording of the cavernous electrical activity was most probably due to the neurological lesions of the patients and not to smooth muscle degeneration. Nevertheless, further electron microscopic studies are required to elucidate the influence of smooth muscle degeneration on SPACE.

In the patients who had had insulin-dependent diabetes for over 20 years and who had shown signs of extensive cavernous smooth muscle degeneration in the work-up, significant changes of cavernous electrical activity were found. Desynchronization of cavernous electrical activity seems to indicate peripheral autonomic dysfunction, whereas the low amplitude and the slow depolarization of the potentials are suggestive of cavernous smooth muscle degeneration. This assumption correlates well with electron microscopic findings in patients with venous leakage [8].

Our findings in normal patients suggest that during flaccidity, the contractions of many cavernous smooth muscle cells are synchronized by the sympathetic tone. This results in a potential of high amplitude and long duration. During sexual arousal and with increasing tumescence and rigidity, the sympathetic tone is dramatically reduced, resulting in non-synchronization of the smooth muscle cells. This results in potentials of decreased amplitude and length, but increased frequency. In contrast to this physiological erection, erection induced by vasoactive drugs is accompanied by electrical silence at the amplification used (50 μV/unit). Further examinations with higher signal amplification (5 μV/unit) must determine whether or not there is any electrical activity. Our study showed abnormal SPACE findings in 51% of 154 consecutive patients with erectile dysfunction. Even if we subtract the patients with presumable neurogenic lesions in their clinical history (e.g., after cysto-prostatectomy), we still have abnormal SPACE findings in 34% of impotent patients with normal neurological history. Compared with a rate of about 10% neurogenic factors in the etiology of impotence in the literature, this rate seems surprisingly high. Nevertheless, it must be taken into account that this rate was mostly based on the measurement of BCRL. Comparing the possibility of damage to the autonomic (possibly diagnosed by SPACE) and to the somatosensory system (diagnosed by BCRL), it is well known that damage to the autonomic system may occur much earlier [1]. Furthermore, our own (unpublished) electron microscopic findings showed pathologic findings of cavernous innervation in 40% of patients.

In all patients, the diagnosis of abnormal autonomic innervation could be made by SPACE without using AVSS. Synchronous recording with two needles in each corpus facilitated diagnosis. In our opinion, the individual response to AVSS cannot be standardized due to possible patient disapproval of such methods in general, or to specific parts of the video. In disagreement with Gerstenberg and Wagner [2], we think that dyscoordination of cavernous electrical activity is more likely to be of psychogenic than of organogenic origin.

We consider SPACE to be a minimally invasive and reproducible diagnostic method for evaluating autonomic cavernous innervation. A diagnosis of cavernous smooth muscle degeneration by SPACE seems possible.

References

1. Ellenberg M (1980) Development of urinary bladder dysfunction in diabetis mellitus. Ann Internal Med 92:321–324
2. Gerstenberg TC, Nordling J, Hald H, Wagner G (1989) Standardized evaluation of erectile dysfunction in 95 consecutive patients. J Urol 141:857–861
3. Jevtich MJ (1983) Non-invasive vascular and neurogenic tests in use for evaluation of angiogenic impotence. Inter Angio 3:964–969
4. Laivas JG, Zayed AA, Labib KB (1981) The bulbocavernous reflex in urology. J Urol 126:197–200
5. Lavoisier P, Proulx J, Courtois F, Carful F (1989) Bulbocavernous reflex. J Urol 141:311–315
6. Lue TF, Hricak H, Marich KW, Tanagho EA (1985) Vasculogenic impotence evaluated by high resolution ultrasonography and pulsed Doppler spectrum analysis. Radiology 155:777–781
7. Lue TF, Hricak H, Schmidt RA, Tanagho EA (1986) Functional evaluation of penile veins by cavernosography in papaverine induced erection. J Urol 135:479–484
8. Persson C, Diederichs W, Lue TF, Yen TS, Fishman I, Mc Lin PH, Tanagho ET (1989) Correlation of altered ultrastructure with clinical arterial evaluation. J Urol 142:1462
9. Siroky MB, Sax DS, Krane RJ (1979) Sacral signal tracing. J Urol 122:661–665
10. Stief CG, Bähren W, Gall H, Scherb W (1988) Functional evaluation of penile hemodynamics. J Urol 139:734–737
11. Wagner G, Gerstenberg T (1988) Human in vivo studies of electrical activity of corpus cavernosum. J Urol 139:327A
12. Wagner G, Gerstenberg T, Levin RJ (1989) Electrical activity of corpus cavernosum during flaccidity and erection of the human penis. J Urol 142:723–727

Therapy

Erectile Disorders: A Psychosexological Review

M.W. Hengeveld

This book mainly describes *organic* aspects of the etiology, diagnosis, and treatment of erectile disorders. It is in this domain that most progress has taken place in recent years: research into the anatomy and physiology of the penis, new diagnostic tests, and modern physical therapies. As a consequence of these developments, it has become clear that organic factors play a role in the etiology of erectile disturbances much more often than was believed for many years. That is why one is justified in paying so much attention to the organic aspects of erectile dysfunctions. Yet, in doing this one should not lose sight of the psychosexological factors, as many erectile disorders are completely psychogenic in origin. Moreover, psychosocial or psychiatric factors *always* play a more or less important role in the pathogenesis and treatment of erectile disturbances, even if one has found a satisfactory organic explanation for the cause of the disorder. This chapter, therefore, presents an up-to-date review of the prevalence, classification, etiology, pathogenesis, diagnosis, and therapy of erectile dysfunction from the point of view of a psychiatrist-sexologist.

Prevalence

Little is known about the prevalence of erectile disorders. Kinseys et al. [18], in their famous report, mentioned an average value of 1.6% of all men interviewed. With increasing age the percentages rose hyperbolically, from 0.1% in under 20-year-olds to 75% in men over 70 years. Their samples, however, were not randomly chosen. Frank et al. [7], reporting on a selected group of 100 men with an average age of 36 years, found that 7% complained of difficulties obtaining an erection and 9% complained of difficulties maintaining an erection. Impotence was reported by 7% of a representative sample of 58 married Swedish men with an average age of 31 years [24]. In a random sample of 250 middle class Dutch men between 18 and 55 years old, moderate to severe erectile problems were reported by 6%, while another 16% mentioned mild erectile problems [8]. The number of men presenting this complaint to a physician has certainly increased because of the enormous growth of diagnostic and therapeutic possibilities in recent years.

U. Jonas et al. (Eds.) Erectile Dysfunction
© Springer-Verlag Berlin Heidelberg 1991

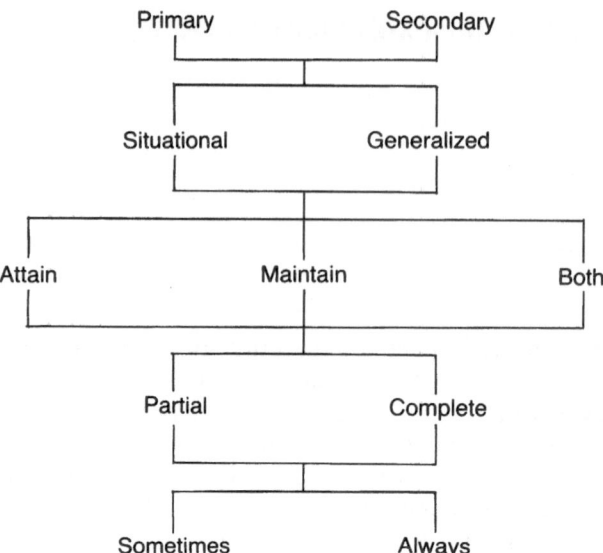

Fig. 1. Classification of erectile disorders. (After Graber and Kline-Graber [8])

The incidence rate is, of course, strongly influenced by the severity of the disturbance. In most relevant literature, however, the nature and seriousness of the erectile dysfunction are not specified, thus hampering comparison of incidence and results of various treatments. It is, therefore, important to distinguish various subgroups of erectile disorders. For this purpose, a modified version of the classification of Graber and Kline-Graber [10] is presented (Fig. 1).

Classification

The first division that can be made is between primary and secondary dysfunction. This division depends upon whether or not the man has previously functioned well sexually. Secondary erectile disorders, often of a transient nature, occur much more frequently than primary erectile disorders, which are generally considered to be indicative of more severe organic or psychiatric pathology. Further specification can be achieved if a division is made between generalized erectile failure (both with intercourse and in noncoital situations) and situational erectile failure (only in specific situations, e.g., coitus or masturbation). This division is diagnostically important, since the presence of full erectile capacity in certain situations strongly points to a psychological origin of the disorder. Nowadays, the differentiation between inability to achieve a sufficient erection and inability to maintain it is more emphasized, because the latter may indicate a vascular cause. The degree of erectile failure should also be established, i.e., complete or only partial failure. Finally, it is relevant to specify whether the dysfunction is always present, or only sometimes. The latter finding implicates a psychological or physical cause that is changing in severity over time. An example would be the man who functions well sexually during his holidays, when his physical and psychological condition is optimal.

The importance of this classification for the differentiation between organic and psychogenic dysfunction will be shown in the paragraph on diagnosis.

Often, disorders of erection and sexual arousal are not clearly distinguished from disorders of sexual desire. Not only patients themselves confound these two sexual dysfunctions, misconception is also repeatedly found in the literature. This is particularly the case in reports of sexual side-effects of medicaments or of sexual disturbances in the physically ill. It is very important to establish whether the male patient complaining of erectile impotence is not actually suffering from inhibited sexual desire. This could save him from further somatic diagnostic or therapeutic endeavors. Also ejaculatory disorders, in particular premature ejaculation, are sometimes wrongly described as a form of impotence. If the patient appears to have such sexual disorder(s) instead of or in addition to erectile failure, the somatic specialist should refer him to a psychosexologist for further diagnosis and treatment. This should also be the case if the patient's partner complains of any sexual dysfunction.

Etiology and Pathogenesis

In general, a distinction is made between *psychogenic* and *organic* erectile failure. This is a theoretically and didactically useful differentiation that is also applied in this book. Yet, in practice, it is often not possible to make this differentiation. In many patients with an undeniable organic etiology, psychological problems play a more or less important role, whether cause or effect. Likewise, an indication of psychogenic impotence does not rule out the concomitant presence of organic factors subtly intertwined in the pathogenesis. Similar to many other physical and mental disorders, erectile failure is a multifactorial syndrome, the pure organic and pure psychogenic forms being the extremes of a continuous spectrum. Diabetes mellitus, a disease accompanied by erectile problems in 30%–50% of all male patients, is a typical example of the interplay between somatic and psychological factors. In addition to the neurological or vascular causes, the following psychological problems may be involved: fear of future complications, the role of a chronically ill person with daily restrictions, poor body image, and fatigue [32].

Table 1. Etiology of erectile disorders

Authors	No. of patients	Etiology (%)			
		Organic	Psychogenic	Mixed	Unknown
Schoenberg et al. (1982) [25]	122	20	69		11
Jacobs et al. (1983) [16]	106	52	38		10
Melman et al. (1988) [23]	406	29	40	25	6
Stief et al. (1989) [28]	67[a]	27	16	58	6

[a] Only patients with primary erectile dysfunction

Traditionally, sexology authors have claimed that 90%–95% of all erectile disturbances are caused by psychological factors. The source of this percentage is not clear; probably it was copied from one author to another. Sufficient evidence to substantiate it, however, has never been produced. Recently, some evaluative studies have been published, using both the organic diagnostic tools described in this book and extensive psychosexological assessments. The results of these studies are summarized in Table 1.

From this table one concludes that organic factors can be found in 20%–85%, and psychological factors in 38%–74% of patients. The wide ranges of these figures may be explained in part by the differences in criteria used to decide whether the cause is organic, psychological, or both. But selection of patients by the diagnostic centers is certainly an important factor, too. Schoenberg et al. [25], for example, compared a group of patients referred to a urology department with a group self-referred to a sex therapy clinic, and found an organic etiology in 26% and 4%, respectively. Age is also an important confounding factor: organic impotence will be found more often in an older than in a younger group of patients. All in all, however, it is nowadays assumed that organic factors play a role in the etiology of far more than 5%–10% of erectile disorders. But that does not alter the fact that it is very important to look for psychological causes in *all* patients with erectile disorders.

Psychological Causes

It is difficult to prove that an erectile disorder is caused by psychological factors, let alone ascertained which specific psychological causes play a role in the etiology or pathogenesis. An erectile dysfunction that is cured by itself or

Table 2. Psychological causes of erectile disorders

Fear	of failure; of sex; of disease; of pregnancy; of lust; of intimacy; of women; of ridicule; of rejection; of inflicting injury; after physical injury
Hostility	towards the partner; towards women
Disgust	of sex; of the female sexual organ
Shame	due to upbringing
Guilt	due to religion; when unfaithful; in widowers
Humiliation	due to unemployment or social failure
Latent homosexuality	
Poor sex education	
Psychiatric disorder	depression; psychosis

following sexological therapy, strongly points to a psychological etiology. The literature is full of descriptions of psychological causes, mainly in the form of case histories. Only recently have criteria for the psychogenesis of erectile disorders been systematically investigated [29]. Reviewing sexological hand- books, however, it is possible to select a number of etiological factors on which there is general agreement [3, 11, 17, 20, 22]. They are presented in Table 2. These are certainly not causes essential to the disorder, but factors that often contribute to its onset or continuation.

In classical sexological literature, a distinction was made between constitu- tional factors, factors from early development, and more immediate causes of erectile dysfunctions [27]. This is still a practical distinction because imme- diate causes are usually easier to treat. The physician should begin with treat- ment directed at these actual causes, and only search for deeper causes when treatment is unsuccessful [17]. In the search for factors causing erectile failure, those that maintain the disorder are often neglected. Thus, in the patho- genesis of erectile disorders, besides predisposing and immediate causes, one encounters vicious circles of organic and psychological causes and their consequences (Fig. 2).

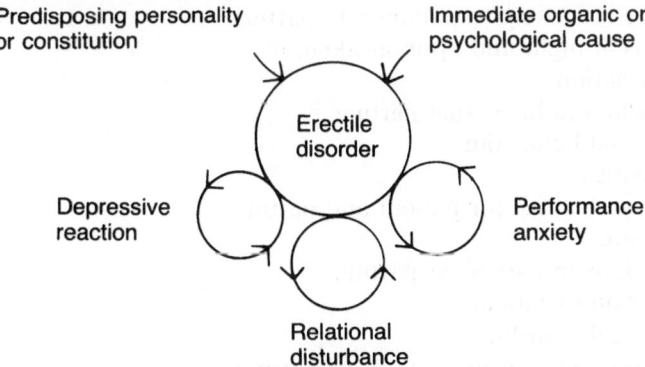

Fig. 2. Vicious circles in the pathogenesis of erectile disorders

Consider, for example, the man who never had a great sexual repertoire. Perhaps he was born with a weak sexual constitution, or had a restricted sexual education. An organic deficit, such as elevated blood pressure, will decrease his erectile potency. The patient's negative reaction to his diminished capacity, such as performance anxiety, exacerbates the problem causing complete dysfunction. His wife, who can only experience an orgasm through straight intercourse, reacts in a reproachful way and refuses to engage in alternative sexual activities. Lack of communication leads to an unspoken marital conflict, which is disastrous for the man's sexual desire and potency. He may react with resentment, guilt or depression, each in its turn reinforcing his erectile disorder.

Diagnosis

The development of new psychosexological and surgical therapies for erectile disturbances has only increased the need for careful assessment of all possible etiological factors. This book presents a comprehensive overview of all new diagnostic techniques. It remains essential to take an accurate and extensive sexual history and biography of the man and, if possible, of his sexual partner. In some cases this in itself will be sufficient to help the patient: the clarifying, informative, and reassuring effects of a detailed discussion of the sexual history can lead to the reduction of anxiety, guilt or inhibition.

The reader is referred to the various sexological handbooks available for details of all the questions that can or should be asked [3, 11, 17, 21]. The most relevant questions regarding the sexual history are as follows:

Severity and duration of erectile disorder
Gradual or sudden onset of disorder
Circumstances in which the disorder occurs
Intrapersonal or interpersonal conflict as an immediate cause
Causes of the disorder according to patient and partner
Erections or emissions at night and upon awakening
Erections with masturbation
Reactions of the patient and his sexual partner
Current erotic and sexual behaviour
Noncoital sexual activities
Meaning of sexuality and coitus for patient and partner
Changes in sexual desire
Other sexual dysfunctions in patient or partner
Complaints of depression or fatigue
Quality of the general relationship
Serious psychosocial problems in the patient or partner
Psychosexual biography of patient and partner

Table 3. Traditional differentiation between organic and psychological etiology of erectile disorders

Item	Organic	Psychological
Onset	Gradual[a]	Sudden
Course	Constant	Varying
Immediate cause	No psychological conflict	Psychological conflict
Circumstances	Dysfunction at all times	Not with all partners
Morning erections	Absent	Present
Masturbation	Erectile failure	Normal erection

[a] Except in traumatic or surgical causes

Traditionally it is assumed that the sexual history of the patient allows differentiation between a psychological and organic etiology. The data that, according to most authors, are essential for this differentiation are presented in Table 3 [13].

All criteria mentioned in Table 3, however, can also point in the other direction. Psychogenic impotence may develop gradually if, for example, negative feelings towards the sexual partner gradually grow stronger. An erectile disorder that seems undoubtedly to have been caused by injury or surgery may also be the consequence of the simultaneous psychological trauma. A varying course, with sufficient erections under certain circumstances, can equally point to a mild organic cause of the disorder. An interesting example is the man who loses his erection at the moment he starts to initiate coitus. Traditionally this is interpreted by psychodynamically oriented sexologists as proof of a psychological cause, because the erection disappears right at the psychological *moment suprême*. We now know it may also be a symptom of the "pelvic steal syndrome" As well as being a cause of impotence, intrapersonal or marital conflicts may also be the consequence of an organic erectile dysfunction. Additionally, the onset of organic impotence may coincidently occur during a time of emotional stress. The sexual history may not be reliable because the patient harbors feelings of shame or guilt. Sexual experiences with other women or masturbation may, therefore, be concealed, or morning erections denied. Finally, a man who is impotent with his wife may experience failure when he desperately tries to prove his sexual potency with another woman.

Psychological tests do not provide much additional information in the area of etiology and diagnosis of erectile disorders. Some pscyhologists have attempted to discriminate between organic and psychogenic erectile dysfunction with such tests, but others have failed to duplicate their results. The research to date, therefore, does not produce convincing evidence that psychological testing is useful in the differentiation of psychogenic and organic impotence [26].

Some studies have been conducted into the validity of sexual sympto-matology for the differential diagnosis of erectile disorders [26]. From this research it appears that the capacity for having firm early morning erections or turgid noncoital erections is the only item that strongly points to the absence of an organic etiology. Preliminary results of our own investigations suggest that the patient's and partner's opinions about the causes of the disorder significantly predict the eventual diagnostic conclusions about etiology [15]. Generally, in most patients it is impossible to make a diagnosis from the sexual history alone. Only in cases where the patient reports firm erections under certain circumstances or when he or his partner strongly suggest a psychological cause, is one justified in forgoing organic diagnostic tests and starting psychosexual therapy.

Since the sexual history will often not disclose the etiology of an erectile problem, clinicians nowadays rely heavily on modern diagnostic techniques to determine the causes of impotence. The problem with these methods, however, is first, defining what is an organic cause and what not, and, second, deciding what test result is sufficiently abnormal to explain the erectile dis-order. There is no absolute standard or benchmark for distinguishing between organic and nonorganic impotence [13]. The main goal, therefore, of the diagnostic process is not to differentiate organic from psychogenic erectile dysfunction, but to track down all the interrelated etiological factors. An extensive sexual history is essential to our understanding of the meaning of the erectile failure at this particular moment in the life of this particular man and his sexual partner. Organic diagnostic procedures are essential to detect organic factors in the etiology that may be suitable targets for treatment.

Choice of Therapy

Is it possible to decide on the appropriate therapy after one has completed all diagnostic pursuits? In many cases the resultant conclusions about the causes of the erectile disorder do not provide sufficient arguments for the correct treatment of the patient to be chosen. Sex therapy is certainly effective in a number of men with so-called organic impotence, and a physical therapy may well be the treatment of choice in a number of men with so-called psychogenic impotence. The patient described in the section "Psychological causes" might be treated equally well with sex therapy, marital therapy, intracavernosal injections or a penile implant. Thus, the choice of therapy is not only deter-mined by the etiology of the disorder. Other factors should play an important role in the decision as to what treatment is offered to the patient. These might be called the *psychosexological (contra)indications*.

Before one starts actively treating a patient, it is sobering to realize that a relatively large proportion of impotent patients improve before the real therapy is carried out. According to some studies, 15% of erectile disorders

remit spontaneously while waiting for the first assessment, and another 15%
get better as soon as treatment begins [30]. Many other patients do not
comply with the physician's recommendations, particularly when there is a
discrepancy between the patient's and the physician's frame of reference. The
high drop-out rate of autoinjection treatment patients mentioned below
indicates the frequent difference between the expectations of the impotent
male and those of the urologist treating him. Thus, the most important
psychosexological factor determining the choice of therapy is what the patient
and his partner wish themselves.

The results of psychosexological therapies of erectile disorders depend
mainly on factors related to the patient [13]. Certain psychosexological
factors appear to decrease the chance of restoring erectile function by psychosexological therapies:

Uncooperative patient or sexual partner
Low sex drive
Homosexual inclinations
Psychosis or major mood disorder
Major interpersonal problems with sexual partner
Failure of previous psychosexological treatment

These factors can be considered as relative contraindications to psychosexological therapy. If one considers offering a patient psychosexological
treatment, one should check whether one or more of these negative factors is
present. For example, it is not useful to prescribe sensate focus exercises for
an old man with a long-lasting erectile disorder, particularly when his wife
refuses to engage in noncoital sexual activities. One or more failures of
psychosexological treatment by an experienced sexologist can also be considered a relative contraindication to making another attempt.

From clinical experience, the psychosexological contra-indications to
physical therapies appear to be:

Unrealistic expectations (of improvement of sexual desire, arousal, ejacu-
    lation, orgasm, or psychological disturbances)
Other sexual dysfunctions prior to erectile disorder
Psychosis or major mood disorder
Somatoform mental disorder (conversion disorder, chronic pain disorder,
    hypochondriasis)
Substance use disorder
Crisis situation (divorce; grief; serious illness; major surgical procedure)
Major interpersonal problems with sexual partner
Sexual partner aversive, sexually dysfunctional, or psychiatrically disturbed

For example, to offer physical therapy to a man with marital problems,
who expects to solve these problems with this therapy, while his spouse states
that she shudders at the very thought of artificial erections, is contra-
indicated. Furthermore, the risk of suggesting autoinjections or implanting a

prosthesis in the penis of a man who has a history of multiple unexplained somatic complaints, particularly in his genital region, must be pointed out. Finally, it can be considered a medical error to combine prosthetic with oncological surgery. One can not expect a patient to make a well-thought-out decision while still struggling with the fact that he is suffering from cancer. A comparable situation is that of the old widower, mourning over his deceased wife, who is impotent with his new sexual partner. One should explain to the man the psychological causes of his erectile failure and wait some time before offering him such a radical remedy. When such contraindications are established, the urologist or surgeon should refer the patient to a sexologist or a psychiatrist.

Psychosexological Therapies

Masters and Johnson [22] showed that many patients with erectile problems suffer from only minor sexual concerns and anxieties, and that such patients can be cured with brief and direct treatment methods. Some time ago there were, broadly speaking, two forms of psychosexological therapy: psychoanalytical individual therapy, and brief, symptom-oriented counseling. The premise in psychoanalytical therapy is that the erectile disorder represents an underlying subconscious conflict. The dysfunction is seen as a neurotic defense against the emergence of this conflict. The therapy, therefore, is aimed at treating the neurosis according to normal principles of psychoanalysis [17]. This matter will not, however, be pursued, particularly because, according to most sexologists, erectile disorder is rarely an indication for orthodox psychoanalytical therapy.

Brief, symptom-oriented treatments have been used for some time by many physicians [6, 12, 20]. They usually involve randomly selected patients, with various causes of erectile dysfunction. The physician may use various techniques, adapted to the patient and his partner. The main elements of such counseling are: an explanation of the causes of the problem, sexual information, reassurance, encouragement, and advice (e.g., to take longer over foreplay). Psychotherapeutic exploration of the background of the symptom (e.g., of any anxieties the patient might have) may also take place. The partner is often included in the therapy with the intention of enhancing communication between her and the patient. Because anxiety often plays a role in the etiology, the therapy may be pharmacologically supported with a low dose of anxiolytic medication, to be taken ½–1 h before coitus. In the case of a depressive disorder, the prescription of an adequate dose of antidepressant is indicated. Endocrine therapy in the absence of demonstrable endocrinopathy is controversial. Possibly, performance anxiety is reduced as a placebo response. Sexual desire may be slightly increased, which could lead to a breakthrough in the negative vicious circle. The effects may, however, be counter productive: an erectile failure when desire is heightened may increase the disappointment. Moreover, there is a risk that the man will be convinced more than ever that he suffers from a physical disorder, which may decrease his acceptance of a psychotherapeutic approach.

Sex Therapy

Masters and Johnson [22] developed a program for the treatment of erectile dysfunctions, which can be characterized as follows: The patient and partner are treated as a couple by a mixed gender couple of cotherapists. The couple stay for 2 weeks in a pleasant motel near the clinic and follow an intensive daily treatment program. The most essential ingredients of their sex therapy are the sensate focus exercises. These are intended to (re)educate the couple to enjoy their bodies, using all senses in a relaxed and erotic way. The aim is to detach sexuality from the atmosphere of inhibition, guilt, and performance anxiety. During this period the couple is ordered to abstain completely from coitus, in an attempt to break through rigid sexual patterns and to prevent disappointing failures. (For a clear description of the sensate focus exercises, see Hawton [11]). In a subsequent phase of the treatment the sexual organs are also involved in the exercises. An erection is not striven after, but may appear and disappear. If this stage is reached, the specific treatment follows. The female partner may then, while astride the man, stimulate him to erection and lower herself onto his phallus, which enters her vagina. The man lies still on his back and does not strive for an orgasm. This exercise is slowly expanded until successful coitus is achieved. Finally, the goal is reached simply by initially distracting all attention from it.

The sex therapy method of Masters and Johnson has attracted many followers within a very short time. All sexologists have been influenced by it. There are very few, however, who apply this technique in its original form. Many variations are applied, e.g., the treatment is carried out on an outpatient basis, with fewer sessions, by one therapist, and with a more random group of patients. Kaplan [17], with her psychoanalytical background, emphasizes the treatment of underlying personal or interpersonal conflicts which can come to light while performing or discussing the sensate focus exercises. Thus many sex therapies develop into couple therapies. Particular attention is paid, nowadays, to inaccurate or distorted beliefs (e.g., "erections should occur on demand", and "my partner will think I am a failure if I don't get an erection") and other so-called cognitive factors (e.g., distraction by performance-oriented thoughts) which play a role in causing or maintaining erectile difficulties [4].

Sex therapy usually entails between 8 and 16 treatment sessions over 3–5 months. The outcome following sex therapy for clearly psychogenic erectile dysfunction is often satisfactory, with approximately two-thirds of couples either having an entirely successful outcome or experiencing considerable improvement. The gains from therapy are maintained in most couples when seen 1–6 years after treatment [12].

Physical Therapies

Alloplastic rods or inflatable cylinders have been implanted in the penises of many thousands of impotent males. The extensive surgical literature mainly discusses technique, complications and functional outcome. Follow-up studies present satisfactory results in over 90% of the patients. However, all studies are of a retrospective nature, follow-up periods are often short or not mentioned at all, criteria for outcome are generally not specified, and little attention is paid to the effects of surgery on the patient and his partner [5, 9]. Only 14 evaluative reports have been published on the subjective, psychosexological results of implantation therapy [14]. All these studies are retrospective and uncontrolled in design, the great majority using mailed questionnaires. Table 4 presents a summary of this literature.

It appears that the majority of male erectile dysfunction patients treated with alloplastic implants are satisfied with the results. The opinions of their partners are less well studied, but according to the patients 60%–100% were satisfied [9]. An early follow-up study, and the only one that interviewed the partners without the patient present, produced a low partner satisfaction rate of 42% [19]. Careful assessment of both the patient and his partner, ruling out other sexual dysfunctions and psychiatric problems, are mandatory, therefore, when prosthesis implantation is being considered.

Intracavernosal autoinjections of vasoactive substances (or smooth muscle relaxants) have very rapidly become the most popular somatic therapy of erectile dysfunction. Analogous to the prosthesis literature, urological evaluative reports of this treatment are often very positive. The only well-designed study, however, prospectively following patients over a 2-year period, found a cumulative drop-out rate of 46%, with patients being most at

Table 4. Psychosexological evaluation of alloplastic implant surgery. Review of 14 publications [14]

	%
Response	24–100
Satisfied	47–100
Dissatisfied	1– 23
Relationship improved	51– 85
Self-esteem increased	70–100
Would do it again	67–100

Follow-up period: 1 month to 8 years; number of respondents: n = 15–137

risk for leaving the program after the diagnostic evaluation or during the trial dose phase. Patients declined therapy because they were unable to accept the idea of injecting themselves or because of potential side effects. They discontinued therapy because of perceived lack of efficacy [2]. Most patients continuing treatment were satisfied. The quality of their erections improved, the frequency of intercourse increased and their partners' sexual arousal during intercourse was enhanced. Moreover, decreases in general psychiatric symptomatology and increases in relationship satisfaction and self-esteem were apparent [1].

It has been suggested that autoinjection therapy might cure long-lasting psychogenic impotence by alleviating performance anxiety and restoring sexual confidence. In a very recent study, in which the sexual and psychosocial outcome of self-injection treatment of psychogenic erectile failure were prospectively assessed, a very high drop-out rate of 60% was found. In the patients who remained, frequency of intercourse and sexual satisfaction increased, but performance anxiety was not alleviated, dependence upon injections for intercourse remained, and capacity for intimacy was not improved [31].

Autoinjection therapy, therefore, appears to be an effective therapy for a well-selected group of impotent patients, improving their sexual, psychological, and marital functioning. It is certainly not the treatment of choice for most men with psychogenic erectile dysfunction, as it does not by itself reverse the potency problem or address the psychological factors underlying the symptom of impotence, and seems to create a dependency upon injections for sexual activity. In some cases, however, the introduction of intracavernous injections in the context of ongoing sex therapy may enhance the benefits of both. It may be of value as an alternative treatment when sex therapy has been unsuccessful.

References

1. Althof SE, Turner LA, Levine SB, Risen CB, Kursh ED, Bodner DR, Resnick MI (1987) Intracavernosal injection in the treatment of impotence: A prospective study of sexual, psychological, and marital functioning. J Sex Marital Ther; 13:155–67
2. Althof SE, Turner LA, Levine SB, Risen CB, Kursh ED, Bodner DR, Resnick MI (1989) Why do so many people drop out from autoinjection therapy for impotence? J Sex Marital Ther 15:121–129
3. Bancroft J (1983) Human sexuality and its problems. Churchill Livingstone, Edinburgh
4. Barlow DH (1986) Causes of sexual dysfunction: the role. of anxiety and cognitive interference. J Consult Clin Psychol; 54:140
5. Collins GF, Kinder BN (1984) Adjustment following surgical implantation of a penile prosthesis: a critical overview. J Sex Marital Ther 10:255–71
6. Finkle PS, Finkle AL (1975) Urological counseling can overcome male sexual impotence. Geriatrics 30:119–29
7. Frank E, Anderson C, Rubinstein D (1978) Frequency of sexual dysfunction in normal couples. N Engl J Med 299:111–5

8. Frenken J (1980) Het vóórkomen van seksuele problemen in man-vrouw relaties. In: Frenken J (ed) Seksuologie, een interdisciplinaire benadering. Van Loghum Slaterus, Deventer, pp 227–250
9. Goldman L, Segraves RT (1985) Psychiatric evaluation of penile prosthesis candidates. In: Segraves RT, Schoenberg HW (eds) Diagnosis and treatment of erectile disturbances. Plenum, New York, pp 197–128
10. Graber B, Kline-Graber G (1981) Research criteria for male erectile failure. J Sex Marital Ther (1981) 7:37–48
11. Hawton K (1985) Sex therapy: A practical guide. Oxford University Press, Oxford
12. Hawton K (1988) Erectile dysfunction and premature ejaculation. Br J Hosp Med 40:428–36
13. Hengeveld MW (1986) Erectile dysfunction: Diagnosis and choice of therapy. World J Urol 3:249–52
14. Hengeveld MW (1987) Erectiestoornissen: somatische therapieën. Tijdschr Seksuologie 11:55–62
15. Hengeveld MW, Gent PG van (1988) A screening test to distinguish psychogenic impotence. In: Proceedings Third World Meeting of Impotence. International Society for Impotence Research, Boston, 129
16. Jacobs JA, Fishkin R, Cohen S, Goldman A, Mulholland SG (1983) A multidisciplinary approach to the evaluation and management of male sexual dysfunction. J Urol 192:35–38
17. Kaplan HS (1974) The new sex therapy. Brunner/Mazel, New York
18. Kinsey AC, Pomeroy WB, Martin CE (1948) Sexual behavior in human male. Saunders, Philadelphia
19. Kramarsky-Binkhorst S (1987) Female partner perception of Small-Carrion implant. Urology 12:545–548
20. Levine SB (1976) Marital sexual dysfunction: erectile dysfunction. Ann Intern Med 85:342–350
21. LoPiccolo J, LoPiccolo L (eds) (1978) Handbook of sex therapy. Plenum Press, New York
22. Masters WH, Johnson VE (1970) Human sexual inadequacy. Little, Brown, Boston
23. Melman A, Tiefer L, Pedersen R (1988) Evaluation of first 406 patients in urology department based center for male sexual dysfunction. Urology 32:6–10
24. Nettelbladt P, Uddenberg N (1979) Sexual dysfunction and sexual satisfaction in 58 married Swedish men. J Psychosom Res 23:141–147
25. Schoenberg HW, Zarins CK, Segraves RT (1982) Analysis of 122 unselected impotent men subjected to multidisciplinary evaluation. J Urol 127:445–447
26. Segraves RT, Schoenberg HW, Segraves KAB (1985) Evaluation of the etiology of erectile failure. In: Segraves RT, Schoenberg HW (eds) Diagnosis and treatment of erectile disturbances. Plenum Press, New York, pp 165–196
27. Steiner M (1907) Die funktionelle Impotenz des Mannes und ihre Behandlung. Wiener Med Presse 42:1535–1540
28. Stief CG, Bähren W, Scherb W, Gall H (1989) Primary erectile dysfunction. J Urol 141:315–319
29. Surridge D, Condra M, Morales A, Fenmore J (1983) Psychogenic impotence: New light on its causation. World J Urol 1:233–238
30. Tiefer L, Melman A (1987) Adherence to recommendations and improvement over time in men with erectile dysfunction. Arch Sex Behav; 16:310–319
31. Turner LA, Althof SE, Levine SB, Risen CB, Bodner DR, Kursh ED, Resnick MI (1989) Self-injection of papaverine in the treatment of psychogenic impotence. J Sex Marital Ther 15:163–176
32. Wagner G, Green R (1981) Impotence: physiological, psychological, surgical diagnosis and treatment. Plenum Press, New York

Intracavernous Pharmacotherapy for Erectile Dysfunction

U. Wetterauer

The accidental discovery of the effect of intracavernous injection of papaverine on penile erection by Virag [51], and systematic research into the effects of the α-adrenergic receptor-blocking drug phenoxybenzamine and various smooth muscle relaxing agents by Brindley [3, 5] have completely changed the treatment modalities of erectile impotence in the last decade.

Vasoactive drugs injected into the corpus cavernosum of the penis imitate the action of endogenous neurotransmitters and lead to changes in penile hemodynamics similar to those obtained by neurostimulation of the cavernous nerves [31]. Changes in penile hemodynamics are the relaxation of sinusoidal smooth muscle, an increase in arterial blood flow, and the restriction of venous drainage. These changes, already postulated, in past, as the physiological mechanism underlying penile erection by the morphologists von Ebner [13], Eckhardt (1863), and Kiss [27], were summarized in the "erection model" by Conti [7].

With the introduction of the intracavernous administration of vasoactive drugs, it was possible to influence penile hemodynamics at a local level and to induce an erection despite disturbances in penile arterial blood flow or innervation. Since the corpus cavernosum is pharmacologically a separate compartment [59] with a volume of 60–160 ml (depending on the size of the penis), very high local drug concentrations can be achieved without severe side effects on systemic blood pressure after dilution of the drug in the central compartment in a volume of about 5000 ml.

In this contribution I will discuss vasoactive drugs and drug combinations that have been used on a long-term basis for intracavernous injection therapy; these are papaverine, the combination of papaverine and phentolamine, and prostaglandin E1 (PGE 1).

Historical Background

In 1974, Klinge and Sjöstrand [28] published in vitro assays on contraction and relaxation of the retractor muscle of the penis and the cavernous artery in animals. They examined different neurotransmitters such as acetylcholine, norepinephrine, dopamine, histamine, substance P, and various prosta-

U. Jonas et al. (Eds.) Erectile Dysfunction
© Springer-Verlag Berlin Heidelberg 1991

glandins. Domer et al. [11] reported that the intravenous injection of α-adrenergic receptor-blocking agents such as phentolamine and phenoxybenzamine induces penile erection in cats.

The American surgeon De la Torre [9] obtained the patent on every form of intracavernous administration of vasoactive substances including neurotransmitters for the treatment of impotence. However, wide publicity of the intracavernous administration of vasoactive drugs for erectile disorders was achieved only after Virag [51] described the effects of papaverine and Brindley [3] those of phenoxybenzamine and phentolamine.

Zorgniotti and Lefleur [63] pioneered the use of a mixture of papaverine and phentolamine for corpus cavernosum autoinjection therapy (CAT) for vasculogenic impotence. Favorable results using this drug combination compared with the effects of papaverine monotherapy were confirmed by many investigators in the following years. In 1986, Ishii et al. [18] published for the first time the intracavernous injection of PGE1 for the pharmacological induction of an erection.

Pharmacology and Mechanism of Action

Papaverine is an opium alkaloid derived from papaver somniferum and is said to act directly on smooth muscle cells by inhibiting phosphodiesterase, which leads to an accumulation of cyclic adenosine monophosphate. Papaverine hydrochloride facilitates erection by two mechanisms: by relaxation of smooth muscles in the sinusoids and by dilatation of helicinal arteries inducing an increase in penile blood flow.

Brindley [3] showed that phenoxybenzamine induces a long lasting erection of up to 24 h. As an alkylating substance it binds firmly to the α-adrenergic receptor, which explains its long-lasting effect. Phentolamine has a plasma half-life of 3–5 min and therefore would seem, for pharmacodynamic reasons, to be the substance of choice for intracavernous injection. However, phentolamine, as all other α-adrenergic receptor-blocking agents, does not generally induce a satisfactory erectile response. In combination with papaverine, however, it showed an additive effect both in vitro [15, 34] and in clinical studies [26, 63].

In the nonerect penis, the helicine arteries show a vasoconstriction mediated by sustained sympathetic stimulation. Both electrical stimulation of the sympathetic chain and systemic application of epinephrine can abolish or decrease the initiation or maintenance of an erection [2]. In the cavernous tissue this effect can be neutralized by the α-adrenergic receptor-blocking agent phentolamine [10]. Therefore, the combination of papaverine and phentolamine has two sites of action; papaverine acts directly on the smooth muscle cells of the sinusoids and helicine arteries, and phentolamine dilates arterial vessels and abolishes sympathetic inhibition of erection.

PGE1 was shown to have a relaxing effect on smooth cavernous muscle in vitro [15]. Ishii et al. [19] were the first to report a clinical study on 88 patients with intracavernous injection of 10 µg and 20µg PGE1 for erectile dysfunction. Its detailed mechanism of action has not been elucidated to date. The clinical response in patients, however, gives evidence that PGE1 has a strong relaxing effect on cavernous arteries [16, 17] and causes a marked restriction of venous outflow.

Pharmacological Treatment

Papaverine

In 1982, Virag [51] reported on the first 15 patients who received intracavernous injections of papaverine for neurogenic and psychogenic impotence. Since the discovery of this treatment for erectile impotence, reports on more than 3000 patients treated by intracavernous papaverine have been published [22]. With repeated saline perfusion after intracavernous administration of 80 mg papaverine, Virag reported an improvement in sexual activity in 68% and cure of erectile impotence in 38% of 125 patients with arterial disease over a period of 3 years.

By visual sexual stimulation in combination with low-dose papaverine (8 mg; [52]), psychogenic impotence can be distinguished from vascular impotence. In 75% of neurogenically or psychogenically impotent patients, a full erection could be achieved after an average dose of 26 mg papaverine [53]. However, Buvat et al. [6] reported that most of the patients with severe arterial or venous impotence failed to respond after intracavernous papaverine injections.

A long-term evaluation was published by Rudnick and Weidner [39] on the use of papaverine alone. They reported on 5127 injections in 126 patients with a mean follow-up of 23 months. The applied mean dose of papaverine was 42 mg with a range of 10–85 mg. For self-injection they recommended the smallest dose necessary to obtain a rigid erection. With this procedure, side effects could be minimized and prolonged erections occurred in 7.8% of patients and in 0.14% of all injections. Scarring and fibrosis of the cavernous body was reported in 3.3% of patients. Although better erections in a higher percentage of impotent men are obtained with the combined administration of papaverine and phentolamine or with PGE1 alone, papaverine mono-substance is still widely used for injection therapy because standard preparations are commercially available.

Papaverine/Phentolamine

The use of the combination of papaverine and phentolamine for intra-cavernous therapy was first propagated by Zorgniotti and Lefleur in 1985 [63].

Table 1. Intracavernous injections for diagosis and therapy of erectile impotence with the combination of papaverine/phentolamine: reports on more than 100 patients

Authors	Year	Number of patients
Robinette et al.	1986	144
Zorgniotti	1986	250
Padma-Nathan et al.	1987	201
Wetterauer et al.	1987	110
Williams et al.	1987	181
Juburi et al.	1987	100
Nellans et al.	1987	200
Trapp	1987	700
Jünemann et al.	1988	115
Bähren et al.	1988	156
Stief et al.	1988	200
Steffens et al.	1988	170
Weiske	1988	300
Levine et al.	1989	280

They used a mixture of 30 mg/ml papaverine and 0.5–1.0 mg/ml phentolamine mesylate. In 59 of 62 patients with impotence due to different causes, penetration was possible after 1 ml of the mixture had been injected as an office procedure and coitus was subsequently attempted at home. In a later report by Zorgniotti [62] on intracavernous autoinjection therapy, a pharmacologically induced erection, sufficient for sexual intercourse was obtained in 71.9% of 250 patients.

Since then, a fixed combination of 15 mg/ml papaverine and 0.5 mg/ml phentolamine has been used by the majority of investigators, resulting in roughly 4000 well-documented cases (see Table 1). Sidi et al. [42] found a response rate of 100% in neurogenic and 65.7% in vascular impotence. They observed a high rate of prolonged erections, especially in cases of neurogenic etiology. This can be explained, assuming that a denervated organ reacts maximally to neurotransmitters and transmitter-like substances.

In a double-blind study, Keogh et al. [24] compared the efficacy of papaverine with that of papaverine/phentolamine in 40 patients. A rigid erection could be obtained in 27% of patients with papaverine alone, and in 48% of patients treated with papaverine/phentolamine. The difference in favor of the combination was significant. This study demonstrated that the addition of phentolamine leads to a much higher response rate, even with a markedly reduced dose of papaverine.

In a comparative study undertaken in our hospital [58], an intraindividual comparison of the efficacy of the single agents papaverine and phentolamine with the combination of both was evaluated in 37 patients. A pathological Doppler sonographic finding of the deep cavernous arteries was found in 19 of 37 patients; pharmacocavernosography showed venous leakage in 18 of the 37 patients.

The solutions compared were:

- 15 mg/ml papaverine plus 0.5 mg/ml phentolamine
- Papaverine 15 mg/ml
- Phentolamine 0.5 mg/ml

After a thorough clinical examination and after written consent had been obtained, that dosage of the combined drug solution which caused a rigid erection of at least 20 min duration was evaluated. The first test dose of 0.25 ml was repeatedly doubled, up to a maximum of 2.0 ml (30 mg papaverine plus 1 mg phentolamine), until a response occurred. The next step was to determine the dose of papaverine alone, varying from 7.5 mg up to a maximum of 80 mg which caused an equivalent response. Finally, the erectile response to 1 mg phentolamine was evaluated.

Full response rates for papaverine were achieved in 46% of patients and for the drug combination in 60% (Fig. 1). Of the men treated with papaverine alone, 54% were nonresponders and did not produce sufficient erections, even when the highest dose of 80 mg was administered. When the drug combination was compared to phentolamine alone (Fig. 2), it was clear that the latter is an inferior treatment for organic impotence.

Table 2 shows that in 21 of 37 patients a sufficient erection cound be induced both by papaverine and the drug combination. In 16 patients the combination was more effective than the corresponding dose of papaverine alone. When using the drug combination, lesser amounts of papaverine are required for the same response. Our study showed that in the same patient, on average, 12 mg papaverine plus 0.4 mg phentolamine were necessary to induce a rigid erection. Using papaverine alone 50 mg had to be injected to induce the same reaction. These results show significantly that the addition of the α-adrenergic receptor-blocker phentolamine, allows a fourfold reduction

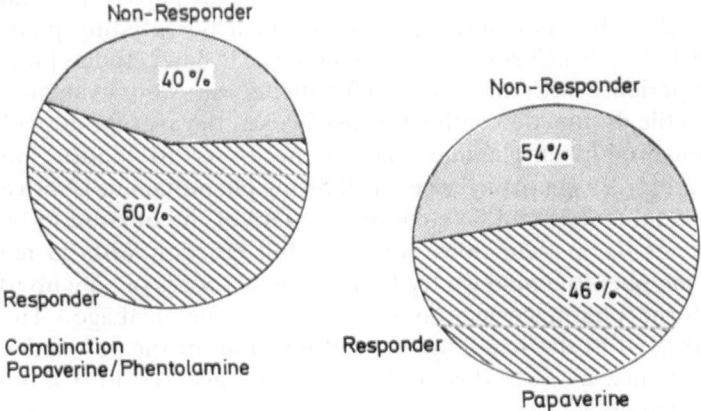

Fig. 1. Response rates for the combination papaverine/phentolamine and for papaverine alone in 37 patients

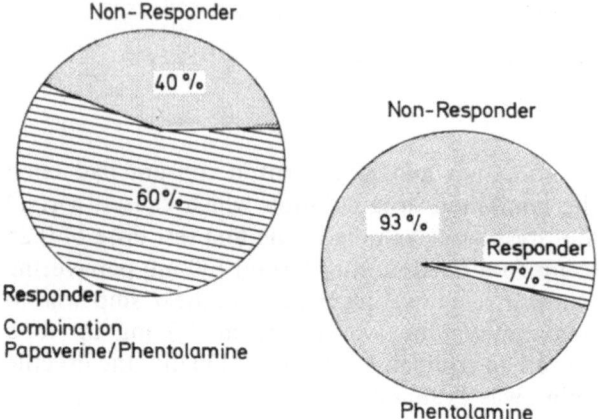

Fig. 2. Response rates for the combination papaverine/phentolamine and for phentolamine alone in 37 patients

Table 2. Comparison of response to the drug combination papaverine/phentolamine with response to the equivalent dose of papaverine and to 1 mg phentolamine in 37 patients

	Combination more effective (n)	Combination equally effective (n)	Combination less effective (n)
Papaverine	16	21	0
Phentolamine	20	17	0

n, number of patients

in the amount of papaverine required. The combination of papaverine and phentolamine therefore has not only an additive but a potentiating pharmacodynamic effect. This conclusion has been confirmed by later studies [46].

In our own experience with more than 500 patients who were evaluated and treated for erectile dysfunction within the last 5 years, the average dose of the standard papaverine/phentolamine solution necessary to induce full erection was 1.15 ml (17.25 mg papaverine and 0.58 mg phentolamine), with a range between 0.05 ml and 2.0 ml. We consider 2.0 ml of the mixture to be the maximal dose. If the patient does not get a full erection with 30 mg papaverine and 1 mg phentolamine we try PGE1 instead (doses of 5 µg up to 40 µg) and perform pharmacocavernography for venous leakage. The patients were instructed in the handling and self-injection of the vasoactive solution; in 155 patients, an 18% dose reduction was registered to 0.95 ml during long-term treatment.

During pharmacotesting, an obvious dose-dependent relationship between erectile response and etiology of impotence was reported by several

Table 3. Recipe for the papaverine/phentolamine solution used in present study

Ingredient	Amounts (g)
Papaverine hydrochloride	1.5
Phentolamine mesylate	0.05
sodium disulfite	0.1
Glucose $\times$ H_2O	4.0
Distilled water	ad 100 ml

Gassed by sterile carbon dioxide stored at 4°C

authors [23, 35, 42]. They were able to differentiate between vasculogenic and nonvascular erectile dysfunction according to the response to papaverine/phentolamine injection with a high degree of accuracy. Therefore, invasive diagnostic procedures, such as phallarteriography or cavernosography, need be performed only in selected patients.

The overall response rate to papaverine/phentolamine is about 50% to 100%, depending on patient selection and underlying etiology. It is superior to that obtained after papaverine alone [25, 58] and almost equal to PGE1 [36].

Drop-out rates during long-term autoinjection therapy vary from 5% [1] to 34% [41]. Levine et al. [29] even experienced a drop-out rate of 41% after 12 months. This might be due to the development of tolerance to the drug, which is supposed to occur in 5% to 10% during self-injection, to the spontaneous improvement of erectile function during therapy, so that further drug injection is no longer required (about 7% in our own experience), and to the changing to other treatment modalities such as penile prostheses.

The pharmaceutical preparation of intracavernously injected drug solutions seems to be important for local side effects and the stability of the solution. The papaverine/phentolamine mixture used by us (Table 3) is isosmolaric and has a pH value of 4.9. This could be responsible for the very low incidence of local pain during injection (2%) and of corporeal fibrosis, which only occurred in one out of 155 patients participating in the long-term injection program. The stability of the solution is guaranteed by the addition of the antioxidant sodium disulfite and carbon dioxide gassing during preparation. This solution remains stable for at least 6 months at storage temperatures of 4°C.

Prostaglandin E1

In vitro studies by Hedlund and Andersson [15] showed PGE1 to have a strong smooth muscle relaxing effect on human erectile tissue and cavernous artery. The first report on 88 patients with organic impotence treated with intracavernous PGE1 injections was published by Ishii et al. [19]. Based on

Table 4. Intracavernous injections with prostaglandin E1 for therapy of erectile impotence

Authors	Year	Number of patients
Stackl et al.	1988	210
Porst	1989	447
Ishii et al.	1989	135
Lue	1989	150
Hwang et al.	1989	80
Schramek et al.	1990	149
Earle et al.	1990	129
Stackl	1990	550

their encouraging results, several groups started to evaluate PGE1 for diagnostic and therapeutic intracavernous injections (Table 4).

Stackl [43] reported on 550 patients who were examined using the prostaglandin test with the injection of 20 µg PGE1 as a standard dose. The test was considered to be positive if an erection of at least 30 min duration occurred. After a positive reaction, the dosage for autoinjection therapy could be estimated according to the reaction to the test dose and was set between 5 µg and 40 µg. With the test dose of 20 µg PGE1, 70% of patients obtained an erection which lasted 0.5–7 h. Five prolonged erections lasting over 7 h and one priapism were recorded.

Porst [37] evaluated 447 patients who underwent pharmacological testing with PGE1. The responder rate was 72% with full erections lasting up to 6 h. He compared PGE1 with papaverine and papaverine/phentolamine in 249 patients and found PGE1 to be clearly superior to papaverine and, less markedly, to papaverine/phentolamine. Ishii et al. [20] observed a response rate of 62% and incomplete erections in 24%. Patients who did not respond well generally had severe vasculogenic disorders. Neither priapisms nor other severe side effects were seen.

In 149 men evaluated by Schramek et al. [40], 79% responded to the intracavernous application of PGE1 in varying doses from 5 to 40 µg with an erection sufficient for intercourse. Surprisingly, four cases of priapism were recorded, one of which occurred after the injection of only 5 µg PGE1.

In a prospective intraindividual comparison of PGE1 and papaverine/phentolamine in 50 patients [59], a response rate of 86% after PGE1 was found compared to 82% following papaverine/phentolamine injection (Table 5).

Especially in patients with venous leakage, PGE1 seems to be superior to the drug combination of papaverine/phentolamine. A disadvantage with PGE1 was the high incidence of discomfort and pain after the injection and during erection. It should be emphasized, however, that in our experience, these side effects are reduced after repeated injections. The efficacy of PGE1 has been demonstrated by several authors and it therefore represents a valid alternative to the use of papaverine/phentolamine solution.

Table 5. Intraindividual comparison of PGE1 and papaverine/phentolamine in 50 patients (Wetterauer et al. 1990)

	PGE1	Papaverine/phentolamine
Response rate	43 (86%)	41 (82%)
Average dose for response	14.7 µg	1.02 ml
Average duration of rigid erection	80.5 min	85.8 min
Prolonged erections (> 3 h)	3	5
Discomfort during erection	15	1
Pain during erection	12	0

Complications of Intracavernous Pharmacotherapy

Systemic side effects associated with vasoactive intracavernous pharmacotherapy are rarely seen. Padma-Nathan et al. [35] reported an elevation of liver enzyme levels in three patients. Other authors such as Zorgniotti and Lefleur [63], Williams et al. [61] and Stief et al. [47] did not detect any changes in hepatic enzyme levels during long-term follow-up of patients treated with papaverine/phentolamine. Orthostatic hypotension and fainting are rarely seen and occur mainly after intracavernous injection of papaverine in doses over 40 mg.

Continuous measurement of blood pressure and heart rate, which was done in a multicenter study [23], did not reveal any significant changes following the intracavernous injection of papaverine/phentolamine. Local side effects of intracavernous pharmacotherapy are ecchymosis, hematoma, temporary paresthesia, and pain; also, severe complications such as priapism and corporeal fibrosis can occur.

Ecchymosis and small local hematomas are often associated with needle puncture; they always resolve within a few days and never require therapy. We do not consider anticoagulation therapy with warfarin to be an absolute contraindication for intracavernous injections. We have two patients on warfarin therapy in our autoinjection program who have regularly used intracavernous pharmacotherapy for 2 and 3 years respectively, without major subcutaneous hematomas. They were advised to apply firm compression to the injection site for at least 3 min.

Pain during the injection is commonly caused by needle trauma and, with papaverine, by the acidic pH of the solution. Discomfort or even severe pain during erection is rarely seen with papaverine, almost never with papaverine/phentolamine, and more frequently following PGE1 injection (see above and Table 6).

Pharmacologically induced prolonged erections are frequently seen during the dose-determination period and, to a lesser extent, during autoinjection therapy and constitute the most serious side effect. With papaverine and papaverine/phentolamine, prolonged erections occur in

Table 6. Pain during erection after PGE1 injection

Incidence	Author
9.4	Porst (1989)
23.8	Hwang et al. (1989)
25.0	Lue (1989)
40.0	Schramek et al. (1990)

Table 7. Antidotes to pharmacologically induced prolonged erections

Drug	Dose (mg)
Metaraminol	2
Epinephrine	0.03
Etilefrine	5–20

5%–10% [22, 56]. During the treatment phase these are less frequent with an incidence of 0.4%.

Early intervention to reverse prolonged erections is strongly recommended because of the tissue damage that might occur after 6–12 h of persistent erection. Lue et al. [32] showed that after 6 h of pharmacologically induced prolonged erections, changes in cavernous blood pH and blood gas values occur indicating inadequate blood supply. Another reason for early intervention in cases of prolonged erection is that the antidote has a success rate of almost 100% when given within 6 h. Generally, α-adrenergic agonists such as metaraminol, epinephrine, etilefrine, and others can be used as antidotes (Table 7).

Metaraminol was first described as a therapeutic agent for priapism by Brindley [4]. Since then, it has been used to reverse prolonged erections by several investigators [48]. Acute, severe arterial hypertension and even resultant death have been reported as side effects of metaraminol [54]. Although mismanagement cannot be ruled out in those cases, one should be very careful when injecting metaraminol or other α-adrenergic agonists intracavernously. A strict dosage regimen should be followed to avoid hypertensive crises.

We still use metaraminol to relieve sustained erections and have treated about 50 patients without severe complication. Two milligrams of the drug (corresponding to 0.2 ml of the commercially available preparation) are injected by a 26G needle into one of the cavernous bodies. If detumescence does not occur within 3 min, a further 2 mg can be injected. Blood pressure has to be monitored continuously; in older, hypertensive men we usually give 10 mg nifedipine sublingually prior to the first intracavernous injection of metaraminol.

In most cases of prolonged erection, aspiration of blood from the corpus cavernosum is not necessary (except for blood gas analysis). It should be using a thick butterfly needle used as a second-line procedure to relieve priapism if the administration of metaraminol fails to induce detumescence.

Prolonged erections predominately occur during the dose-determination period in patients with neurogenic impotence. For this group especially, it is therefore recommended that the first test dose be reduced to 0.25 ml of papaverine/phentolamine or 5 µg PGE1 to reduce the risk of priapism.

Local induration at the injection site and fibrosis of the cavernous body were observed in 5.4% during long-term employment of papaverine or papaverine/phentolamine for the treatment of erectile dysfunction [8, 22]. Small nodules in the tunica albuginea may be caused at the site of injection by the needle trauma, whereas corporeal fibrosis is probably a reaction to the injected pharmacological agent. It is very difficult to compare the data on side effects derived from different authors, since not only the injected agents themselves but differences in drug concentrations, pH values, and pharmaceutical components of the solutions may influence local side effects such as fibrotic lesions of the cavernous tissue.

Summarizing our side effects during long-term treatment on 8000 recorded autoinjections using papaverine/phentolamine (Table 8), we observed seven prolonged erections that could be terminated by metaraminol injections. Two patients arbitrarily increased the dose, one administered a second injection within a short period, and in four patients no explanation exists for the occurrence of prolonged erections. Small hematomas at the site of injections were also observed; on three occasions, bleeding from the urethra was reported due to an inaccurate injection technique. No cases of local inflammation or cavernitis were seen. One patient developed a fibrotic plaque and a corporeal induration leading to penile deviation. In nearly 10% of all injections the resulting erection was incomplete, and therefore, in about 3% coital penetration was not possible.

The reported complications and side effects of intracavernous injections show that a strict selection of patients, a detailed informed consent of the patient, and thorough instruction on injection technique are necessary. None

Table 8. Complications of CAT in 8000 recorded injections

Complication	Number of injections
Prolonged erection	7
Hematoma at site of injection	128
Bleeding ex urethra	3
Inflammation	0
Fibrosis	1
Incomplete rigidity	884
Intercourse not possible due to lack of rigidity	254

of the above-mentioned drugs used for intracavernous pharmacotherapy has been approved by any national health authority for this type of administration. Therefore a strict surveillance is mandatory to detect and register possible side effects.

Conclusions

Intracavernous pharmacotherapy has become a cornerstone in the therapy of erectile dysfuction within the last 5 years. Most of the patients suffering from chronic organic impotence can now be treated successfully and can be offered the chance to lead an adequate sexual life. Compared to other drugs used for intracavernous injections, papaverine has only a moderate response rate. In animal experiments, a high rate of cavernous fibrosis following repeated papaverine injections was observed. The major advantage of the combination of papaverine and phentolamine is a fourfold reduction in the amount of papaverine required. Addition of the α-adrenergic receptor-blocking agent phentolamine not only has an additive but a potentiating effect on induced erections. With the combination of both drugs a significantly higher response rate and a better diagnostic discrimination of patients with venous leakage can be obtained.

Concerning efficacy and side effects, the fixed combination of 15 mg/ml papaverine and 0.5 mg/ml phentolamine constitutes the best documented form of therapy that has been applied and recorded in over 4000 patients since 1985.

PGE1 has an equivalent response rate and seems, especially in patients with venous leakage, to be superior to the combination. With PGE1 prolonged erections are seldom seen and corporeal fibrosis seems to be exceptionally rare. However, long-term follow-up in large trials with PGE1 is still lacking. A disadvantage of PGE1 for intracavernous therapy is a high rate of discomfort and pain during erection in up to 50% of patients.

Based on the experience with different agents and their known efficacy and side effects, the combination of papaverine and phentolamine as well as PGE1 alone seem to be choices of equal value for intracavernous pharmacotherapy. However, research is continuing to test other drugs and neurotransmitters with perhaps even fewer complications and side effects.

References

1. Bähren W, Scherb WH, Gall H et al. (1988) Effects of intracavernous self-injection therapy on self-esteem and partnership in patients with chronic erectile dysfunction. Third Biennial World Meeting on Impotence, Boston, Mass, Oct. 6–9

2. Bénard F, Stief CG, Bosch R, Diederichs W, Lue TF, Tanagho EA (1988) Systemic infusion of epinephrine: its effect on erection. Third Biennial World Meeting on Impotence, Boston, Mass, Oct. 6–9
3. Brindley GS (1983) Cavernosal alpha-blockage: A new technique for investigating and treatig erectile impotence. Br J Psychiatry 143:332–337
4. Brindley GS (1984) New treatment for priapism. Lancet I:220–221
5. Brindley GS (1986) Pilot experiments on the actions of drugs injected into the human corpus cavernosum penis. Br J Pharmacol 87:495–500
6. Buvat J, Lemaire A, Marcolin G et al. (1987) Intracavernous injection of papaverine (ICIP). Assessment of its diagnostic and therapeutic value in 100 impotent patients. World J Urol 5:150–155
7. Conti G (1952) L'érection du penis humain et ses bases morphologico-vasculaires. Acta Anatomica 14:217–262
8. Corriere JN, Fishman IJ, Benson GS, Carlton CE (1988) Development of fibrotic penile lesions secondary to the intracorporeal injection of vasoactive agents. J Urol 140:615–617
9. De la Torre (1978) US Patent no 4.127.118
10. Diederichs W, Lue TF (1989) Reduktion der Sympathikuswirkung auf die Erektion durch Phentolamin. 41. Kongreß der Dtsch Ges für Urologie, Freiburg, 4. – 7. Okt.
11. Domer FR, Wessler G, Brown RL et al. (1978) Involvement of the sympathetic nervous system in the urinary bladder internal sphincter. Invest Urol 15:404
12. Earle CM, Keogh EJ, Wisniewski ZS, Tulloch GS et al. (1990) Prostaglandin E1 therapy for impotence, comparison with papaverine. J Urol 143:57–59
13. Ebner V von (1900) Über klappenartige Vorrichtungen in den Arterien der Schwellkörper. Anatom Anzeiger (Ergänzungsheft 7) 18:79–81
14. Goldstein I, Payton TR, de Tejada IS, Krane RJ (1985) Pharmacologic erections: Role in the treatment of neurologic impotence. J Urol 133:261
15. Hedlund H, Andersson KE (1985) Contraction and relaxation induced by some prostanoids in isolated human penile erectile tissue and cavernous artery. J Urol 134:1245–1250
16. Hwang T, Lue TF, Yang CR, Chang CL (1989) Drug-induced penile blood flow study: effect of papaverine versus prostaglandin E1. J Urol 141:261 A
17. Hwang T, Yang CR, Wang SJ et al. (1989) Impotence evaluated by the use of prostaglandin E1. J Urol 141:1357–1359
18. Ishii N, Watanabe H, Irisawa C, Kikuchi Y (1986) Therapeutic trial with prostaglandin E1 for organic impotence. Second World Meeting on Impotence, Prague
19. Ishii N, Watanabe H, Irisawa C et al. (1986) Studies on male sexual impotence. Jap J Urol 77:954
20. Ishii N, Watanabe H, Irisawa C et al. (1989) Intracavernous injection of prostaglandin E1 for the treatment of erectile impotence. J Urol 141:323–325
21. Juburi AZ, O'Donnell PD (1987) Experience with a new impotence therapy: penile self-injection. J Urol 37:208A
22. Jünemann K-P, Alken P (1989) Pharmacotherapy of erectile dysfunction: a review. Int J Impotence Res 1:71–93
23. Jünemann K-P, Jecht E, Müller-Mattheis V et al. (1988) Offene Multicenterstudie zur Differentialdiagnostik der erektilen Dysfunktion mit einer Papaverin-Phentolamin-Kombination (By 023). Urologe A 27:2–7
24. Keogh EJ, Earle CM, Wisniewski ZS, Lord PJ, Tulloch AGS (1988) Comparison of vasoactive agents for impotence. Third Biennial World Meeting on Impotence, Boston, Mass Oct 6–9
25. Keogh EJ, Watters GR, Earle CM et al. (1989) Treatment of impotence by intrapenile injections. Am comparison of papaverine versus papaverine and phentolamine: a double-blind, crossover trial. J Urol 142:726–728
26. Kiely EA, Ignotus P, Williams G (1987) Penile function following intracavernosal injection of vasoactive agents or saline. Br J Urol 59:473–476
27. Kiss F (1921) Anatomisch-histologische Untersuchungen über die Erektion. Z Anat 61:455–521

28. Klinge E, Sjöstrand, HO (1974) Contraction and relaxation of the retractor penis muscle and the penile artery of the bull. Acta Phys Scand (Suppl) 420
29. Levine S, Althof S, Turner L et al. (1989) Side effects of self-administration of intracavernous papaverine and phentolamine for the treatment of impotence. J Urol 141:54–57
30. Lue TF (1989) Editorial comment on Ishii et at. (1989) Intracavernous injection of prostaglandin E1. J Urol 141:325
31. Lue TF, Takamura T, Schmidt RA et al. (1983) Hemodynamics of erection in the monkey. J Urol 130:1237–1240
32. Lue TF, Hellstrom WJ, McAninch JW, Tanagho EA (1986) Priapism: a refined approach to diagnosis and treatment. J Urol 136:104–108
33. Nellans RE, Leland RE, Kramer-Levien D (1987) New treatment for impotence: pharmacologic erection. Medical Aspects of Human Sexuality, March 20–28
34. Padma-Nathan H, Goldstein J, Azadzoi R et al. (1986) In vivo and in vitro studies on the physiology of penile erection. Semin Urol 4:209–216
35. Padma-Nathan H, Goldstein I, Payton T, Krane RJ (1987) Intracavernosal pharmacotherapy: the pharmacologic erection program. World J Urol 5: 160–165
36. Porst H (1988) Stellenwert von Prostaglandin E1 (PGE1) in der Diagnostik der erektilen Dysfunktion (ED) im Vergleich zu Papaverin und Papaverin/Phentolamin bei 61 Patienten mit ED. Urologe A 27:22–26
37. Porst H (1989) Prostaglandin E1 bei erektiler Dysfunktion. Urologe A 28:94–98
38. Robinette MA, Moffat MJ (1986) Intracorporeal injection of papaverine and phentolamine in the management of impotence. Br J Urol 58:692–695
39. Rudnick J, Weidner W (1990) Schwellkörper-Autoinjekionstherapie mit Papaverin-Monosubstanz — eine mittelfristige Verlaufsbeobachtung. In: Wetterauer U, Stief CG (Hrsg) Diagnostik und Therapie der erektilen Dysfunktion mit vasoaktiven Substanzen. de Gruyter, Berlin New York, S 75–80
40. Schramek P, Dorninger R, Waldhauser M et al. (1990) Prostaglandin E1 in erectile dysfunction. Efficiency and incidence of priapism. Br J Urol 65:68–71
41. Sidi AA, Chen KK (1987) Clinical experience with vasoactive intracavernous pharmacotherapy for the treatment of impotence. World J Urol 5:156–159
42. Sidi AA, Cameron JS, Duffy LM, Lange PH (1986) Intracavernous drug-induced erections in the management of male erectile dysfunction: experience with 100 patients. J Urol 135:704–706
43. Stackl W (1990) Prostaglandin E1 zur Therapie der erektilen Dysfunktion. In: Wetterauer U, Stief CG (Hrsg) Diagnostik und Therapie der erektilen Dysfunktion mit vasoaktiven Substanzen. de Gruyter, Berlin New York, S 91–96
44. Stackl W, Hasun R, Marberger M (1988) Intracavernous injection of prostaglandin E1 in impotent men. J Urol 140:66–68
45. Steffens J, Postma H, Steffens L (1988) Ergebnisse und Akzeptanz der Schwellkörper-autoinjektionstherapie (SKAT) bei organischer erektiler Dysfunktion. Urologe A 27:14–16
46. Stief CG, Wetterauer U (1988) Erectile Responses to intracavernous papaverine and phentolamine: Comparison of single and combined delivery. J Urol 140:1415–1416
47. Stief CG, Thon W, Scherb W et al. (1987) Zwei Jahre Erfahrungen mit der Schwellkörper-Autoinjektionstherapie (SKAT). Urologe A 26:294–296
48. Stief CG, Gilbert P, Wetterauer U et al. (1987) Metaraminol – ein Antidot bei SKAT-bedingter prolongierter Erektion. Urologe A 25:164–166
49. Stief CG, Bähren W, Gall H, Scherb W (1988) Functional evaluation of penile hemodynamics. J Urol 139:734–737
50. Trapp JD (1987) Pharmacologic erection program for the treatment of impotence. South Med J 80:426–427
51. Virag R (1982) Intracavernous injection of papaverine for erectile failure. Lancet II:938
52. Virag R, Bouilly R, Daniel C, Virag H (1985) Intracavernous injection of papaverine and other vasoactive drugs: a new era in the diagnosis and treatment of impotence. In:

Virag R, Virag H (eds) Proceedings of the First World Meeting on Impotence. Ceri, Paris, pp 187–194
53. Virag R, Daniel C, Sussman H, Bouilly P, Virag H (1986) Self-intracavernous injection of vasoactive drugs for the treatment of psychogenic and neurologic impotence (late results in 109 patients). Proc 2nd World Meeting Impotence, Prague
54. Watters GR, Keogh EJ, Carati CJ et al (1988) Prolonged erections following intracorporeal injection of medications to overcome impotence. Br J Urol 62:173–175
55. Weiske WH (1988) Prolonged erection by vasoactive drugs. Third Biennial World Meeting on Impotence. Boston, Mass, Oct. 6–9, p 89
56. Wetterauer U, Zentgraf M (1988) Impotenz: Komplikationen der Autoinjektionstherapie – eine Übersicht. Akt Urol 19:315–320
57. Wetterauer U, Stief CG, Sommerkamp H (1987) Intracavernous application of papaverine and phentolamine for erectile dysfunction. Experience with 110 cases. Proceedings 5th Int Forum of Andrology, Paris
58. Wetterauer U, Weiske WH, Stief CG, Zentgraf M (1988) Intraindividual comparison of the efficacy of the intracavernously injected single agents papaverine and phentolamine with the combination of both. Third Biennial World Meeting on Impotence, Boston, Mass, Oct. 6–9
59. Wetterauer U, Koppermann U, Lühmann R, Hakenberg O, Sommerkamp H (1990) Pharmakokinetik von Papaverin und Phentolamin bei intracavernöser Applikation. 11th Int Symposium Ludwig-Boltzmann-Institut, Vienna, Febr. 22–24
60. Wetterauer U, Koppermann U, Bischoff R, Sommerkamp H (1990) Intraindividueller Vergleich von Prostaglandin E1 und einem Papaverin-Phentolamin-Gemisch zur Erektionsauslösung bei Patienten mit erektiler Dysfunktion. 11th Int Symposium Ludwig-Boltzmann-Institut, Vienna, Febr. 22–24
61. Williams G, Mulcahy MJ, Kiely EA (1987) Impotence: treatment by autoinjection of vasoactive drugs. Br Med J 295:595–596
62. Zorgniotti AW (1986) Corpus cavernosum blockade for impotence: practical aspects and results in 250 cases. J Urol 135:306A
63. Zorgniotti AW, Lefleur RS (1985) Auto-injection of the corpus cavernous with a vasoactive drug combination for vasculogenic impotence. J Urol 133:39–41

Andropen – Intracavernous Self-Injection Pen for Pharmacotherapy in Erectile Dysfunction

W.F. Thon

Intracavernous injection of vasoactive drugs is a safe and effective treatment in patients with erectile dysfunction [1, 2, 5–7, 9–11]. Cavernous autoinjection therapy (CAT) is an accepted method of treatment for patients with neurogenic and arterial etiologies of erectile dysfunction. CAT is also used as an adjuvant treatment to psychotherapy in cases of psychogenic erectile dysfunction.

Commonly used drugs for vasoactive intracavernous pharmaco-therapy are papaverine hydrochloride alone [12] or in combination with phetolamine [14] and prostaglandin E1 [13]. One major disadvantage encountered by the patient is the filling of the syringe, which is a precarious maneuver for the average patient. Since this procedure must be carried out just prior to the injection into one cavernous body, it can interfere with sexual foreplay.

To improve drug administration, a pen similar to an insulin pen has been developed for intracavernous self-injection therapy. The Andropen consists of a diaposable single injection cartridge containing the vasoactive drug and the driver mechanism (Fig. 1).

The drug used for pharmacological testing and treatment of erectile dysfunction is a combination of 15 mg/ml papaverine hydrochloride and 0.5 mg/ml phentolamine mesylate (Androskat, Tosse, Hamburg, FRG). The physico-chemical stability of this vasoactive mixture was recently reported to be 6 months at room temperature with a reasonable storage interval of 2 months if exposure to higher temperatures cannot be excluded [4]

In each patient the effective individual dosage for an erection sufficient for vaginal penetration and intercourse is determined using RigiScan real-time penile tumescence and rigidity monitoring during visual erotic stimulation [3]. The smallest intracavernous test dosage is 0.25 ml. If necessary, this dosage is increased until a rigidity of at least 70% that lasts for more than 10 min is achieved. Once the proper dosage has been determined the patient learns the injection technique and is required to perform self-injections with the pen during medical supervision.

After the dosage titration phase has been concluded, patients are generally able to handle the pen after only two self-injections. The injection volume of 0.25 to 2.0 ml is predetermined and controlled by a safety key, which only the physician has access to, in order to avoid involuntary overdosage. The cartridge and the driver can be screwed together without

U. Jonas et al. (Eds.) Erectile Dysfunction
© Springer-Verlag Berlin Heidelberg 1991

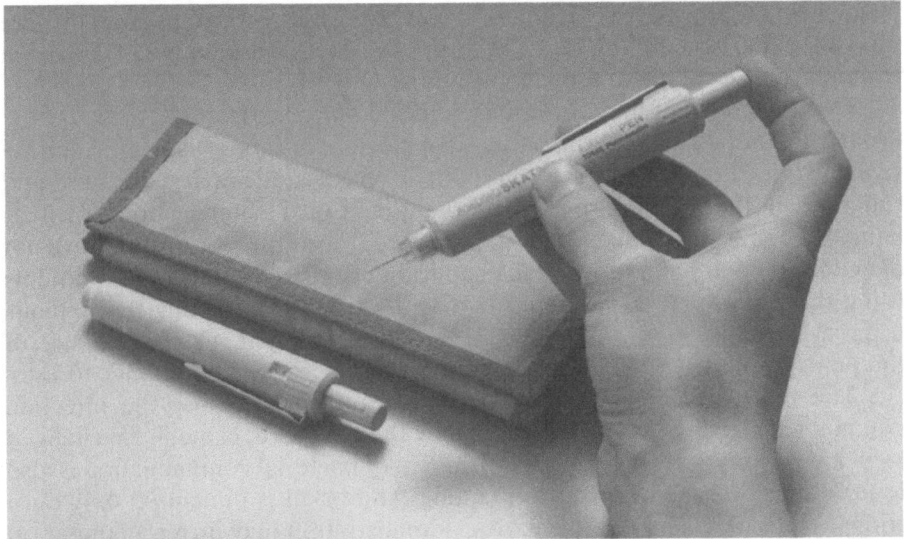

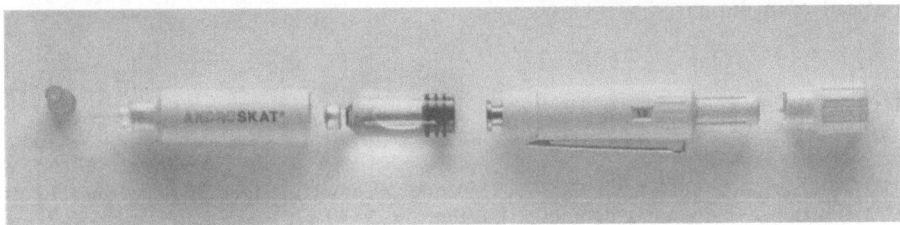

Fig. 1. Intracavernous safety autoinjection pensystem: Andropen

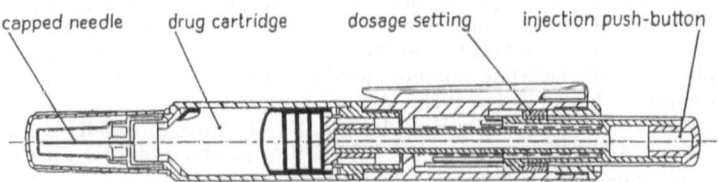

Fig. 2. Construction outline of Andropen

compromising the sterility of the vasoactive solution. Upon application, the front end of the Insuject needle pierces the rubber cartridge cap and thus prepares the pen for injection (Fig. 2). The maximum excursion of the plugger driver is preset with the key. The preset volume can only be expelled once even if the patient inadvertently, or on purpose, presses the injection button again.

Andropen, Androskat cartridges, and ultrafine 26G needles are prescribed in quantities sufficient for a 5-week interval at a given application frequency of one to two injections weekly. Follow-up appointments are scheduled at 5-week intervals in order to monitor possible changes in response and to perform a penile examination.

Complications of intracavernous autoinjection therapy are avoided if the dosage is cautiously determined by RigiScan real-time monitoring during visual erotic stimulation and if the patient receives adequate education and training on the proper injection technique. Local complications such as hematoma, infection, inadvertent injection of the urethra, or fibrosis have not been observed in patients using the pen for more than 12 months [8]. Patients using the Andropen do not need more education and training tha patients using syringes for CAT. Patients are enthusiastic about the convenience of the pen system and prefer the pen to a syringe because it is simpler to use.

The risk of an involuntary overdose is reduced because the injection volume, which has been predetermined by the physician, can only be changed by using the physician's safety key. The risk of bacterial contamination is also reduced because the cartridge containing Androskat is punctured only once and is disposable. The improved drug administration may increase long-term patient compliance.

References

1. Al-Juburi AZ, O'Donnell PD (1987) Penile self-injection for impotence in patients after radical cystectomy-ileal loop. Urology 30:29–30
2. Gasser TC, Roach RM, Larsen EH, Madsen PO, Bruskewitz RC (1987) Intracavernous self-injection with phentolamine and papaverine for the treatment of impotence. J Urol 137:678–680
3. Giesbers AAGM, Bruins JL, Kramer AEJL, Jonas U (1987) New methods in the diagnosis of impotence: RigiScan penile tumescence and rigidity monitoring and diagnostic papaverine hydrochloride injection. World J Urol 5:173–176
4. Hadzija BW, Mattocks AM, Stahl GM (1988) Physicochemical stability of papaverine hydrochloride-phentolamine mesylate mixtures used for intracavernous injection: a preliminary evaluation. J Urol 140(1):64–65
5. Ishii N, Watanabe H, Irisawa C, Kikuchi Y, Kubota Y, Kawamura S, Suzuki K, Chiba R, Tokiwa M, Shirai M (1989) Intracavernous injection of prostaglandin E1 for the treatment of erectile impotence. J Urol 141(2):323–325
6. Kiely EA, Williams G, Goldie L (1987) Assessment of the immediate and long-term effects of pharmacologically induced penile erections in the treatment of psychogenic and organic impotence. Br J Urol 59:164–169
7. Kursh ED, Bodner DR, Renick MI, Althof SE, Turner L, Risen C, Levine SB (1988) Injection therapy for impotence. Urol Clin North Am 15(4):625–629
8. Seidl E, Thon WF, Kramer AEJL, Jonas U (1989) The use of a preset self-injection pen for intracavernous auto-injection therapy in erectile impotence. J Urol 141:273 A
9. Sidi AA, Cameron JS, Duffy LM, Lange PH (1986) Intracavernous drug-induced erections in the management of male erectile dysfunction: experience with 100 patients: J Urol 135(4):704–706
10. Stackl W, Hasun R, Marberger M (1988) Intracavernous injection of prostaglandin E1 in impotent men. J Urol 140(1):66–68
11. Stief CG, Gall H, Scherb W, Baehren W (1988) Mid-term results of autoinjection therapy for erectile dysfunction. Urology 31(6):483–485

12. Virag R (1982) Intracavernous injection of papaverine for erectile failure. Letter of the editor. Lancet 2:938
13. Virag R, Adaikan PG (1987) Effects of prostaglandin E1 on penile erection and erectile failure (letter). J Urol 137(5):1010
14. Zorgniotti AW, Lefleur RS (1985) Auto-injection of the corpus cavernosum with a vasocative drug combination for vasculogenic impotence. J Urol 133:39–41

Reconstructive Vascular Surgery for Impotence

F.J. Levine and I. Goldstein

Erectile function is dependent not only upon the hemodynamic interaction of arterial inflow and perfusion pressure but also on the development of an adequate venous outflow resistance [1–3]. Functional impairment of either arterial inflow, or veno-occlusive function, or both may result in erectile dysfunction. Vascular reconstructive procedures aim to correct any existing abnormalities identified in penile arterial and veno-occlusive hemodynamics in order to restore adequate erectile function. Though both of these hemodynamic processes interact during erection, for purposes of clarity this article will discuss separately arterial reconstructive procedures designed to increase perfusion pressure and flow to the corpora cavernosa and procedures designed to increase resistance to corporal venous outflow.

Arterial Reconstructive Procedures for Impotence

Arterial Hemodynamics of Erection

The cavernosal artery, running medially within each corpus, provides arterial inflow to the erectile tissue. Branching from each artery are the helicine arterioles that serve as the primary resistance vessels to arterial inflow. During erection, arteriolar smooth muscle relaxation occurs. The resultant lowered arteriolar resistance allows transmission of the systemic blood pressure from the cavernosal artery to the lacunar spaces. The corporal body pressure that exists during erection is equal to the cavernosal artery perfusion pressure minus the pressure loss from corporal venous drainage [4]. Transient increases in corporal body pressure will occur from contraction of the striated perineal muscles or from externally squeezing the penis [3].

In the flaccid state, arteriolar smooth muscle tone is increased and penile corporal hemodynamics reflect a state of low arterial inflow. The contracted helicine arterioles produce a resistance bed to arterial inflow shielding the lacunar spaces from the systemic arterial pressure in the cavernosal artery [1–3, 5–7]. The corporal body pressure in the flaccid state approximates systemic venous pressure [8].

U. Jonas et al. (Eds.) Erectile Dysfunction
© Springer-Verlag Berlin Heidelberg 1991

Hemodynamics of Arterial Impotence

Organic erectile dysfunction appears to occur frequently as a consequence of abnormal corporal arterial hemodynamics [4]. The common result is a corporal body pressure during erection that develops slowly and is too low to produce an erection sufficiently rigid for successful coitus (Fig 1).

Atherosclerotic vascular disease and traumatic arterial occlusion are the most common pathologic mechanisms affecting arterial inflow in the hypogastric-cavernous pathway. Atherosclerotic disease tends to be more diffuse and is associated with a history of vascular risk factors such as cigarette smoking, hypertension, hypercholesterolemia, diabetes mellitus, or a family history of vascular disease [9–13]. Traumatic occlusion tends to be more focal in nature and is associated with a history of pelvic fracture or blunt perineal trauma such as a fall or sports injury [14–18]. Occlusive arterial lesions may lead to a reduction in inflow, limiting the rate of corporal body filling, and diminished perfusion pressure, decreasing the maximal corpoal body pressure attainable with sexual stimulation.

Evaluation of Arterial Hemodynamics

Our evaluation of the patient complaining of erectile dysfunction begins initially with a thorough history and physical examination. The history details present and premorbid sexual activity and investigates possible medical, pharmacologic, and traumatic causes of impotence. The physical examination is performed to identify any genital, endocrine, neurologic, or vascular abnormalities. Following this, noninvasive studies, if indicated, are performed. Such studies may include dorsal nerve biothesiometric testing, somatosensory evoked potential testing, sacral latency testing, Doppler ultrasonographic determination of the penile-brachial index, endocrine screening, nocturnal penile tumescence and rigidity monitoring, office intracavernosal injection testing, and psychological interviews. If this initial

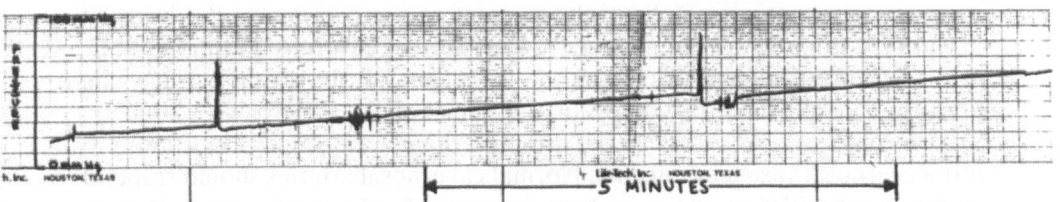

Fig. 1. Pharmacocavernosometry in a patient with organic erectile dysfunction secondary to abnormal corporal arterial hemodynamics. There is a slow rise in corporal body pressure (scale 0–100 mmHg) in response to intracavernosal smooth muscle relaxing agents, resulting in an erection that develops too slowly and is not adequately rigid for successful coitus. BP: 148/75 mmHg, MAP: 115 mmHg

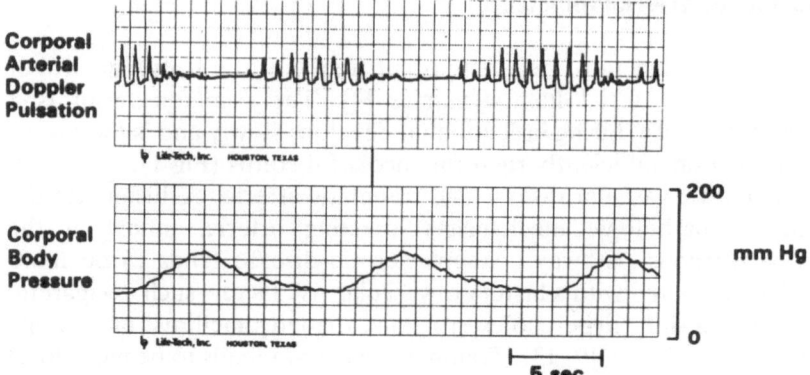

Fig. 2. Cavernosal artert systolic occlusion pressure determination in a patient with a lesion proximal to this artery. Brachial artery systolic pressure was 130 mm Hg. Doppler pulsations (*above*) are absent when the corporal body pressure is raised above 80 mm Hg (*below*), and return when corporal body pressure again drops below 80 mm Hg. The pressure gradient between the brachial and cavernosal arteries is, therefore, 50 mm Hg

evaluation leads to a suspicion of nonendocrinologic, nonneurologic organic impotence, and if the patient wishes to consider a possible vascular reconstructive procedure, invasive erectile function studies are considered.

The initial invasive study of erectile function that we perform is dynamic infusion pharmacocavernosometry and pharmacocavernosography (DICC) [19]. Two phases of this four-phase study assess the corporal arterial response to intracavernosal injection of papaverine hydrochloride (45 mg) and phentolamine mesylate (2.5 mg). In phase one of this study, the rise from baseline corporal body pressure, measured in mm Hg, is evaluated in response to these intracavernosal pharmacologic agents. Cavernosal artery hemodynamics are evaluated in phase three by determining both the right and left cavernosal artery systolic occlusion pressures which are compared with the brachial artery systolic pressure.

Normal values for the DICC study have been published [19]. The normal corporal body pressure response to the intracavernosal pharmacologic agents approximates at least 90% of the mean systemic arterial blood pressure, and the cavernosal artery systolic occlusion pressure approximates the brachial artery systolic pressure. In patients with abnormal cavernosal artery systolic occlusion pressures, focused, pulsed Doppler ultrasonography may be performed as the next stage in evaluating the cavernosal arteries [3, 20] (Fig. 2). This procedure records arterial flow and diameter changes in response to intracavernosal vasoactive agents. Normal cavernosal arteries should respond with at least a 75% increase in diameter and a flow rate of at least 25 cm/s [20]. Atherosclerotic cavernosal arteries will show only minimal dilation and a low blood flow velocity. Cavernosal arterial dilation may be normal, however, despite significant proximal arterial occlusive pathology. This may be seen especially in the patient felt to be the optimal revascularization

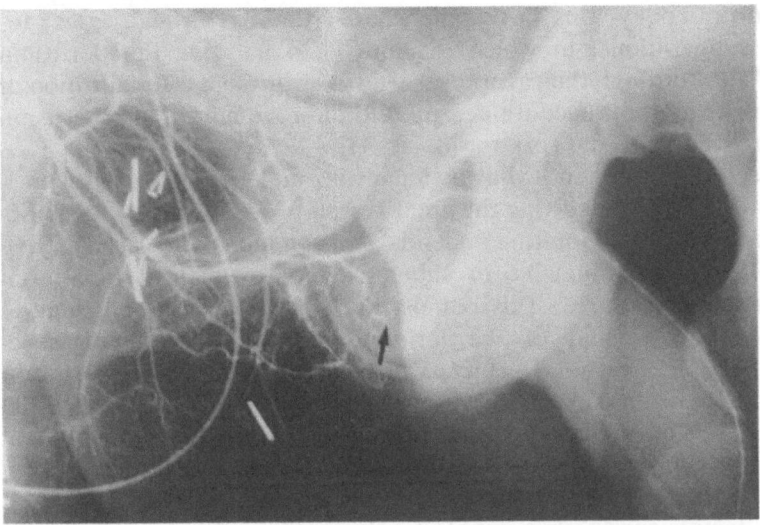

Fig. 3. Pharmacoangiography in an impotent patient with an abnormal right cavernosal artery systolic occlusion pressure. The arteriogram shows an occluded cavernosal artery (*arrow*) inferior to the pubic symphysis

candidate, that is, the young man with traumatic occlusive injury to the internal pudendal or common penile artery.

At our institution, selective internal pudendal pharmacoarteriography is considered only in those revascularization candidates whose response to intracavernosal pharmacologic agents and whose cavernosal artery systolic occlusion pressures during DICC show abnormalities, and who show only absent or focal, proximal veno-occlusive dysfunction on cavernosography. Selective injection of the internal pudendal artery is performed following intra-arterial and intracavernosal injection of vasoactive agents in order to optimally visualize the hypogastric-cavernous arterial bed [21, 22]. This study is utilized to defined the anatomic pattern of occlusive arterial disease and allows the planning of appropriate vascular surgical repair (Fig. 3).

Penile Arterial Revascularization

Occlusive pathology diminishing the perfusion pressure and arterial flow to the lacunar spaces may exist anywhere along the arterial supply to the corpora. This includes the proximal large vessels, the aorta and the iliac arteries, as well as the distal arteries of the hypogastric-cavernous bed, and may result in diminished rigidity of the erect penis and increased time to maximal erection [9]. The aim of all penile arterial revascularization procedures is to increase the arterial inflow and perfusion pressure to the corpora during sexual stimulation, thus improving the corporal body pressure during erection. Today, this is accomplished primarily through artery-to-artery bypass operations, in which the aim is to improve the perfusion pressure and flow through the cavernosal artery, or through arterialization of the deep dorsal vein, a procedure designed to improve inflow and perfusion pressure retrograde into the corpora [8, 23–33].

It has been our experience that patients with multiple sites of atherosclerotic arterial occlusion involving the great vessels as well as the hypogastric-cavernous bed, such as the internal pudendal and common penile artery, have not realized long-term objective or subjective improvement with arterial revascularization procedures. This is most likely the result of concomitant atherosclerotic involvement of the terminal artery of the hypogastric-cavernous bed, the cavernosal artery, which prevents increased perfusion pressure and flow to the lacunar spaces as a result inadequate distal arterial run-off. It has also been our experience that these patients have concomitant corporal veno-occlusive dysfunction presumed secondary to a loss of compliance of the fibroelastic frame of the penis as a result of aging or vascular risk factors such as hypercholesterolemia [34–38].

There are patients who on arteriography show occlusive lesions that are focal in nature and proximal to the cavernosal artery in the internal pudendal or common penile artery. This has most often been found in young men who report a history of pelvic fracture or perineal trauma from a sporting or straddle injury [14–16, 18]. These patients may present with impotence immediately following the injury or may present several years after the blunt traumatic episode. The injury may cause arterial endothelial injury which may itself, or in combination with other vascular risk factors, cause plaque formation at the site of the trauma and lead to focal arterial occlusion [39–40]. We consider treating these patients with an anastomosis of the inferior epigastric artery to the proximal dorsal penile artery if a communication between the dorsal and cavernosal arteries is shown to exist distal to the occlusion. In these selected patients, the rationale for this bypass surgical procedure is to increase perfusion pressure and inflow to the cavernosal artery retrograde from the proximal dorsal artery with the presumption that there will be adequate arterial run-off.

There are also young patients with a history of blunt perineal trauma who are shown to have occlusive cavernosal artery disease localized to its origin off the common penile artery or in its proximal third [14–18]. We consider treating these patients with an inferior epigastric artery or dorsal artery anastomosis to an isolated deep dorsal vein segment that communicates with several emissary veins. The rationable for this surgical procedure is an attempt to establish retrograde arterial flow through the emissary veins to the subtunical venules and ulitmately to the corporal lacunar spaces. We have seen that in more than 50% of patients emissary vein valves, as distinguished from dorsal vein valves, have impeded the retrograde recovery of methylene blue from the corpora following its injection into the isolated dorsal vein segment.

Proximal Procedures

Proximal arterial revascularization procedures may be considered in the unique situation where the occlusive pathology exists exclusively in the larger vessels such as the distal aorta, common iliac artery, or the origin of the hypogastric artery and where normal cavernosal arteries also exist. Aortoiliac or iliacohypogastric bypass operations using saphenous vein or synthetic graft material may improve distal arterial inflow and perfusion pressure. Endarterectomies may be performed to remove occlusive arterial plaque at the origin of the internal iliac artery or in the proximal internal pudendal artery [24, 41].

Distal Procedures

Microsurgical arterial revascularization procedures for the treatment of erectile dysfunction were first introduced in 1973 with the creation of an end-to-side anastomosis between the inferior epigastric artery and a defect made in the tunica albuginea of the corpus cavernosum (Michal I) [42]. Initial results of this operation showed success rates of 60%–70% which subsequently decreased to 40% after 1 year, possibly due to inadequate arterial run-off [23]. One series reported a 100% failure rate at 1 year due to graft thrombosis, though many patients had initially improved [25]. Priapism and corporal fibrosis were additional complications of this procedure which now is rarely performed.

The success of any type of distal microvascular repair in restoring potency is dependent upon several factors including adequate flow and perfusion pressure in the neoarterial inflow source, a technically sound anastomosis, and sufficient arterial run-off into the distal penile vessels. If care is not taken to ensure that these principles are specifically attended to anastomotic thromboses may occur.

Today, microvascular arterial revascularization procedures performed for erectile dysfunction primarily use a neoarterial inflow source anastomosed to the dorsal artery or isolated dorsal vein segment [23–27]. The neoarterial source is usually the inferior epigastric artery or an arterialized saphenous vein [23]. If preoperative arteriography demonstrates an occlusive lesion in the internal pudendal or common penile artery, and the dorsal and cavernosal arteries are shown to bifurcate from the common penile artery, then the neoarterial source can be anastomosed end-to-end to the proximal dorsal artery allowing retrograde arterial flow from the dorsal to the cavernosal artery. If there exist cavernosal artery branches coming directly off the dorsal artery distal to the site of arterial occlusion, a neoarterial anastomosis to the distal dorsal artery can be performed allowing improved flow into the corpora via these branches. Careful attention to a properly performed arteriogram will guide the surgeon toward the proper anastomoses to achieve the goal of bypassing proximal arterial lesions.

Surgical Technique for Isolation and Preparation of the Neoarterial Source.
It is important to adequately isolate and prepare the neoarterial inflow source
to insure that it is of appropriate length and is not injured during harvesting.
Most commonly the inferior epigastric artery is used as the neoarterial inflow
source. In our technique the inferior epigastric artery is harvested through a
paramedian abdominal incision. Alternative incisions include a midline or
transverse incision. In all cases, the rectus muscle is reflected to identify the
artery and its accompanying two veins. The decision to use the right or left
inferior epigastric artery is dependent upon sufficient arterial length, absence
of occlusive lesions especially at the origin, and the presence of distal arterial
branching. An arterial segment 14–16 cm in length is isolated beginning at the
vessel's origin at the external iliac artery and extending distally towards the
umbilicus. Microbipolar cautery or fine silk ties are used to control the small
proximal branches to the pelvis, rectus muscle, or abdominal side wall. No
attempt is made to separate the artery from its veins so as to prevent arterial
injury and vasospasm. Distally, near the umbilicus, the inferior epigastric
artery commonly bifurcates and both branches should be preserve if more
than one microsurgical anastomosis is planned.

Alternatively, the saphenous vein may be used as the neoarterial inflow
source. In this case, a segment 14–16 cm long may be harvested either
subinguinally in the thigh or at the medial malleolus in the lower calf. Dorsal
veins of the foot, hand, or forearm have also been used. The vessel is reversed
to prevent valvular obstruction to arterial flow. The proximal anastomosis is
usually performed to the femoral artery but may be fashioned end-to-end to
the proximal third of a previously ligated inferior epigastric artery.

The potential advantage of using an arterialized saphenous vein from the
femoral artery as the neoarterial inflow source is its ability to allow high flow
through the anastomosis. The use of the saphenous vein is also controversial
in this elective procedure as it precludes its later use for coronary artery
bypass grafting. The advantage of the inferior epigastric artery is that no
proximal anastomosis is required. The inferior epigastric artery also has a
diameter that is approximately the same size as the dorsal artery and it is also
usually free of atherosclerotic disease.

After fashioning an infrapubic incision the neoarterial inflow source is
transferred through the inguinal canal to the base of the penis, under Buck's
fascia, in the plane of the dorsal neurovascular bundle. It may be brought
through a window in the aponeurosis of the external oblique muscle or passed
subcutaneously to this location, especially in cases where a previous
herniorrhaphy has been performed. An arterialized saphenous vein, after
having been anastomosed to the femoral artery, is tunnelled subcutaneously
to this location.

Microsurgical Technique of Distal Arterial Revascularization. In our experience, the most frequent anastomosis has been a unilateral or bilateral
end-to-end anastomosis between the inferior epigastric artery and the

proximal dorsal penile artery. A unilateral anastomosis to the dorsal artery is typically performed when only one dorsal artery communicates to its ipsilateral cavernosal artery in the presence of occlusive proximal arterial disease. A bilateral anastomosis, using two inferior epigastric artery branches, is typically performed when both dorsal arteries communicate with their respective cavernosal arteries. If the inferior epigastric artery has no branches of sufficient caliber, the contralateral dorsal artery may be anastomosed end-to-side to the inferior epigastric artery or end-to-side to the contralateral neoarterialized dorsal artery.

Under microscopic control at a ×5 magnification, the distal adventitia of the neoarterial inflow source is removed for 1–2 cm to prevent its being sutured into the lumen and causing an anastomotic thrombosis. One or both dorsal arteries are freed for approximately 3 cm from any attachments to the tunica albuginea and from fibers of the ipsilateral dorsal nerve. If an end-to-end anastomosis is planned, the artery is transected and the segment of artery not used is either cauterized or suture ligated. Next, 1–2 cm of adventitia is removed from the transected end of the dorsal artery segment used for the anastomosis. The inferior epigastric artery and the dorsal artery are approximated with a temporary sliding bar microvascular clamp and the anastomosis is created, usually over a 2 F Silastic stent using interrupted 10–0 nylon sutures under ×10 magnification.

When one or both cavernosal arteries are occluded, bypass procedures to the dorsal artery are unlikely to be successful. Direct anastomoses of the neoarterial source to the cavernosal artery distal to a proximal occlusion have also been performed [25, 26, 31]. At our institution, in one case of proximal cavernosal artery occlusion secondary to blunt trauma, the ipsilateral dorsal artery was utilized as the neoarterial inflow source. Anastomoses to the cavernosal artery involve incising the tunica albuginea and separating the surrounding trabecular smooth muscle to approach the cavernosal artery. In our experience, trabecular smooth muscle injury has occurred in the area surrounding the anastomosis. This injury has led to corporal scarring with subsequent focal corporal veno-occlusive dysfunction. In one study, potency was initially improved in six of nine patients undergoing direct cavernosal artery revascularization. This improvement declined, however, to only two of nine on long-term follow-up, possibly as a result of iatrogenic corporal veno-occlusive dysfunction [31]. In our institution, cavernosal artery surgery has been discontinued because of the possibility of worsening erectile function, a complication not appreciated utilizing dorsal artery revascularization procedures.

In the presence of cavernosal artery occlusion, arterialization of a deep dorsal vein segment may be considered if retrograde flow through a deep dorsal vein segment into the corpora can be established. In our experience, retrograde flow through the dorsal vein segment could not be predicted preoperatively and, thus, cannot be depended upon as a primary treatment form. For this reason, we perform dorsal vein arterialization primarily to treat

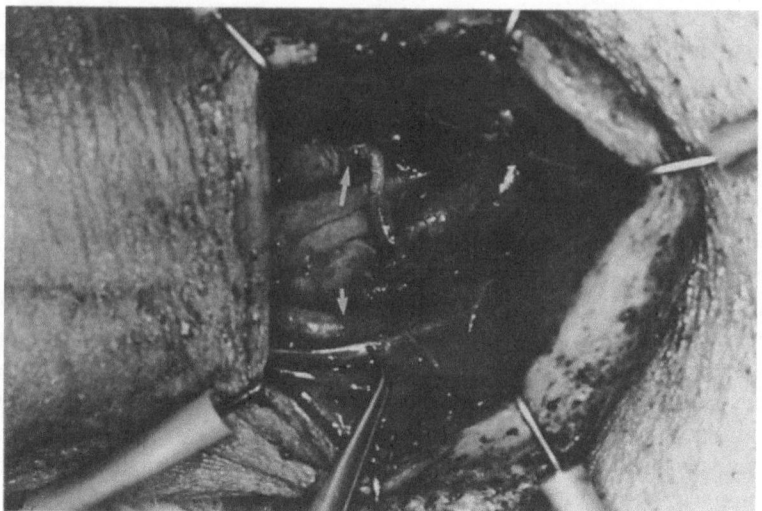

Fig. 4. Distal microvascular penile revascularization in a patient with a lesion in both the right cavernosal and left common penile arteries. There are two inferior epigastric artery branches. Dorsal vein arterialization is performed with one branch (*narrow arrow*) and an anastomosis to the left dorsal artery is performed with the other branch (*bold arrow*)

unilateral cavernosal artery occlusion in association with contralateral common penile artery occlusion. In these cases, as discussed above, the inferior epigastic artery is also anastomosed to the contralateral dorsal artery (Fig. 4).

The deep dorsal vein is identified at the base of the penis and a 3- to 4-cm segment of vein including several emissary vein branches is temporarily isolated and occluded with vessel loops. This segment begins distally at approximately midshaft and extends proximally under the pubic symphysis to the midsuspensory ligament. To establish the capability of retrograde arterial flow through the deep dorsal vein, one corpus is first cannulated with a 19-gauge butterfly needle and free flow of corporal blood is established. A dilute methylene blue solution is then injected into this isolated venous segment using a 25-gauge butterfly needle and the corporal effluent is observed. In cases where the effluent turns blue, arterialization of the dorsal vein segment is performed using the inferior epigastric artery or the ipsilateral dorsal artery as the neoarterial inflow source. Prior to performing the anastomosis, suture ligatures on the deep dorsal vein are placed distally to prevent glans hypervascularization, and proximally to complete the isolated segment. The neoarterial source is placed over the dorsal vein segment and the location for the venotomy is chosen. Typically this is in a dorsolateral location on the vein wall. The dorsal vein adventitia overlying the region of the proposed venotomy is removed for a distance of approximately 2 cm. An end-to-side anastomosis is performed between the neoarterial inflow source and the dorsal venous segment using 10–0 interrupted nylon sutures.

In the event that retrograde flow cannot be established, the use of a direct fistula from the arterialized venous segment to the tunica albuginea has been described [28, 30, 33]. Using 6–0 nylon suture, a fistula between the deep dorsal vein and the corporal bodies is fashioned after making both a posterior venotomy and a 2-cm defect in the adjacent tunica albuginea of one corpus. In patients with organic impotence, dorsal vein arterialization, with or without the creation of a fistula to the tunica albuginea, has a reported success rate of 40%–75% [23, 25, 29, 30, 33, 43].

Hauri described an anastomosis between the inferior epigastric artery, dorsal artery, and dorsal vein. The dorsal artery and deep dorsal vein are isolated at the base of the penis and two 1-cm longitudinal incisions are made in both vessels. The medial walls of both vessels are anastomosed, leaving a common arteriovenous lumen; the inferior epigastric artery is then anastomosed to this common lumen. Both anastomoses are made with 7–0 nylon sutures. Results in 44 consecutive patients have shown an 89% success rate including all seven patients with diabetes [32].

Corrective Procedures for Veno-Occlusive Dysfunction

Veno-Occlusive Hemodynamics of Erection

Subtunical venules lying in the potential space between the periphery of the erectile tissue and the tunica albuginea provide venous drainage from the lacunar spaces [2–4]. In the pendulous penis, these venules coalesce to form emissary veins that pierce the tunica albuginea to drain either directly into the deep dorsal vein or first into circumferential veins which then enter the deep dorsal venous sytem. Proximally in each crus, an independent drainage system exists in which the multiple emissary veins enter directly into cavernosal veins along the length of the crus. The cavernosal veins originate at the penile hilum [2, 44, 45]. Though independent, the cavernsoal and deep dorsal venous drainage systems may communicate via small connecting branches.

During erection, trabecular smooth muscle relaxation occurs. Trabecular smooth muscle relaxation allows lacunar space engorgement, increasing corporal volume. The expanded lacunar spaces compress the subtunical venules between them and the tunica albuginea increasing venous outflow resistance [1–3, 46–49]. The corporal body pressure that exists during erection is equal to the cavernosal artery perfusion pressure minus the pressure loss from corporal venous drainage [4].

In the flaccid state, trabecular smooth muscle tone is increased and penile corporal hemodynamics reflect minimal venous outflow resistance. Trabecular smooth muscle contraction leads to minimal corporal veno-occlusion providing unimpeded venous outflow via the subtunical venules. The corporal body pressure in the flaccid state approximates systemic venous pressure [8].

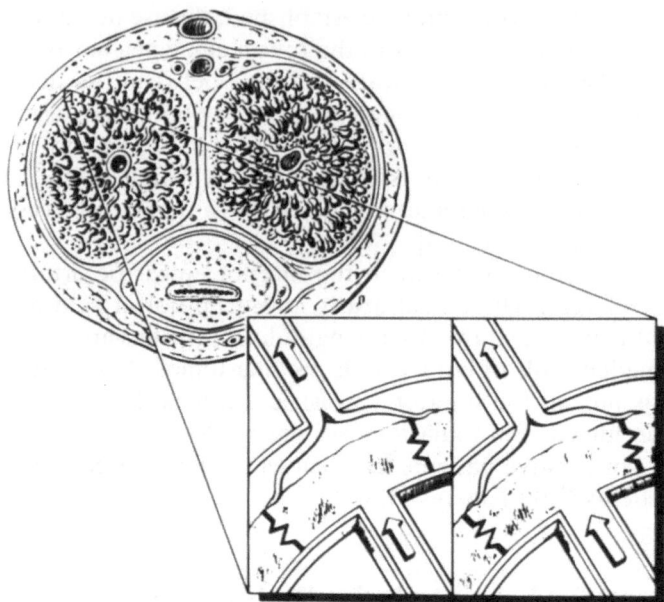

Fig. 5. Pathophysiology of corporal veno-occlusive dysfunction. In the flaccid state, there is low arterial inflow, the trabeculae are contracted and there is minimal compression of subtunical venules (*left*). With sexual stimulation, arterial inflow increases but the trabeculae are not able to adequately compress the subtunical venules either due to insufficient smooth muscle relaxation or decreased erectile tissue compliance (*right*). This causes inadequate venous outflow resistance, excessive venous drainage, and a failure to sustain maximal corporal body pressure

Hemodynamics of Corporal Veno-Occlusive Dysfunction

Organic erectile dysfunction appears to occur frequently as a consequence of abnormal corporal veno-occlusive hemodynamics [4]. The result is a corporal body pressure during erection that is inadequately sustained and insufficiently rigid for successful coitus.

Insufficient trabecular smooth muscle relaxation and decreased erectile tissue compliance are the most frequent pathologic mechanisms affecting corporal veno-occlusive function. Insufficient trabecular smooth muscle relaxation may occur secondary to excessive adrenergic constrictor tone, as seen in anxious individuals, or from damaged parasympathetic dilator nerves, as seen in neurogenic impotence [4, 50–53]. It has been suggested that decreased erectile tissue compliance results from structural alterations in the fibroelastic components of the trabeculae. This loss of compliance appears to be associated with aging, trauma, priapism, prior penile surgery, and vascular risk factors [34–38]. Corporal veno-occlusive dysfunction results from inadequate compression of the subtunical venules causing inadequate venous

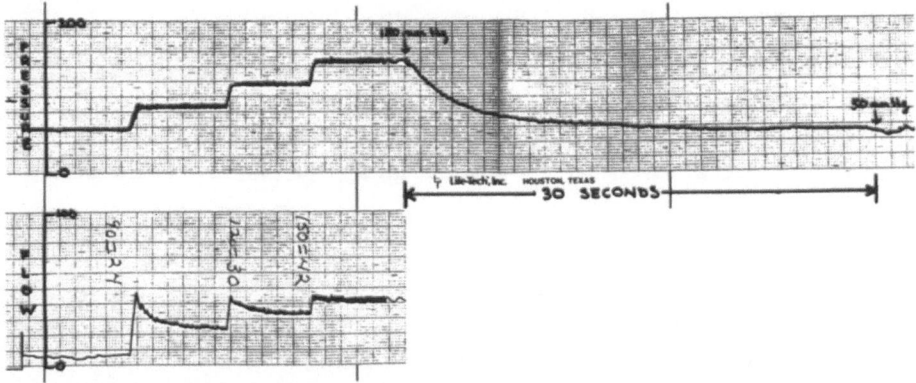

Fig. 6. Phase 2 DICC study of corporal veno-occlusive function. The flows of heparinized saline necessary to maintain corporal body pressures increase progressively from 6 ml/min at 60 mm Hg to 42 ml/min at 150 mm Hg. Following termination of the heparinized saline infusion, the corporal body pressure falls from 150 mm Hg to 50 mm Hg over a 30-period

outflow resistance, excessive venous drainage, and a failure to sustain maximal corporal body pressure (Fig. 5).

Diagnosis of Corporal Veno-Occlusive Function

After performing the initial history, physical examination, and noninvasive erectile function tests, DICC is performed [9]. Three of the four phases of the study assess the veno-occlusive mechanism following the intracavernosal injection of papaverine hydrochloride (45 mg) and phentolamine mesylate (2.5 mg). Following the phase-one response to these intracavernosal pharmacologic agents, provocative tests of corporal veno-occlusive function performed in phase two. The flow of heparinized saline necessary to maintain various corporal body pressures is determined in increasing intervals of 30 mm Hg, to a pressure of 150 mm Hg. Once this level is reached, the flow of heparinized saline is terminated and the fall in corporal body pressure over a 30-s period is determined (Fig. 6). Phase two tests are repeated in the presence of perineal compression to examine if this maneuver will reduce the maintenance flow rates or the pressure fall over 30 s. In phase four, the radiologic examination of the corporal venous drainage system during erection is performed. The various patterns of drainage may be described as either absent visualization or as visualization of the dorsal, cavernosal, or crural veins, the glans, or the corpus spongiosum.

Normal values for phase two of the DICC study have shown the flow of heparinized saline necessary to maintain various corporal body pressures to be equal to or less than 3 ml/min and the fall of corporal body pressure over a 30 period from a suprasystolic pressure of 150 mm Hg to be less than 45 mm Hg (Fig. 7). During cavernosography, there is virtually no visualization of any

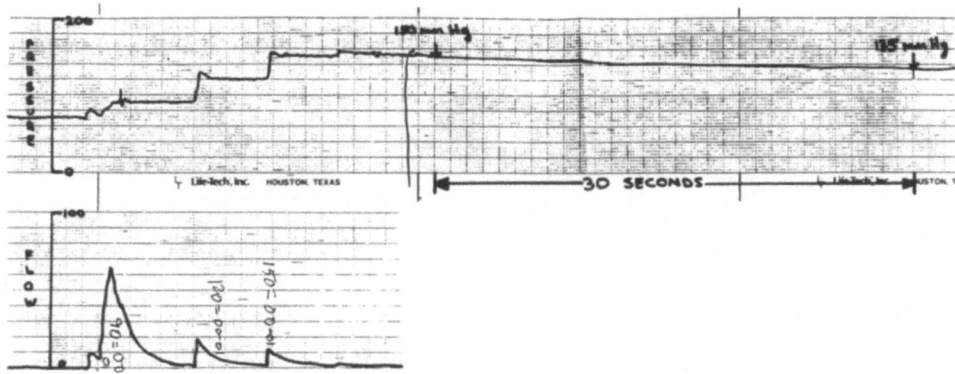

Fig. 7. Normal phase 2 DICC study of corporal veno-occlusive function. The flow of heparinized saline necessary to maintain corporal body pressures of 60, 90, 120, and 150 mm Hg is, in each case, 3 ml/min or less. The corporal body pressure falls only 15 mm Hg over a 30 period, from 150 mm Hg to 135 mm Hg

venous drainage. In our experience, those patients who have cavernosometric evidence of corporal veno-occlusive dysfunction, but whose phase two studies normalize during perineal compression show only focal, proximal cavernosal/ crural venous drainage on cavernosography.

Vascular Procedures for Corporal Veno-Occlusive Dysfunction

Patients demonstrating corporal veno-occlusive dysfunction may undergo vascular reconstructive procedures with the aim of increasing venous outflow resistance. In the early 1900's, Wooten first reported improvement in the erectile function of impotent men treated with deep dorsal vein ligation [54] In 1936, Lowsely and Bray described similar improvement with dorsal vein ligation coupled with plication of the ischiocavernosus muscles [55]. Today, in patients who have evidence of abnormal veno-occlusion, as demonstrated by cavernosographic visualization of multiple veins, the glans, or the corpus spongiosum, corrective surgical procedures in the literature include ligation or excision of penile veins draining the corpora with or without spongiolysis [56–60]. Success rates describing subjective improvement following venous ligation surgery have ranged from 28%–76% with an average follow-up, when indicated, of 3–26 months [60–63]. In our experience, such procedures have not resulted in long-term subjective improvement or objective changes on postoperative pharmacocavernosometry and pharmacocavernosography. This may be secondary either to inadequate surgical technique or to the underlying pathophysiology of corporal veno-occlusive dysfunction in these patients, that is, diffuse structural alterations in the fibroelastic components of the tabeculae resulting in loss of corporal tissue compliance, inadequate compression of the sub-tunical venules, inadequate venous outflow resist-

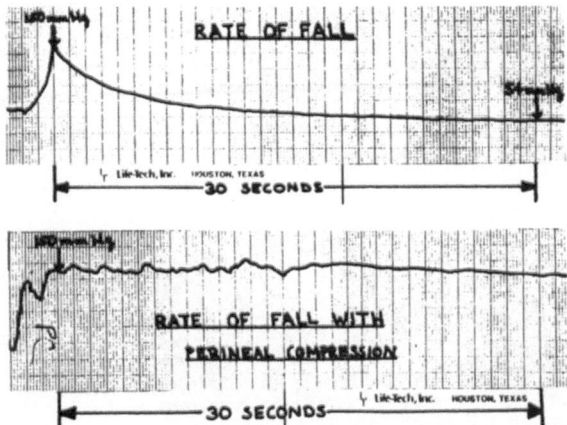

Fig. 8. A patient with corporal veno-occlusive dysfunction demonstrated on a phase 2 pharmacocavernosometric study (*top*) by a fall in corporal body pressure of 96 mm Hg (from 150 mm Hg to 54 mm Hg). This abnormality corrected easily with perineal compression (*bottom*). Cavernosography revealed focal drainage from the proximal cavernosal vein

ance, and excessive venous drainage from the corporal bodies via multiple draining veins.

There are patients, however, with corporal veno-occlusive dysfunction whose cavernosometric abnormalities correct easily with perineal compression, and whose cavernosograms reveal focal drainage primarily into the proximal cavernosal or crural veins (Fig. 8). We consider treating these patients with crual plication, proximal dorsal vein excision, and cavernosal vein ligation. The surgical rationale for this type or procedure is based upon the hypothesis that corporal veno-occlusive dysfunction in such patients has resulted not from a diffuse abnormality of erectile tissue compliance but rather from focal, proximal erectile tissue fibroelastic abnormalities possibly the result of perineal or pelvic trauma. In such situations, this focal compliance change diminishes the ability of the affected erectile tissue to adequately compress its surrounding subtunical venules. Treatment designed to increase venous outflow resistance consists of decreasing the circumferential crural volume and creating more effective compression of the subtunical space (Fig. 9).

Surgical Technique of Crural Plication, Dorsal Vein Excision, and Cavernosal Vein Ligation. After placing a Foley catheter, access to the crura is gained through a curvilinear inguinal-scrotal incision beginning two fingerbreadths lateral to the base of the penis and ending two fingerbreadths inferior to the base of the penis on the midline scrotal raphe. The ipsilateral crus is exposed laterally at its attachment to the ischiopubic ramus. Medially the crus is separated from the corpus spongiosum. In order to properly plicate the crus,

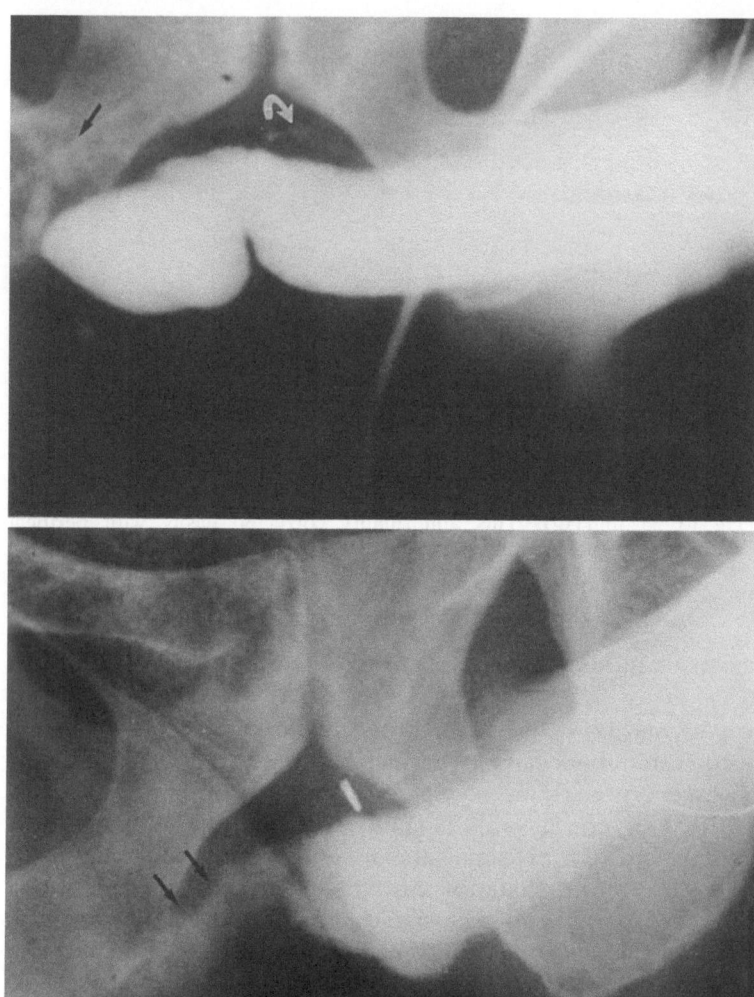

Fig. 9a,b. Patient with focal, proximal veno-occlusive dysfunction. **a** Abnormal venous drainage is seen from the crural veins (*straight arrow*) and proximal dorsal vein (*curved arrow*). **b** Following crural plication, cavernosal vein ligation and proximal dorsal vein excision there is no further cavernosographic evidence of veno-occlusive dysfunction. Circumferential crural volume is significantly decreased (*arrows*)

we have found it useful to identify the tunica albuginea both medially and laterally. Tunical exposure is accomplished by making two longitudinal scarifying incisions through the overlying ischiocavernosus muscle from the proximal tip of the crus to the penile hilum. Using several O-PDS sutures the crus is subsequently plicated from its proximal tip to the penile hilum by joining the exposed lateral and the medial aspects of the tunica albuginea.

The ischiocavernosus muscle is preserved but is buried in the plication. Plication is terminated at the level of the hilum to avoid injury to the dorsal neurovascular bundle. We have recently advanced the plication several centimeters distal to the hilum, under direct vision of the dorsal neurovascular bundle. The penis is then inverted through the incision and the contralateral crus is identified and is similarly plicated.

The origin of the cavernosal veins is not affected by crural plication because of their location at the penile hilum. In order to access and identify the origin of these veins so that they may be ligated, we have found it useful to first excise the proximal dorsal vein in the region of the suspensory and proximal fundiform ligaments. To perform dorsal vein excision and cavernosal vein ligation, the fundiform ligament connecting Scarpa's fascia of the abdominal wall to Buck's fascia of the penis is first retracted. The fundiform ligament helps prevent retraction of the penis and also contains branches of the dorsal (sensory) nerve and, therefore, efforts should be made to preserve this structure. At the proximal aspect of the fundiform ligament is the suspensory ligament which is divided as much as necessary to gain exposure to the dorsal aspect of the penis underneath the pubic symphysis. Here, the deep dorsal vein is isolated and divided. The proximal portion of the vein is then followed toward the urogenital diaphragm and excised. Deep to the excised proximal deep dorsal vein is fascial plane, and deep to this fascial plance lies the hilum of the penis where the cavernosal arteries, nerves, and veins are identified. Cavernosal veins are carefully suture ligated both at the level of the hilum and proximally toward the urogenital diaphragm.

In our experience, postoperative cavernosometric and cavernosographic improvement has been objectively demonstrated only in patients with focal, proximal corporal veno-occlusive dysfunction.

Results of Vascular Reconstructive Surgery at Boston University

Questionnaires were mailed to 77 patients who underwent reconstructive vascular surgery in 1988 and 1989 and 29 (38%) have responded, Follow-up in this group ranges from 6 months to 2 years. In all, 72% of patients reported an improved erectile quality including rigidity and/or sustaining capability. The rigidity of their erections both preoperatively and postoperatively was subjectively compared either to the rigidity of their previously normal erection or to the rigidity of a rigid object. The preoperative rigidity of 30% quality improved to a postoperative rigidity of 80% quality. Improved satisfaction of erections and increased spontaneity of erections were each seen in 61%. Intercourse quality was also graded by determining what percentage of coital episodes were satisfying to the patient. Coital episodes were satisfactory in 25% of patients preoperatively and this improved to satisfactory coitus in 78% of patients postoperatively. An increased frequency of intercourse was claimed by 74%, 69% stated an increase in self-confidence and/or self-image, and 63% noted increased partner satisfaction. When asked if they would undergo the same procedure again if necessary, 93% side they would. Complications were reported in five patients (17%) including two claiming a minor loss of sensation, two noting some loss of erectile length, and one with glans hypervascularization.

We have performed DICC studies 6 months postoperatively in approximately 50% of patients in 1988 and 1989. Objective postoperative improvements have been recorded, as evidenced by increased corporal body pressure responses to intracavernosal vasoactive agents, diminished falls in corporal body pressure following termination of heparinized saline infusion, improved cavernosal artery systolic occlusion pressures, and absence of venous drainage on cavernosography. In our series, a direct correlation is seen between failures of the reconstructive surgical procedure to improve erections and the presence of visualization of the corpus spongiosum on the postoperative cavernosogram.

Conclusion

Many impotent patients would prefer the possibility of surgical restoration of normal hemodynamic conditions if this could be performed in a reliable, reproducible, and objective fashion without significant morbidity. The ideal arterial vascular reconstructive candidates, in our expereince, have been young men with occlusive arterial disease found in a focal location proximal to the cavernosal artery. An arterial vascular reconstructive procedure, such as the anastomosis of the inferior epigastric artery to the proximal dorsal penile artery, may bypass such a proximal occlusive arterial lesion. Similarly, in our experience, the ideal venous reconstructive candidates appear to be young men with corporal veno-occlusive dysfunction that also is focal and proximal involving primarily the crura. Crural plication, dorsal vein excision, and cavernosal vein ligation may improve such localized corporal veno-occlusive dysfunction and increase the overall resistance to venous outflow during erection. Utilizing the vascular surgical principles and techniques discussed above, objective improvements in inflow and perfusion pressure to the corpora have been documented and subjective improvements in erectile quality, satisfaction, and frequency of intercourse have been demonstrated in 72%, 61%, and 74%, respectively.

References

1. Saenz de Tejada I Goldstein I Blanco R et al. (1985) Smooth muscle of the corpora cavernosa: Role in penile erection. Surg Forum 36:623-624
2. Lue TF Tanagho EA (1988) Functional anatomy ad mechanism of penile erection. In: Tanagho EA, Lue TF, McClure RD (eds) Contemporary management of impotence and infertility. Williams & Wilkins, Baltimore, pp 39–50
3. Lue TF, Tanagho EA (1987) Physiology of erection and pharmacological management of impotence. J Urol 137:829–836
4. Krane RJ, Goldstein I, Saenz de Tejada I (1989) Impotence. NEJM 321:1648–1659
5. Padma-Nathan H, Goldstein I, Azadzoi K, Blanco R, Saenz de Tejada I, Krane RJ (1986) In vivo and in vitro studies on the physiology of penile erection. Semin Urol 4:209–216
6. Yanagisawa M, Kurihara H, Kimura S et al. (1988) A novel potent vasoconstrictor peptide produced by vascular endothelial cells. Nature 332:411–415
7. Saenz de Tejada I, Carson MP, Traish A, Eastman EH, Goldstein I (1989) Role of endothelin in the local control of penile smooth muscle tone. J Vasc Med Biol 1:112 (abstract)
8. Levine FJ, Gasior BL, Goldstein I (1989) Reconstructive arterial surgery for impotence. Sem Int Rad 6:220–226
9. Padma-Nathan H, Azadzoi K, Blanco R, Goldstein I, Faxon D, Krane RJ (1986) Development of an animal model of atherosclerotic impotence. Surg Forum 37:640–642
10. Rosen MP, Greenfield AJ, Walker TC et al. (Submitted for publication) Cigarette smoking: an independent risk factor for atherosclerosis in the hypogastric-cavernous bed of men with arteriogenic impotence.
11. Virag R, Bouilly P, Frydaman D (1985) Is impotence an arterial disorder? A study of arterial risk factors in 400 impotent men. Lancet 1:181–184
12. Ruzbarsky V, Michal V (1977) Morphologic changes in the arterial bed of the penis with aging: relationship to the pathogenesis of impotence. Invest Urol 15:194–199
13. Michal V (1982) Arterial disease as a cause of impotence. Clin Endocrinol Metab 11:725–748
14. Levine FJ, Greefield AJ, Goldstein I (1990) Arteriographically-determined occlusive disease within the hypogastric-cavernous bed in impotent patients following blunt perineal ad pelvic trauma. J Urol
15. Rosen MP, Greenfield AJ, Walker TG et al. (1990) Arteriogenic impotence: findings in 195 impotent men examined with selective internal pudendal angiography. Radiology 174:1043–1948
16. Lurie AL, Bookstein JJ, Kessler WO (1988) Angiography of post traumatic impotence. Cardiovasc Interven Radiol 11:232–236
17. St. Louis EL, Jewett MAS, Gray RR et al. Basketball-related impotence. NEJM 308:595–596
18. Sharlip ID (1981) Penile arteriography in impotence after pelvic trauma. J Urol 126:477–479
19. Goldstein I, Krane RJ, Greenfield AJ, Padma-Nathan H (1989) Vascular diseases of the penis: impotence and priapism. In: Pollack H M (ed) Clinical urography. Saunders, Philadelphia, pp 2231–2252
20. Lue TF (1988) Functional evaluation of penile arteries with papaverine. In: Tanagho EA, Lue TF, McClure RD (eds) Contemporary management of impotence and infertility. Williams & Wilkins, Baltimore, pp 57–64
21. Rosen MP, Greenfield AJ (1988) Selective pudendal arteriography for evaluation of arterial impotence. Sem Int Rad 6:198–204
22. Bookstein JJ, Valji K, Parsons L, Kessler W (1987) Pharmacoarteriography in the evaluation of impotence. J Urol 137:333–337
23. Goldstein I (1986) Arterial revascularization procedures. Semin Urol 4:252–258

24. Goldstein I (1988) Overview of types and results of vascular surgical procedures for impotence. Cardiovasc Intervent Radiol 11:240–244
25. Sharlip ID (1988) Surgical treatment of cavernous artery insufficiency. In: Precongress clinical teaching session of the Sixth Biennial International Symposium for Corpus Cavernosum Revascularization & Third Biennial World Meeting on Impotence. International Society for Impotence Research (ISIR), Boston, pp 75–79
26. Crespo E, Soltanik E, Bove D (1982) Treatment of vasculogenic sexual impotence by revascularizing cavernous and/or dorsal arteries. Urology 20:271–275
27. McDougal WS, Jeffery RF (1983) Microscopic penile revascularization. J Urol 129:517–521
28. Bennett AH (1988) Venous arterialization for erectile impotence. Urol Clin North Am 15:111–113
29. Furlow WL, Fisher J, Knoll LD (1988) Penile revascularization: experience with deep dorsal vein arterialization – the Furlow-Fisher modification with 27 patients. In: Proceedings of the Sixth Biennial International Symposium for Corpus Cavernosum Revascularization & Third Biennial World Meeting on Impotence. International Society for Impotence Research (ISIR), Boston, p 139
30. Virag R, Zwang G, Dermange H, Legman M (1981) Vasculogenic impotence: a review of 92 cases with 54 surgical operations. Vasc Surg 15:9–17
31. Konnak JW, Ohl DA (1989) Microsurgical penile revascularization using central corporeal penile artery. J Urol 142:305–308
32. Hauri D (1986) A new operative technique in vasculogenic erectile impotence. World J Urol 4:237–249
33. Virag R (1982) Revascularization of the penis. In: Bennett AH (ed) Management of male impotence. Williams & Wilkins, Baltimore, pp 219–233
34. Cerami A, Vlasssara H, Brownlee M (1987) Glucose and aging. Sci Am 256:90–96
35. Hayashi K, Takamizawa K, Nakamura T, Kato T, Tsushima N (1987) Effects of elastase on the stiffness and elastic properties of arterial walls in cholesteol-fed rabbits. Atherosclerosis 66:259–267
36. Fischer GM, Swain ML, Cherian K (1980) Increased vascular collagen and elastin synthesis in experimental atherosclerosis in the rabbit. Atherosclerosis 35:11–20
37. Montague DK (1988) Penile prostheses. In: Montague DK (ed) Disorders of male sexual dysfunction. Year Book Medical Publishers, Chicago, pp 154–191
38. Hinman F (1960) Priapism: reasons for failure of therapy. J Urol 83:420–428
39. Moore S (1981) Responses of the arterial wall to injury. Diabetes 30(Suppl 2):8–13
40. Moore S, Friedman RJ, Gent M (1977) Resolution of lipid-containing atherosclerotic lesions induced by injury. Blood Vessels 14:193–203
41. Dewar ML, Blundell PE, Lidstone D, Herba MJ, Chiu RC (1985) Effects of abdominal aneurysmectomy, aortoiliac bypass grafting and angioplasty on male sexual potency: A prospective study. Can J Surg 28:154–159
42. Michal V, Kramar R, Pospichal J, Hejhal L (1973) Direct arterial anastomosis on corporal cavernosa penis in therapy of erectile impotence. Rozhl Chir 52:587–590
43. Sharlip ID (1988) Treatment of arteriogenic impotence by penile revascularization. In: Proceedings of the Sixth Biennial International Symposium for Corpus Cavernosum Revascularization & Third Biennial World Meeting on Impotence. Internation Society for Impotence Research (ISIR), Boston, p 135
44. Peuch-Leao P, Reis JMSM, Glina S Reischelt AC (1987) Leakage through the crural edge of the corpus cavernosum. Diagnosis and treatment. Eur Urol 13:163–165
45. Peuch-Leao P, Chao S (1988) Venous drainage of the crura — an anatomic study. In: Proceedings of the Sixth Biennial International Symposium for Corpus Cavernosum Revascularization & Third Biennial World Meeting on Impotence. International Society for Impotence Research (ISIR), Boston, p 2
46. Saenz de Tejada I, Blanco R, Goldstein I et al. (1988) Cholinergic neurotransmission in human corpus cavernosum. I. Responses of isolated tissue. Am J Physiol 254:H459–H467
47. Blanco R, Saenz de Tejada I, Goldstein I et al. (1988) Cholinergic neurotransmission in human corpus cavernosum. II. Acetyline synthesis. Am J Physiol 254:H468–H472

48. Furchgott RF, Zawadski JV (1980) The obligatory role of endothelial cells in the relaxation of arterial smooth muscle to acetycholine. Nature 288:373–376
49. Vanhoutte PM, Rubanyi GM, Miller VM Houston DS (1986) Modulation of vascular smooth muscle contraction by the endothelium. Annu Rev Physiol 48:307–320
50. Saenz de Tejada I, Goldstein I, Azadzoi K, Krane RJ, Cohen RA (1989) Impaired neurogenic and endothelium-mediated relaxation of penile smooth muscle from diabetic men with impotence. NEJM 320:1025–1030
51. Ellenberg M (1971) Impotence in diabetes: The neurologic factor. Ann Intern Med 75:213–219
52. Kolodny RC, Kahn CB, Goldstein A et al. (1974) Sexual dysfunction in diabetic men. Diabetes 23:306–309
53. Lehman TP Jacobs JA (1983) Etiology of diabetic impotence. J Urol 129:291–294
54. Wooten JS (1902/3) Ligation of the dorsal vein of the penis as a cure for atonic impotence. Texas Med J 18:325–328
55. Lowsley OS Bray JL (1936) The surgical relief of impotence. JAMA 107:2029–2034
56. Wespes E, Schulman CC (1985) Venous leakage: surgical treatment of a curable cause of impotence. J Urol 133:796–798
57. Lue T (1988) Treatment of venogenic impotence. In: Tanagho EA, Lue TF, McClure RD (eds) Contemporary management of impotence and infertility. Williams & Wilkins, Baltimore, pp 175–177
58. Lewis RW, Pauyau FA (1986) Procedures of decreasing venous drainage. Semin Urol 4:263–272
59. Gilbert P Steif C (1987) Spongiolysis: a new surgical treatment of impotence caused by distal venous leakage. J Urol 138:784–786
60. Lewis RW (1988) Venous surgery for impotence. Urol Clin North A 15:115–121
61. Lue TF (1988) Surgery for venogenic impotence. In: Proceedings of the Sixth Biennial International Symposium for Corpus Cavernosum Revascularization & Third Biennial World Meeting on Impotence. International Society for Impotence Research (ISIR), Boston, p 140
62. Melman A, Mieza M, Singh V, Pedersen (1988) Results of surgical correction of impaired drainage from the corpora cavernosum of impaired males. In: Proceedings of the Sixth Biennial International Symposium for Corpus Cavernosum Revascularization & Third Biennial World Meeting on Impotence. International Society for Impotence Research (ISIR) Boston, p 141
63. Wespes E, Delcour C, Prejzerowicz L, Struyven J, Schulman CC (1988) Long term follow-up of patients operated for venous leakage. In: Proceedings of the Sixth Biennial International Symposium for Corpus Cavernosum Revascularization & Third Biennial World Meeting on Impotence. International Society for Impotence Research (ISIR), Boston, p 193

Revascularization in Arteriogenic Erectile Impotence

D. Hauri

Introduction

After overcoming the Freudian quagmire and applying advanced techniques to the evaluation of erectile dysfunction, we have come to the realization that the vast majority of erectile impotence cases (80%–90%) have a morphologic cause. Up to 80% of these cases, in turn, can be linked to vascular disease, with arterial lesions playing a predominant role. The poor long-term results of venous surgery for impotence suggest that "venous leakage" is not strictly a venous disease; our experience indicates that arterial pathology also has causal significance in these cases.

The arterial lesions generally consist of a luminal narrowing or occlusion involving the large pelvic vessels or, more commonly, the proximal (internal pudendal artery) or distal (dorsal and deep) penile arteries. Occasionally it may happen that, even with radiographically intact distal penile arteries, inflow is insufficient for a full erection because those vessels are supplied by incompetent collaterals (e.g., by the obturator artery).

Diagnostic Studies

Diagnostic studies for the evaluation of vasculogenic impotence are described elsewhere in this volume. At present we are convinced that selective penile angiography is an indispensable study in the selection of patients for a revascularization procedure. The typical arterial lesions can be identified (Figs. 1–3) and appropriate conclusions drawn with regard to operative tactics. Digital subtraction angiography (DSA) can provide reliable information at reasonable expense. Although color-coded ultrasound duplex scanning may replace DSA in the future, it can demonstrate the peripheral penile arteries but not the equally important proximal vascular channels.

A final comment on intracavernous drug testing with "vasoactive agents": the drugs currently available are primary musculotropic compounds which act primarily on the smooth trabecular muscle of the cavernous tissue and only secondarily upon the vessel wall. Thus the procedure tests the

U. Jonas et al. (Eds.) Erectile Dysfunction
© Springer-Verlag Berlin Heidelberg 1991

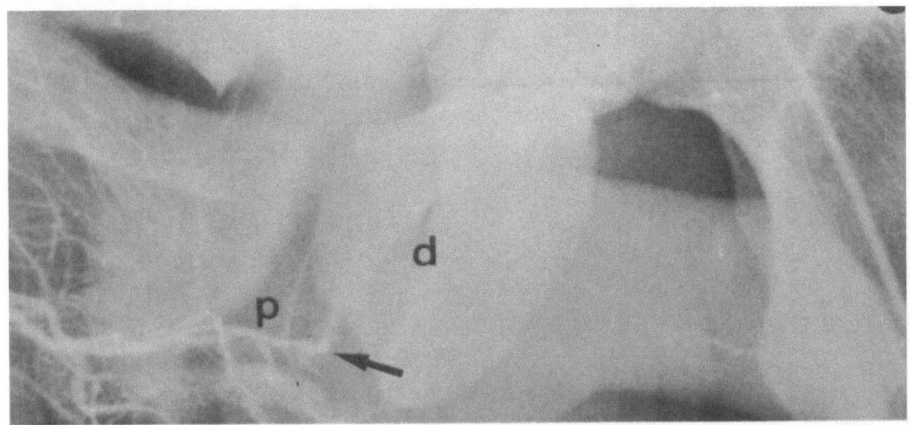

Fig. 1. Occlusion of the deep penile artery at its origin from the internal pudendal artery (→). Typical finding in diabetes mellitus. *p*, internal pudendal artery; *d*, dorsal penile artery

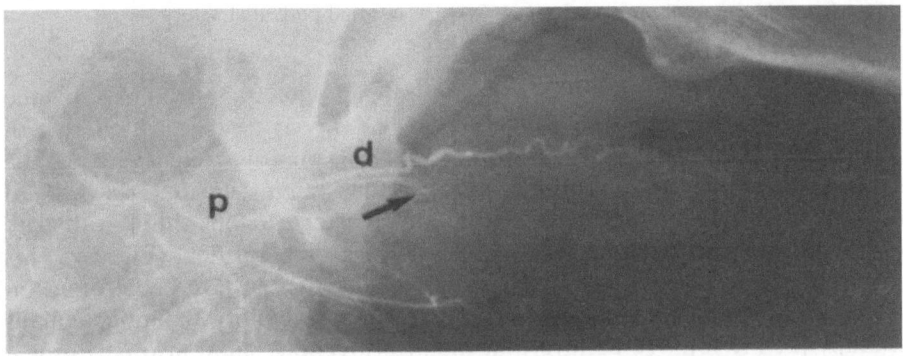

Fig. 2. Occlusion of the deep penile artery distal to its origin (›). *p*, internal pudendal artery; *d*, dorsal penile artery

functional competence of the corpora cavernosa and of their arterial supply. A negative test does not preclude subsequent successful revascularization. Neither does a positive response preclude surgical correction in men who find self-injection an unacceptable option.

Surgical Concept

Earlier attempts [3, 4, 10, 30, 33–37, 48–50] have failed to yield convincing results. While the direct anastomosis of the inferior epigastric artery to the

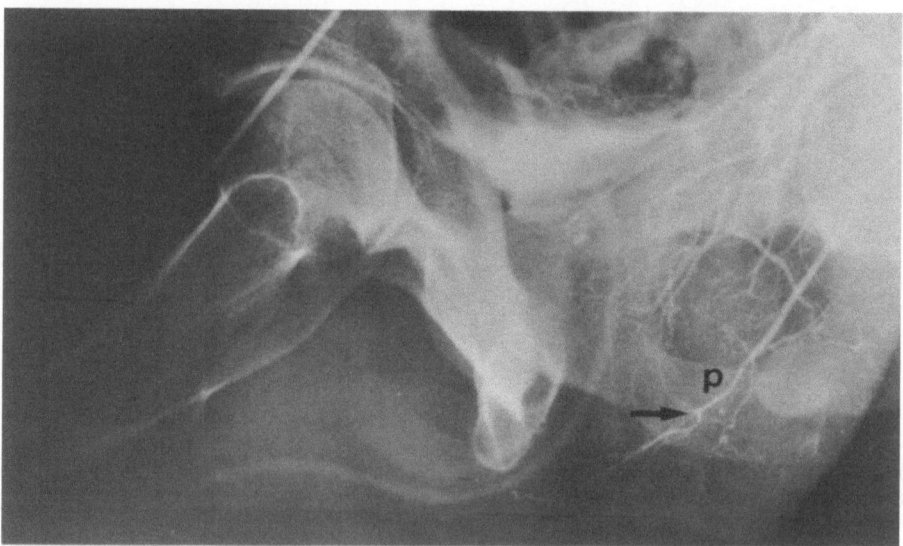

Fig. 3. Impotence secondary to pelvic trauma. Both penile vessels are occluded at their origin from the internal pudendal artery (→). *p*, internal pudendal artery

corpus cavernosum (Fig. 4) is unphysiologic, direct anastomosis of the inferior epigastric artery to a dorsal artery (Fig. 5) carries a high risk of thrombosis at the site of the arterioarterial anastomosis. Experience in the surgery of peripheral vessels [20, 23, 27] has taught us that the risk of thrombosis can be reduced by constructing an arteriovenous shunt at the site of the arterioarterial anastomosis to improve peripheral flow (Fig. 6). This phenomenon has been known for more than 200 years [19], but was forgotten because of poor clinical results due to the unavailability of anticoagulant therapy [2, 14, 46]. We believe that the arteriovenous shunt also performs a more important task: it ensures that the arterioarterial anastomosis is continuously perfused with blood, even in the hazardous low-flow phase of detumescence, so that the risk of thrombosis is further reduced (Fig. 7).

These discoveries prompted us to develop a modified penile arterial revascularization procedure that incorporates an arteriovenous shunt [15, 16] (Fig. 8). One of the inferior epigastric arteries is dissected free through a pararectal incision, divided at the level of the umbilicus, and transposed inguinally to the base of the penis. One of the dorsal penile arteries and the deep dorsal penile vein are exposed at the base of the penis and incised longitudinally for a length of about 2 cm. The median borders of the incisions are approximated with a continuous nonabsorbable 7/0 suture. Then about a 2-cm longitudinal incision is made in the inferior epigastric artery, and the mouth-like opening of the vessel is anastomosed to the common arteriovenous lumen, again using nonabsorbable 7/0 thread. The procedure is performed using about a 4 × binocular loupe. The patient is heparinized

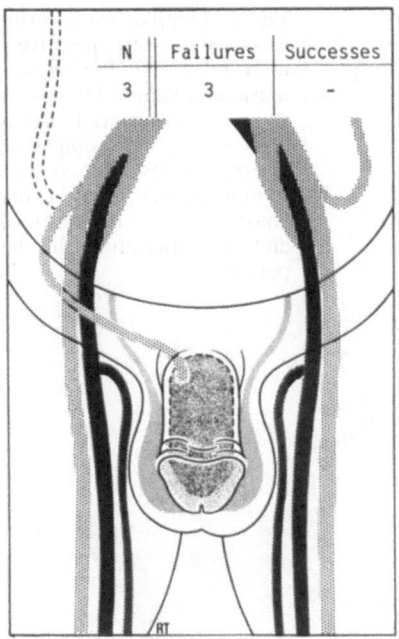

N	Failures	Successes
3	3	-

Fig. 4. Direct implantation of the inferior epigastric artery into the corpus cavernosum (Michal I procedure)

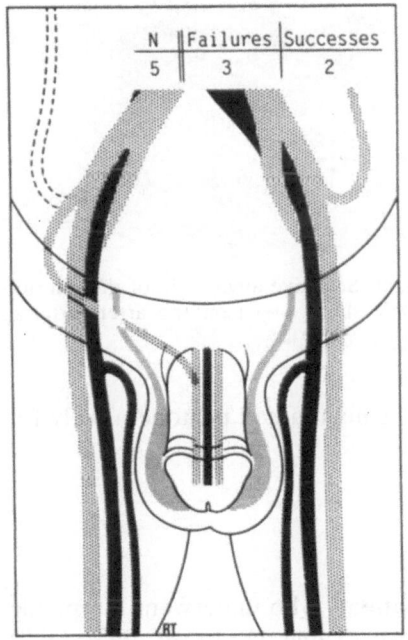

N	Failures	Successes
5	3	2

Fig. 5. Anastomosis of the inferior epigastric artery to the dorsal penile artery (Michal II procedure)

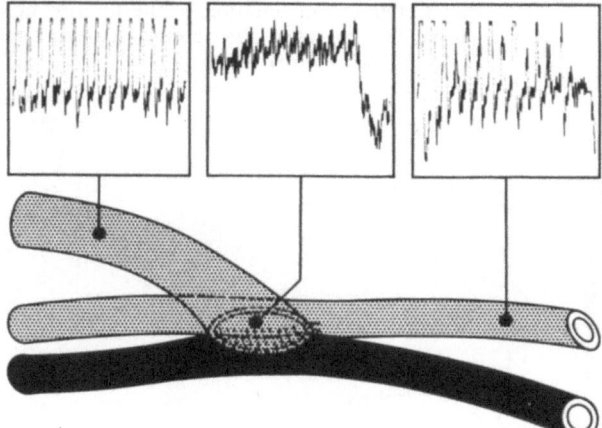

Fig. 6. Doppler wave forms recorded intraoperatively after release of the anastomosis and shunt. The traces show normal arterial signals in the inferior epigastric artery, accessory venous sounds in the area of the anastomosis and shunt, and good pulsations in the periphery

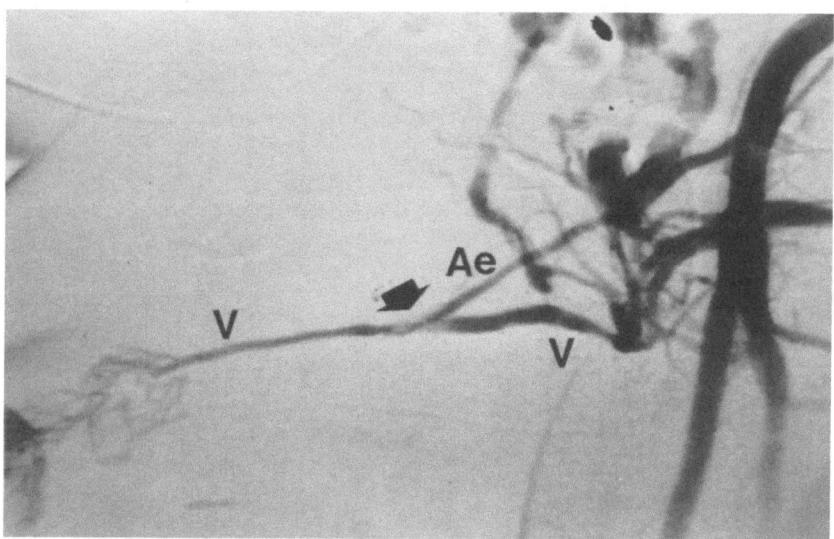

Fig. 7. Venous perfusion of the arterioarterial shunt. Selective angiogram of the inferior epigastric artery (*Ae*) plainly demonstrates the AV shunt (→) near the arterioarterial anastomosis and the venous drainage (*V*)

perioperatively, and anticoagulant therapy is maintained postoperatively for about 6 months.

Results

Since 1983, we have followed 130 of our patients who underwent the penile revascularization procedure described above (Table 1). In all, 79% (102)

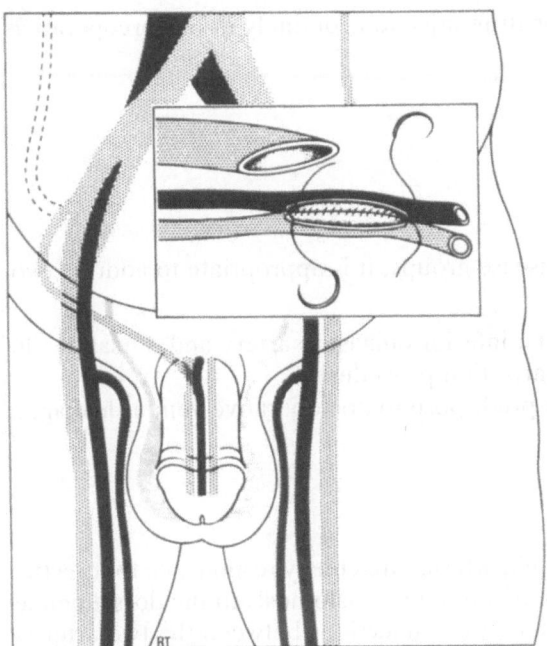

Fig. 8. Our technique for penile revascularization

Table 1. Statistical results for the period 1983–1989

Vasculogenic impotence	No. of patients (n)	Surgery successful (n)	Surgery failed (n)
Idiopathic	58	48	10
Diabetes mellitus	21	14	7
Nicotine abuse	33	28	5
Secondary to pelvic trauma	8	6	2
Secondary to radiotherapy	1	1	–
Secondary to proctectomy	2	1	1
Secondary to radical prostectomy	5	3	2
Secondary to renal transplantation	1	1	–
Secondary to aortic aneurysm surgery	1	–	1
	130	102[a]	28

[a] 79%

developed satisfactory erectile function between several days and 6 months following the surgery. The unsuccessful cases may have included a few patients who had a preexisting venous leak that we did not diagnose before surgery. Because our studies have convinced us that venous leakage is very likely based on an insufficient arterial flow to the corpora cavernosa, since 1988 we have included selective penile angiography and dynamic cavernosography with intracavernous drug injection routinely in our preoperative diagnostic workup.

Discussion

Before discussing the various disease groups, it is appropriate to address two basic questions:

1. Is an anastomosis between the inferior epigastric artery and dorsal penile artery justified in a revascularization procedure?
2. Does the installed AV shunt predispose to postoperative venous leakage?

The Arterioarterial Anastomosis

If it is accepted that the deep penile arteries are chiefly responsible for erectile function, we can justify revascularization by anastomosis to the dorsal penile artery only if we assume that there are connections between the two arterial systems. There is some disagreement as to the existence of these connections in the current literature [1, 7, 9, 17, 38, 39, 41, 42, 45]. To resolve this question, we [26] prepared our own corrosion specimens and were able to demonstrate the presence of myriad fine anastomoses interconnecting the superficial and deep penile arterial systems (Fig. 9). The proposed surgical concept is feasible, therefore. Occasionally these anastomoses can even be demonstrated in selective penile angiograms (Fig. 10).

Venous Leakage Through the AV Shunt?

It is obvious and appropriate to ask whether there is venous leakage through the AV shunt. But if we consider the normal mechanism that prevents venous leak, i.e., compression of the veins in the trabeculae by progressive cavernosal filling (Fig. 11a, b), we must assume that the same process occurs to an enhanced degree following a successful revascularization procedure. We have been able to reproduce this intraoperatively and demonstrate that tumescence causes a drastic flow reduction in the venous system (Fig. 12a). This effect can also be produced by artificial erection depending on the intracavernous pressure (Fig. 12b). In very rare cases, however, leakage through the AV shunt can still occur. So dynamic cavernosography with intracavernous drug injection is the first study that should be performed after an unsuccessful revascularization. If a leak is confirmed, it can be surgically repaired after 6 months of anticoagulant therapy, and the patient has a good chance of acquiring satisfactory erectile function.

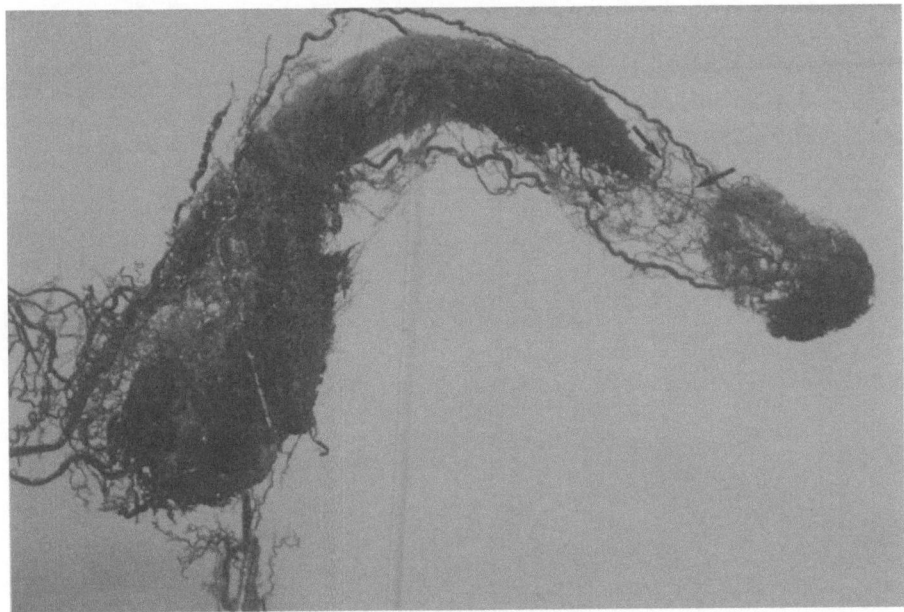

Fig. 9. Corrosion preparation of the penile vessels, demonstrating a rich anastomotic network between the superficial and deep penile arteries (→)

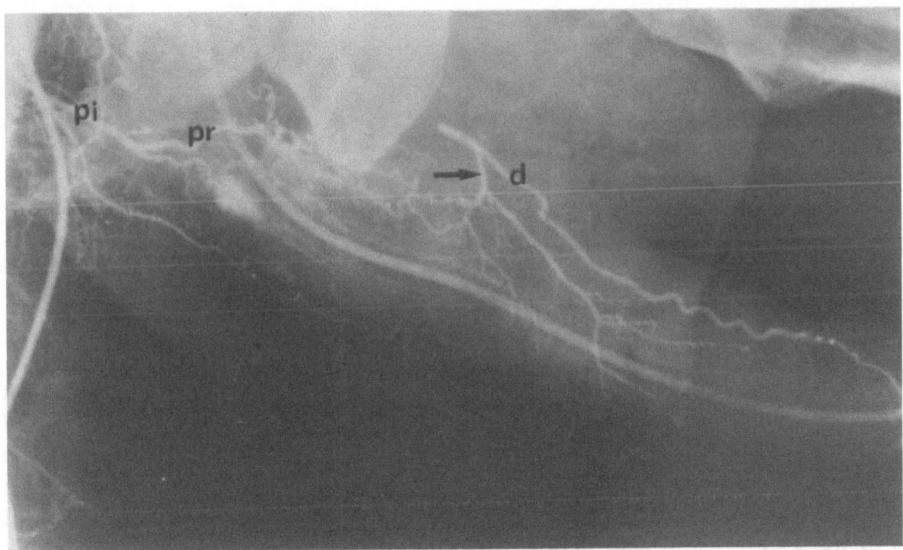

Fig. 10. Selective penile arteriography. The dorsal penile artery, showing proximal segmental occlusion, is supplied distally by an anastomosis to the deep penile artery (→). *pi*, internal pudental artery; *pr*, deep penile artery; *d*, dorsal penile artery

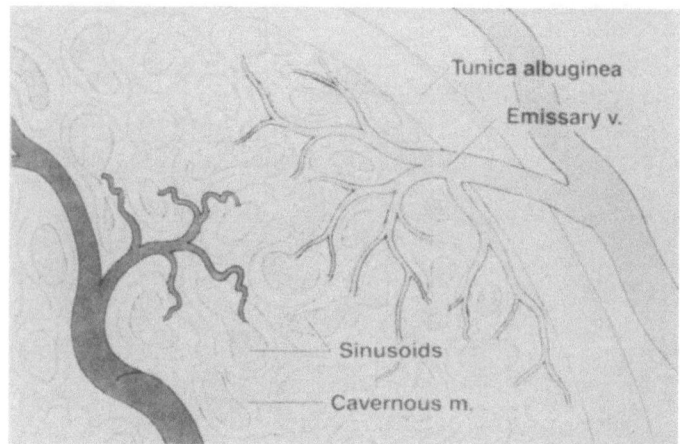

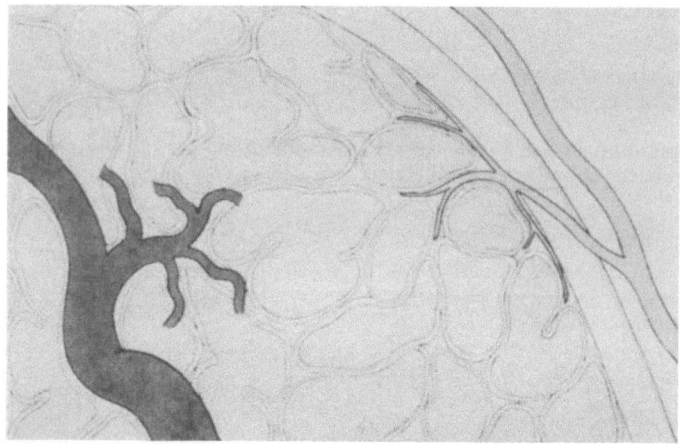

Fig. 11a,b. The veins coursing in the trabeculae are compressed and occluded by penile tumescence, preventing venous leakage. **a** Detumescence, **b** tumescence

Postoperative Hyperemia of the Glans Penis

Postoperative hyperemia of the glans penis is a troublesome complication which occurred in less than 5% of our patients. It involves an acute painful swelling and reddening of the glans penis (Fig. 13), which can compress the external urethral meatus sufficiently to interfere with micturition. This complication may arise in the first postoperative days or may not appear until 4–8 weeks after surgery. Angiography (Fig. 14) shows that the bulk of the new blood supply flows directly into the glans due to complete or partial closure of the anastomosis between the superficial and deep arterial systems. In the first two patients with this complication, we cured the hyperemia by

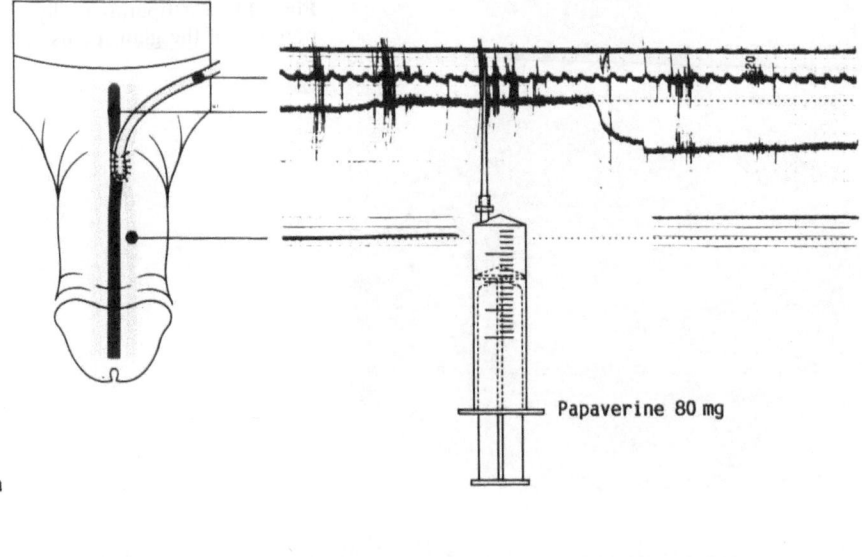

a

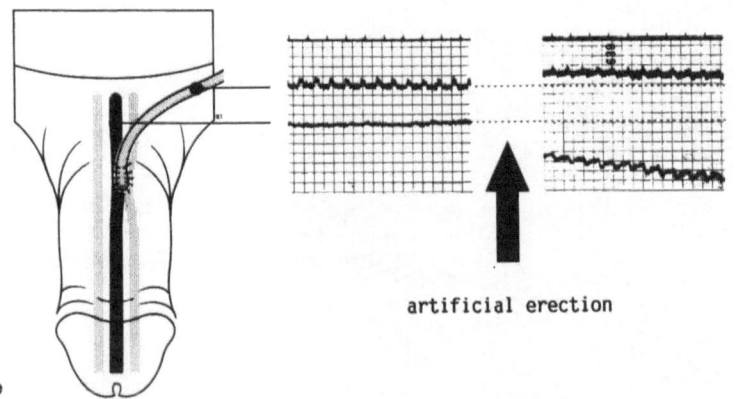

b

Fig. 12a,b. Flow measurements. The points of measurement are indicated (●). **a** Intraoperative papaverine-induced erection (80 mg papaverine). Clinical erection occurs 6 min after the intracavernous injection of papaverine. As tumescence proceeds, a drastic decrease of flow values is recorded in the deep dorsal penile vein proximal to the AV shunt. A full rigid erection ensues. **b** Flow measurements during an artificial erection produced by the infusion of physiologic NaCl solution. Again, a decrease of venous flow proximal to the AV shunt, dependent on the intracavernous pressure, is recorded

ligating all the arterial and venous vessels, except for one artery, in the region of the coronary sulcus (Fig. 15). The main problem in this technique is deciding how many vessels should be left patent to avoid necrosis of the glans. In our remaining three patients with glans hyperemia, we limited treatment to local ice wraps and analgesics to await or accelerate opening of the anastomoses.

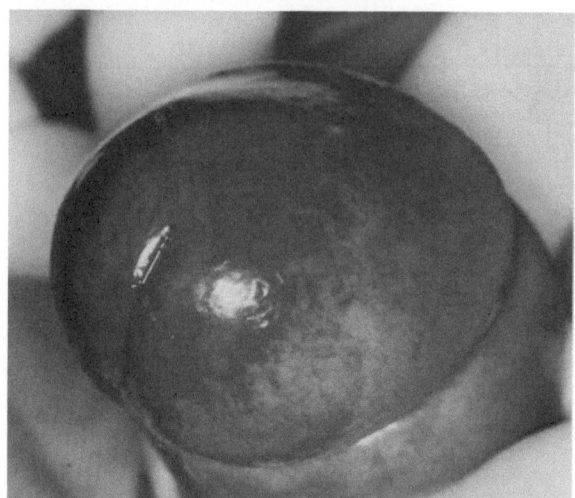

Fig. 13. Postoperative hyperemia of the glans penis

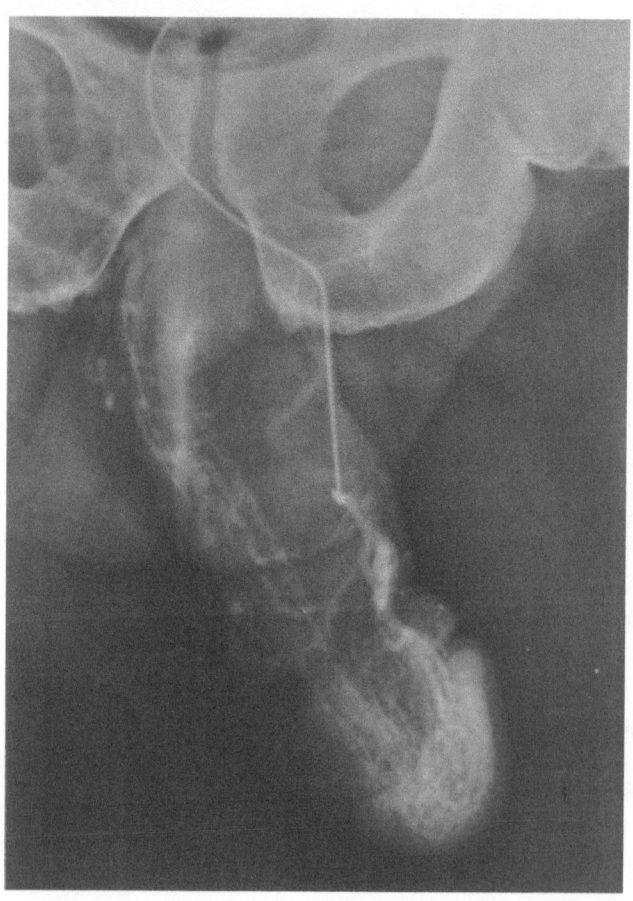

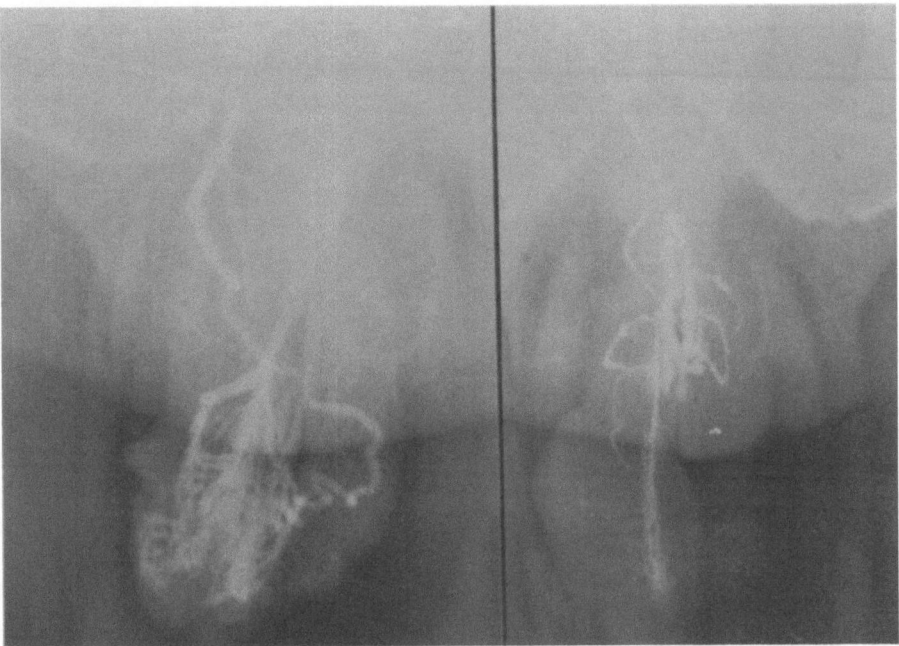

Fig. 15. Vascular ligatures have been placed in the coronary sulcus for glans hyperemia. It is unclear how many vessels should be ligated

"Idiopathic" Arterial Impotence

The group of patients with "idiopathic" arterial impotence was very heterogeneous and there was no demonstable pathogenesis, presumably relating to an incomplete diagnostic workup. This may also account for the relatively high failure rate in this group (initially we did not perform cavernosography routinely). It is also possible that some of these patients may have had unrecognized psychogenic impotence. This group includes several young men with congenital vascular malformations. The more we deal with arteriogenic impotence, the more convinced we are that the coronary arteries of the heart and the penile arteries are similar and are therefore prone to a similar fate. Indeed, the relationship between coronary artery disease and penile arterial insufficiency is becoming increasingly apparent.

◀ **Fig. 14.** Contrast injection into the AV shunt in postoperative glans hyperemia shows most of the arterial inflow spurting into the glans penis with little entering the corpora cavernosa. Drainage is via the corpus spongiosum urethrae

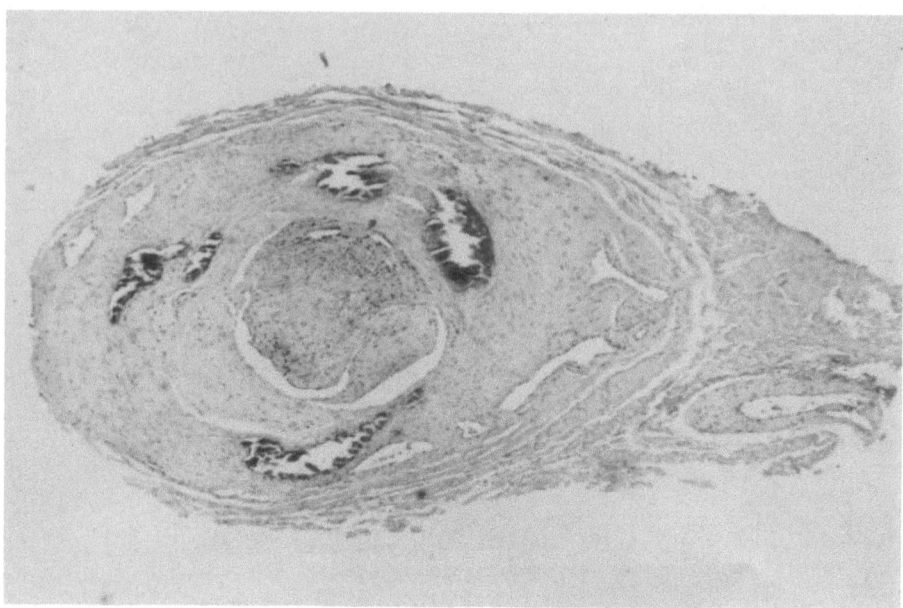

Fig. 16. Typical diabetic vasopathy in a peripheral penile artery. The lumen is almost completely occluded by a heavily fibrosed intima, which has formed an obstructive plug. The media is thickened and contains focal calcifications that partially involve the internal elastic membrane, which is heavily fragmented and no longer present at several sites. The calcifications extend to the intima

Diabetes Mellitus and Impotence

There are still claims in the internal-medical literature [6, 11, 12, 18, 24, 25, 32, 42, 47] that erectile impotence is caused by peripheral neuropathy. But in the examination of juvenile diabetics, who are highly prone to erectile dysfunction, it is consistently found that the small peripheral penile arteries show pathologic changes before any evidence of nerve damage can be recognized (Figs. 16, 17). This peripheral vasopathy is manifested by typical vascular lesions on penile angiograms (Fig. 1). The onset of this angiopathy can be plainly documented by electron microscopy (Fig. 18).[1] We believe, then, that a rationale for penile revascularization exists in the early stage of diabetes mellitus, and we would hope that the improved arterial perfusion might prevent or at least delay the onset of neuropathy, which would unquestionably improve the quality of life in young patients.

It remains to be asked whether it is contradictory to transplant autologous arteries to correct a demonstrably arterial disease. It has been our experience

---

[1] I am indebted to Dr. M. Spycher, Institute of Pathology, Zurich University hospital, for furnishing the electron photomicrographs.

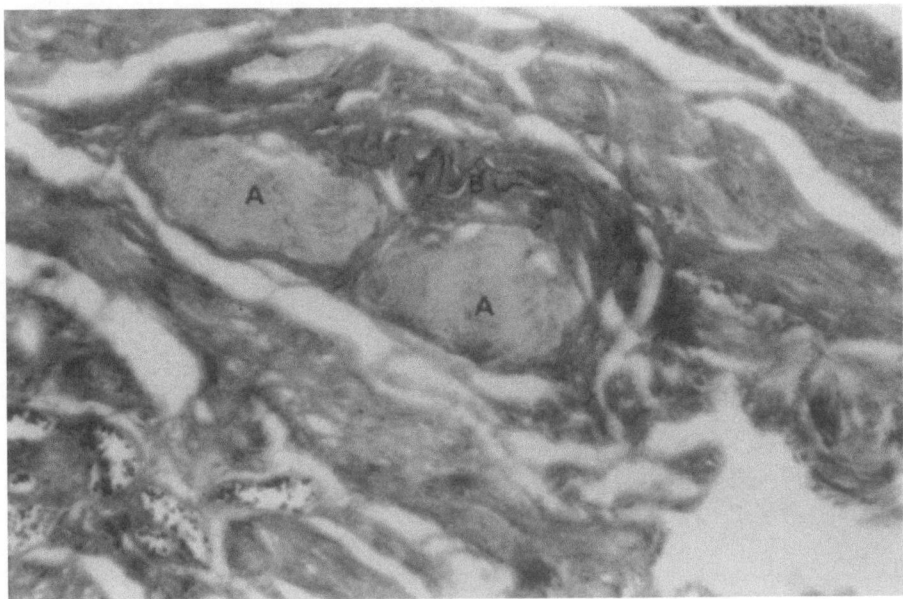

Fig. 17. Nerve preparation from the patient in Fig. 16, taken concurrently with the arterial specimen. There is no evidence of pathology, either in the form of fibrosis or morphologic alterations in the nerve fibers, and there is no excessive fibrosis in the perineural sheath

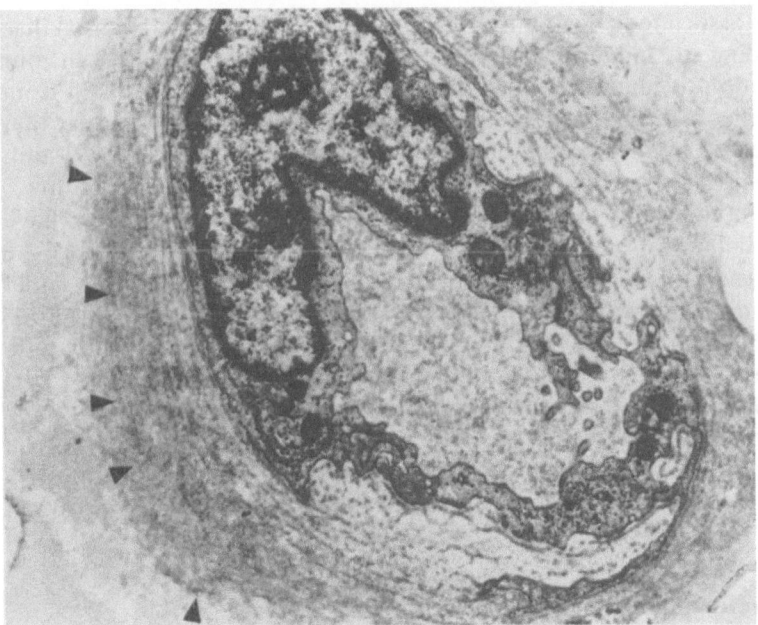

Fig. 18. Detail from an electron micrograph (×20 000) showing an endothelial cell nucleus from a peripheral helicine artery. The nucleus is enveloped by a thickened basement membrane of collagen IV (→)

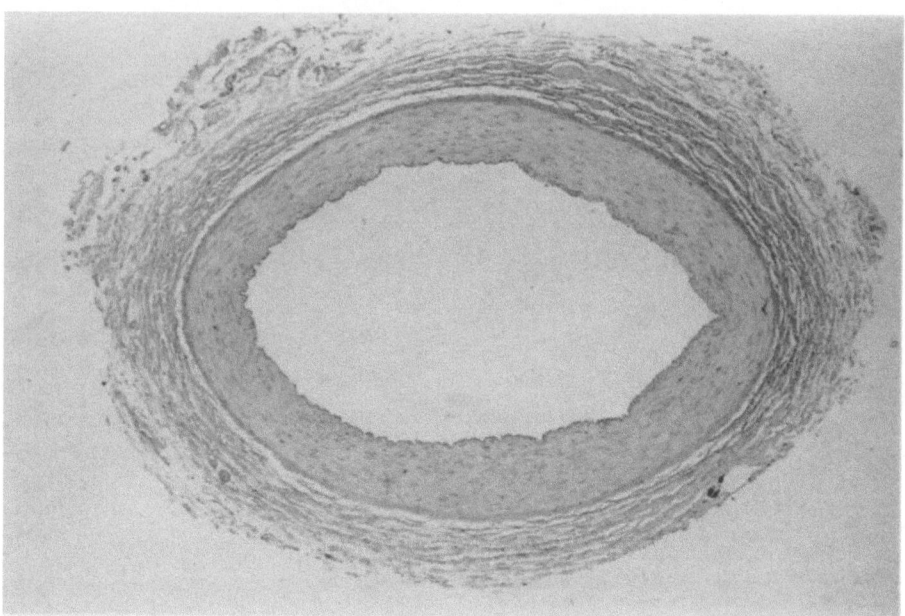

Fig. 19. Normal inferior epigastric artery taken concurrently from the patient in Fig. 16

that diabetes-associated angiopathy generally appears first in the internal iliac system, leading to underperfusion of the penile arteries. But in our revascularization technique, we use the inferior epigastric artery taken from the external iliac arterial tree. The inferior epigastric is a muscular artery that is still unaffected by diabetic lesions at the time of operation (Fig. 19) and, when anastomosed, contributes to the improvement of penile arterial flow.

Despite preoperative evaluation for peripheral neuropathy, we have experienced failures after revascularization. Routine biopsies taken from the corpora cavernosa during operation have alerted us to the fact that the initial changes of diabetic neuropathy may not be detectable by clinical or electrophysiologic methods, largely because our methods are still quite limited in their capacity to evaluate the autonomic nervous system (Fig. 20).

Based on our discoveries to date, we find it disturbing that many internists writing for highly respected publications [47] still espouse an unjustified nihilism by asserting that diabetic erectile failure is a primarily "irreversible" condition. We find some support for our views in the recent literature [21, 28, 43].

Impotence in Heavy Smokers

With impotence in heavy smokers, once again, peripheral angiopathy is the principal causative lesion. Experimental evidence [22] for direct effects of

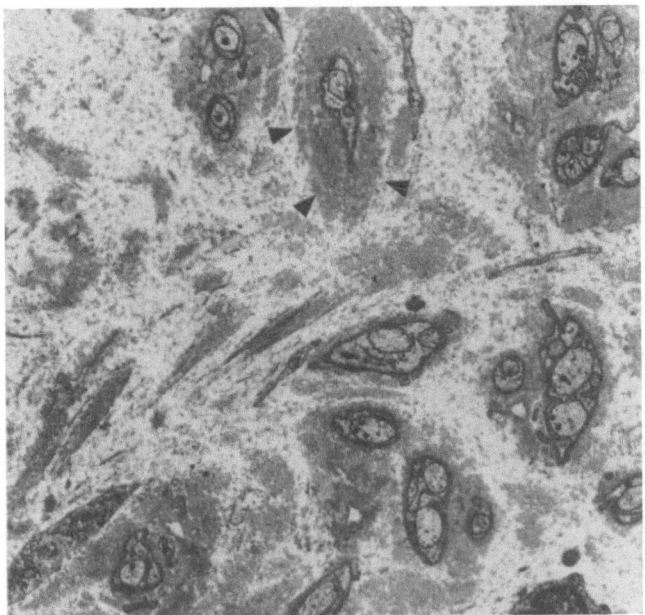

Fig. 20. Biopsy from the corpus cavernosum of a diabetic with no clinical or electro-physiologic signs of neuropathy. Nonmyelinated nerve fibers are clustered, atypically, in a heavily thickened basement membrane (→). This layer of collagen IV will subsequently prevent normal perfusion and lead to neuropathy

nicotine on the venous system covers only the secondary impact of diminished arterial perfusion. The question of whether revascularization should be offered to a patient who refuses to quit smoking is at present a philosophical issue, and long-term results are still needed.

Impotence After Pelvic Trauma

Until a few years ago, it was assumed with fatalistic certainty that erectile failure following pelvic trauma and posterior urethral injuries was strictly neurogenic [5, 8, 31]. Although the possibility of a vascular cause was suggested some years ago [13], it was not until the advent of improved diagnostic procedures, most notably selective penile angiography, that greater attention was paid to the vascular system [44]. The vascular lesions are characteristic (Fig. 3). Revascularization is worthwhile, though we must admit that a coexisting neurogenic lesion is very difficult to evaluate and sometimes can be excluded only by a successful operative revascularization. In some cases an intact nerve supply can be deduced by noting, say, the preservation of ejaculatory function or the occurrence of penile tumescence without rigidity.

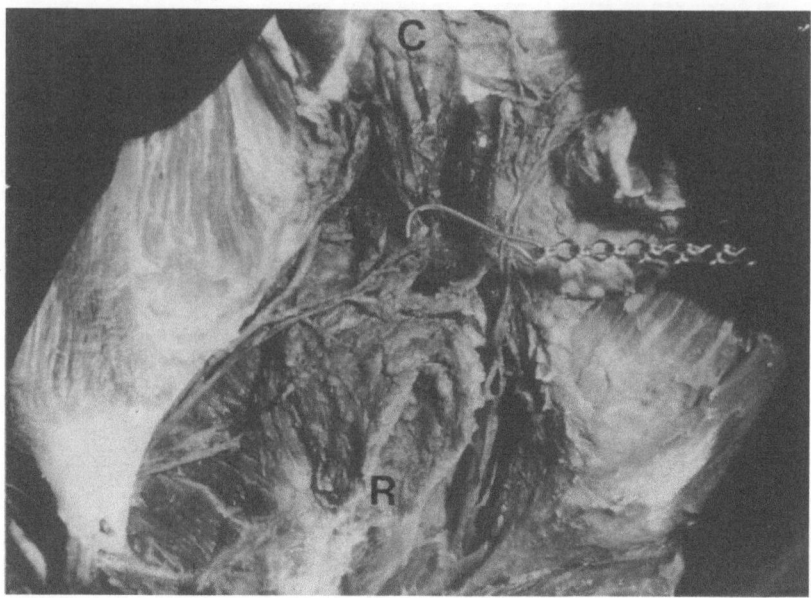

Fig. 21. View into the lesser pelvis with the bladder removed, showing the corpora cavernosa (*C*) superiorly, and inferiorly the site of emergence of the rectum (*R*) through the pelvic floor. The small hook encircles the arteries responsible for penile erection. Their close proximity to the rectum makes them vulnerable during rectal operations

Impotence After Proctectomy

It has been common practice in the past to ascribe impotence after proctectomy to a neurogenic cause. However, our anatomic studies (Fig. 21[2]) have shown that isolated vascular lesions can be inflicted by operations upon the rectum, making revascularization an option for these cases.

Impotence After Radical Prostatectomy

The development of nerve-sparing operating technique has focused new attention on the problem of impotence ofter radical prostatectomy. We have repeatedly been struck by cases in which patients became impotent despite the fact that nervous structures were left intact by the surgery. Our anatomic studies in this area (Fig. 22) and routine selective penile angiograms (Figs. 23, 24) directed our attention to the possibility of isolated arterial lesions. These can be successfully revascularized.

---

[2] I am grateful to Prof. St. Kubik, Institute of Anatomy, University of Zurich, for his assistance and for furnishing Figs. 21 and 22.

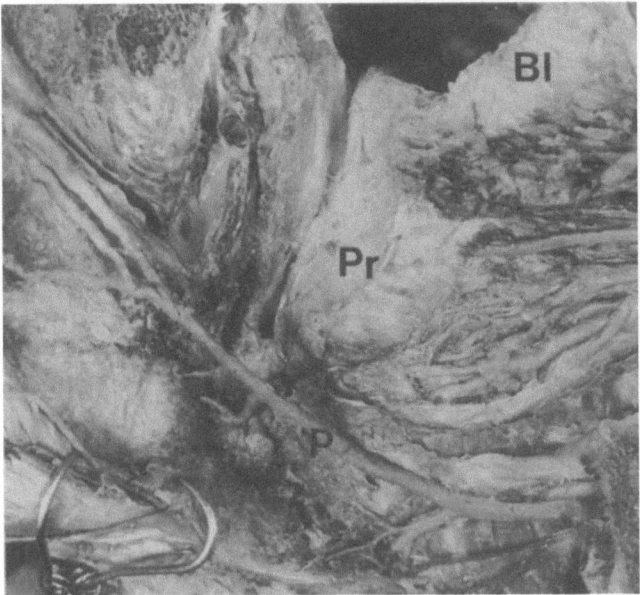

Fig. 22. Preparation of the penile arteries. *P*, common penile artery, which divides into the deep and dorsal penile arteries; *Bl*, bladder; *Pr*, prostate. The proximity of the penile arteries to the prostatic apex accounts for their high vulnerability in radical prostat-ovesiculectomy. Impotence following this operation is not always caused by nerve lesions; approximately one-third of cases are due to isolated vascular injuries

Concluding Remarks

Primary psychogenic impotence is a far less common entity than was once believed. Secondary psychological reactions to a primary organic impotence are understandable and also common. But the most these patients can gain from psychotherapy is the ability to accept their unhappy and inescapable life situation. We have an obligation, therefore, to look for primary organic causes. In undertaking this search, we must substantially improve the diagnostic options now available, and we must extend our investigations to include cellular biology and the nervous system.

The manner in which current therapeutic options are to be utilized is partly a philosophical question and ultimately must be determined by the patient. We believe, however, that the ability to count on a spontaneous erection at the desired time without resorting to technical tricks is an elegant therapeutic concept, and that the surgical cost is worth the gain.

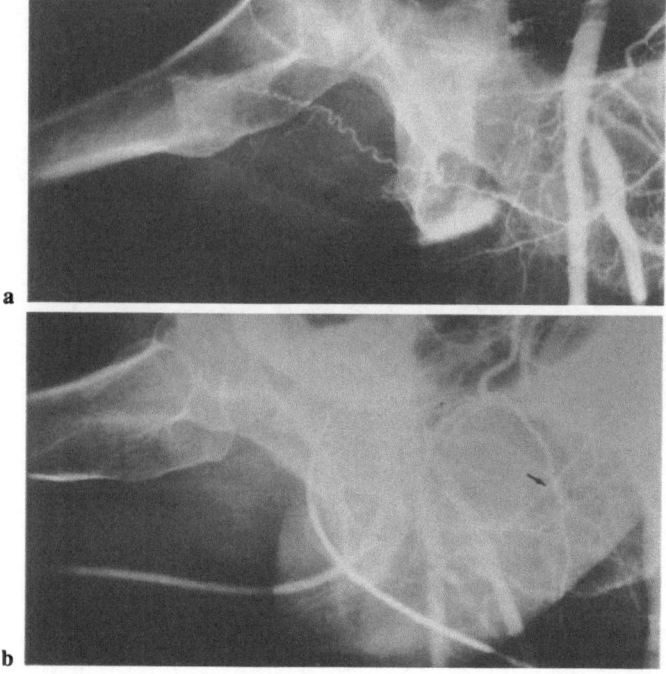
a

b

Fig. 23a,b. Selective penile angiograms in a patient who developed erectile impotence after radical prostectomy. **a** Preoperative view demonstrates a normal arterial supply. **b** Postoperative view shows occlusion of the internal pudendal artery (→) with no peripheral supply

References

1. Alvarez-Morujo A (1967) Terminal arteries of the penis. Acta Anat 67:387
2. Carrel A, Guthrie CC (1906) Reversal of circulation in a limb. Ann Surg 203
3. Casey WC (1979) Revascularization of corpus cavernosum for erectile failure. Urology 14:135
4. Cerespo L, Bove D, Farrell G, Soltanik E (1983) Cinq ans d'expérience dans la révascularisation des corps caverneux avec une nouvelle technique micro-chirurgicale pour le traîtement de l'impuissance sexuelle vasculaire. J Urol (Paris) 89:587
5. Chambers HL, Balfour J (1963) The incidence of impotence following perlvic fracture with associated urinary tract injury. J Urol 89:702
6. Clarke BF, Ewing DJ, Campbell JW (1979) Diabetic autonomic neuropathy. Diabetologia 17:195
7. Cockett ATK, Koshiba K (1979) Manual of urologic surgery. Springer, New York
8. Coffield KS, Weems W (1977) Experience with management of posterior urethral injury associated with pelvic fracture. J Urol 117:722
9. Colleen S, Holmquist B, Olin T (1981) An angiographic study of erection in the dog. Urol Res 9:297

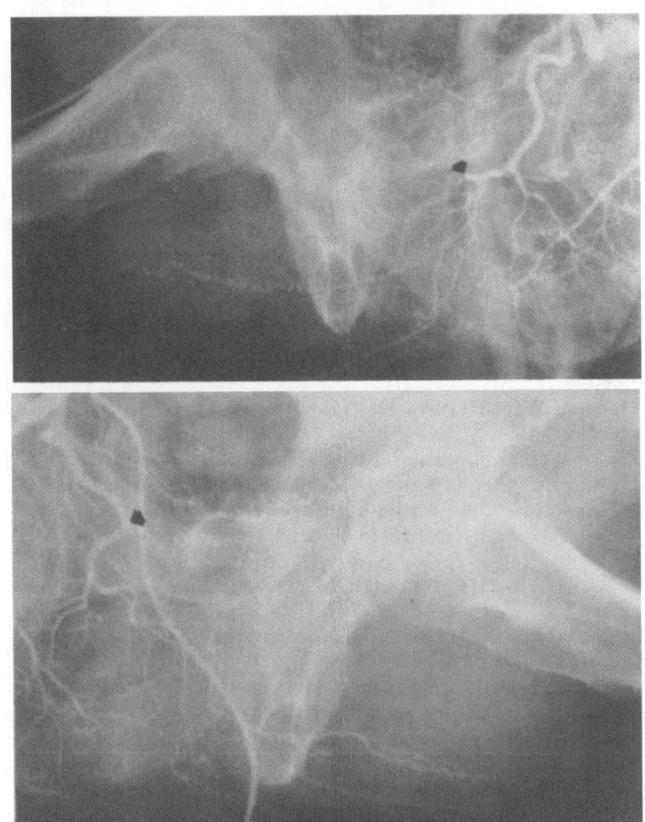

a

b

Fig. 24a,b. Selective penile angiograms in a patient who developed erectile impotence after radical prostectomy. **a** (*left*) Occlusion of the internal pudendal artery with no peripheral arterialization; **b** (*right*) Occlusion of the internal pudendal artery. The peripheral penile arteries are perfused insufficiently through an anastomosis with the obturator artery

10. Crespo E, Soltanik E, Bove D, Farrell G (1982) Treatment of vasculogenic sexual impotence by revascularizing cavernous and/or dorsal arteries using microvascular techniques. Urology 20:271
11. Ellenberger M (1971) Impotence in diabetes: The neurologic factor. Ann Intern Med 75:213
12. Faerman J, Glocer L, Fox D, Jadzinsky MN, Rapaport M (1974) Impotence and Diabetes: Hostologicals studies of the autonomic nervous fibers of the corpora cavernosa in imptent diabetic males. Diabetes 23:971
13. Gibson GR (1970) Impotence following fractured pelvis and ruptured urethra. Br J Urol 42:86
14. Halstead AE, Vaughn RT (1912) A-V anastomosis in the treatment of gangrene of the extremity. Surg Gynecol Obstet 14:1

15. Hauri D (1984) Therapiemöglichkeiten bei der vaskulärbedingten erektilen Impotenz. Akt Urol 15:350
16. Hauri D (1986) A new operative technique in vasculogenic erectile impotence. World J Urol 4:237
17. Hayek H von (1969) Der Penis. In: Alken CE, Goodwin WE, Dix VW, Wildbolz E (Hrsg) Handbuch der Urologie, Bd I: Anatomie und Embryologie. Springer, Berlin Heidelberg New York, S 357–388
18. Heurichs HR (1985) Störung der Potenz als Folge des Diabetes mellitus. Sexualmedizin 5:162
19. Hunter W (1757) The history of an aneurysm of the aorta, with some remarks with aneurysms in general. Medical observations of the Society of Physicians of London 1:323
20. Ibrahim JM, Sussman B, Dardik J, Kalm M, Israel M, Kenny M, Dardik H (1980) Adjunctive arteriovenous fistula with tibial and peroneal reconstruction for limb salvage. Am J Surg 140:246
21. Jevtich MJ, Edson M, Jarman WD, Herrera HH (1982) Vascular factor in erectile failure among diabetics Urology 19:163
22. Jünemann, KP (1986) Personal communication. Symp Exp Urologie, Mainz
23. Kalm M, Sussman B, Ibrahim JM, Dardik J, Israel M, Goldqarb H, Dardik H (1981) Tibial arteriovenous fistula: successful use for limb salvage. Am Surg 47:329
24. Karacan J (1980) Diagnosis of erectile impotence in diabetes mellitus. Ann Intern Med 92:334
25. Kolodny RC, Kahn CB, Goldstein HH, Barnett DM (1974) Sexual dysfunction in diabetic men. Diabetes 23:306
26. Kubik St, Lang E, Hauri D (unpublished) Darstellung der arteriellen Penisversorgung mittels Korrosionspräparaten.
27. Largiadèr J (1983) Arterienrekonstruktion am Unterschenkel: Indikation und Technik. Helv Chir Acta 50:133
28. Lehman TP, Jacobs JA (1983) Etiology of diabetic impotence. J Urol 129:291
29. Lue TF, Müller SC, Jünemann KP, Fournier jr GR, Tanagho EA (1987) Hämodynamische Veränderungen während der Erektion und funktionelle klinische Diagnostik der penilen Gefässe mittels Ultraschall und gepulstem Doppler. Akt Urol 18:115
30. MacGregor RJ, Kormak JW (1982) Treatment of vasculogenic erectile dysfuntion by direct anastomosis of the inferior epigastric artery to the central artery of the corpus cavernosum. J Urol 127:136
31. McAnich JW (1981) Traumatic injuries to the urethra. J Trauma 21:291
32. McCulloch DK, Campbell JW, Wu FC, Prescott RJ, Clarke BF (1980) The prevalence of diabetic impotence. Diabetologia 18:279
33. McDougal WS, Jeffery RF (1983) Microscopic penile revascularization. J Urol 129:517
34. Metz P, Frimodt-Møller C (1983) Epigastrico-cavernous anastomosis in the treatment of arteriogenic impotence. Scand J. Urol Nephrol 17:271
35. Michal V, Kramar R, Pospichal J (1974) Femoro-pudendal by-pass, internal iliac thromboendarterectomy and direct arterial anastomosis to the cavernous body in the treatment of erectile impotence. Bull Soc Int Chir 33:341
36. Michal V, Kramar R, Pospichal J, Hejkal L (1976) Gefässchirurgie erektiler Impotenz. Sexualmedizin 5:15
37. Michal V, Kramar R, Pospichal J, Hejkal L (1977) Arterial epigastricocavernous anastomosis for the treatment of sexual impotence. World J Surg 1:515
38. Nath RC (1981) The multidisciplinary approach to vasculogenic impotence. Surgery 89:124
39. Newman HF, Northup JD (1981) Mechanism of human penile erection: An overview. Urology 17:399
40. Paturet G (1958) Traîté d'anatomie humaine, Tome III. Masson, Paris
41. Rouvière H (1932) Anatomie humaine, 3ème édition. Masson, Paris
42. Rubin A, Babbott D (1958) Impotence and diabetes mellitus. JAMA 168:498
43. Ruzbarsky F, Michal V (1977) Morphologic changes in the arterial bed of penis with aging. Relationship to the pathogenesis of impotence. Invest Urol 15:194

44. Sharlip JD (1981) Penile arteriograpl y in impotence after pelvic trauma. J Urol 126:477
45. Shirai M, Ishh N, Mitsukawa S, Naki mura M (1978) Hemodynamic mechanism of erection in the human penis. Arch An(lrol 1:345
46. Szilagyi DE, Jay GD, Murrel ED (19 }1) Femoral arteriovenous anastomosis in the treatment of occlusive arterial disease. Arch Surg 63:435
47. Tattersal R (1982) Sexual problems of diabetic men. Br Med J 285:911
48. Virag R, Zwang G, Dermange H, l egman M, Peuven JP (1980) Exploration et traîtement chirurgical de l'impuissance vasculaire. J Mal Vasc 5:205
49. Zaorgniotti AW, Rossi G, Padula G, Makovsky RD (1980) Diagnosis and therapy of vasculogenic impotence. J Urol 123:67 l
50. Zorgniotti AW (1980) Diagnosis and herapy of vasculogenic impotence. Ann Urol 14:28

Diagnostic and Surgical Approach to Impotent Patients with Cavernovenous Leakage

E. Wespes

Introduction

The precise mechanism of the venous system during human erection is not completely understood. Recent studies based on isotopic [29], radiological [7, 23, 24, 36, 37] or ultrasonographic [6] examinations of venous return during physiological erection or after papaverine-induced erection have confirmed the existence of a venous blockage. It appears to function due to compression of the emissary veins between the dilated sinusoidal spaces and the tunica albuginea at rigidity [9]. However, if there is complete blockage of the venous return through the emissary veins, venous outflow through the cavernous veins is reduced, but still persists and allows circulation of blood for oxygenation of the erectile tissues during erection [35].

Penile venous return takes place through the deep and superficial dorsal veins of the penis: the cavernous, crural, and bulbis veins. The cavernous veins are located at the bifurcation of the corpora cavernosa. The crural veins drain the most proximal part of the penis. The deep dorsal and cavernous veins terminate in Santorini's vesico-prostatic plexus. The skin and prepuce are drained by the superficial dorsal veins that communicate with the external pudendal vein. The external pudendal vein terminates in the internal saphenous vein. The superficial and deep venous systems are interrelated by multiple anastomoses. The venous system of the penis is thus in communication with the internal iliac vein, the spermatic venous plexus, and the saphenous vein [26].

Static cavernosography has been utilized in the past to study the venous plexus in prostatic and vesical diseases. As it provides a radiological image of the corpora cavernosa, it has also been utilized to demonstrate the abnormal anatomy of the corpora cavernosa in priapism, perineal trauma. Peyronie's disease, and congenital abnormalities.

More recently dynamic cavernosography has been developed for the investigation of male sexual dysfunction by creating a passive erection with physiological saline [31] and a radio-opaque [23, 24, 36] substance. This allows the simultaneous recording of intracavernous pressure and demonstration of venous leakage. These studies were performed after perfusion of the corpora cavernosa either in fresh male cadavers or in patients with a

U. Jonas et al. (Eds.) Erectile Dysfunction
© Springer-Verlag Berlin Heidelberg 1991

tourniquet placed at the base of the penis in order to prevent outflow of the perfused solution [20]. Since the role played by venous outflow was not taken into account in the latter case, however, the different values for the erectile flow obtained in the respective studies can be explained.

In a further series of studies the inflow necessary to produce a passive erection, together with the intracavernous pressure and penile circumference were measured in normal patients [31] and in patients with psychogenic and organic impotence [36] without any artificial mechanism of retention. In normal patients, the perfusion rate necessary to produce an erection was found to range between 80 and 120 ml/min [31]. Intracavernous pressure was weak but remained steady in spite of the increased perfusion rate, while penile diameter increased and reached its maximum circumference before the penis became completely rigid. The circumference during passive erection was the same as during physiological erection. This study demonstrates how difficult it is to quantify erection.

Once complete rigidity had occurred, the intracavernous pressure rapidly increased to reach values up to 90 mm Hg. When the perfusion rate was sustained, the pressure in the corpora cavernosa rapidly increased to values of 200–300 mm Hg while the patient rapidly complained of acute penile pain. The perfusion rate necessary to maintain erection varied between 20 and 40 ml/min. At the beginning of the infusion, the corpora cavernosa appeared clearly opacified and the deep dorsal vein and Santorini's plexus could also be seen. However, in normal individuals they were no longer visible once an erection was obtained since the contrast material remained trapped in the corpora.

The results obtained with psychogenically impotent patients were similar to those obtained with normal patients [36]. In patients with organic impotence, however, two groups were identified; those with normal values and others [17, 18, 23, 24, 32]. Who required perfusion rates varying between 160 and 300 ml/min to create an erection and between 60 and 140 ml/min to maintain the erection. The pressure in the flaccid state varied between 5 and 9 mm Hg and in the erectile state between 93 and 110 mm Hg. There was no significant difference in age between the two groups with organic impotence. In the patients with normal values on cavernosometry, at fluoroscopy under the standardized flow rate (120 ml/min) contrast medium opacified the deep dorsal vein and Santorini's plexus during the initial filling phase, but when erection was obtained, it could no longer be seen in these veins. In the patients for whom a much higher flow rate was necessary to induce a passive erection, the deep dorsal vein and Santorini's plexus were seen under standardized flow rate (120 ml/min) and the intracavernous pressure was around 40 mm Hg. These patients were considered to have cavernovenous leakage [32, 36].

The cavernosometry–cavernosography did not take into account the role of arterial inflow and relaxation of the intracavernous smooth musculature. Moreover, the psychogenic state of the patient could influence the results of cavernosometry by provoking contraction of the intravenous musculature. Therefore, this examination was performed after intracavernous vasoactive drug injection [16, 18, 28, 37].

The flow rate necessary to obtain and maintain an erection was always reduced after papaverine injection, even in patients with venous leakage, but in this latter group it still remained higher than normal most of the time. However, in some patients considered to have venous leakage, intracavernous papaverine injection provoked a return to normal flow rates and therefore a venous leak could not be confirmed. Phentolamine, a vasoactive drug, was also injected prior to cavernosometry but did not influence the venous return [39]. The question concerning pharmacocavernosometry remains as to which drug in which dosage should be injected.

All the surgical procedures for the treatment of a cavernovenous leak are designed to improve the trapping of arterial blood during erection. None of them treat the underlying physiopathological mechanism because this has not yet been established. This article reports the experience of different surgical teams in the treatment of this pathology.

Materials and Methods

Surgery involves the deep dorsal, cavernous, and crural veins, or all of them. The choices of incision and technique are described.

Type of Incision

- Circumferential incision
- Infrapubic incision
- Penoscrotal incision
- Lateral incision
- Circumcision and penoscrotal incision

Type of Surgery

Simple Ligature of the Deep Dorsal Vein

After an infrapubic incision under Buck's fascia, the deep dorsal vein, which is situated between the two dorsal arteries in the intracavernosal groove, is isolated, cut, and ligated. Before dividing the vein, the Doppler stethoscope can be used to ensure that the arteries will not be injured. After ligature of the deep dorsal vein, the small veins around the tunica albuginea are also isolated and ligated.

Resection of the Deep Dorsal Vein

After a circumcision or an infrapubic incision, the deep dorsal vein is resected with ligation or coagulation of the circumflex or emissary veins. Dissection is extended proximally to the level of the suspensory ligament. Distally, the vein is removed to the point at which it begins to fan out under the edge of the glans penis. Tributaries seen to feed into interconnecting veins on the lateral shaft of the penis are also ligated.

Ligature of the Cavernous Veins

After an oblique inguinoscrotal incision made about 3 cm lateral to the root of the penis along the course of the spermatic cord, the root and the entire penile pendulous portion are isolated. The suspensory ligament is completely detached from the pubic bone. The deep dorsal vein is resected under the pubic bone. Incision of the deep layer of Buck's fascia is performed using an operative microscope to expose the cavernous veins, which are ligated. Care must be taken not to injure the cavernous arteries and nerves. Afterwards, the suspensory ligament is reattached to the pubic bone.

Ligature of the Crural Veins

The crural veins come posteriorly from the crural edges and cannot be reached. For that reason, surgical treatment consists of exclusion of the crural edges by ligation of the corpora 1 cm below the point of their union.

Spongiolysis

After circumcision, the skin of the penis is drawn back to the root of the organ and the spongiosum is dissected completely in its distal half. The spongiosum is separated from the corpus cavernosa and the dissection is continued to the glans penis where the tips of the corpora are isolated entirely from the glans.

Results

It should be stressed that follow-up of the various surgical procedures is very short in most of the reported series. A larger number of patients and a long-term follow-up are necessary to appreciate the relative importance of this treatment of impotence. Few recent papers describe the long-term efficacy of surgery that potentially restores spontaneous flaccidity and erection of the penis (Table 1).

In our experience, failures were mainly observed in patients with arterial disease. Some patients complained of loss of penile sensation due to surgical dissection. Relapses or incomplete ligature were also responsible for the nonresponder patients. In other patients, intracavernous papaverine injection

Table 1. Results of venous surgery according to the data reported in the literature

Reference	Number of patients	Type of surgery	Patients cured n (%)	Average follow-up (months)
Our series	67	DDV ligature-resection	31(46)	24–72
Wespes and Schulman [32]	20	DDV ligature	16(80)	3–24
Parrott et al. [21]	10	DDV resection	1(10)	
Lewis [16]	25	DDV resection	10(40)	2–29
Lewis et al. [17]	50	DDV resection	12(24)	15
Bennet et al. [4]	8	DDV resection	6(75)	6–18
Lunglmayr et al. [19]	29	DDV resection	(31)	4–24
Willams et al. [40]	13	DDV resection	9(69)	2–11
Austoni et al. [1]	234	DDV ligation	55(23)	9
Treiber and Gilbert [25]	115	DDV ligature-resection	67(58)	12.9
Buvat et al. [5]	10	DDV ligature-resection	1(10)	–
Puech-Leâo et al. [22]	8	Crural edge ligation	7(88)	short
Bar Moshe and Vandendris [3]	12	Crural edge ligation	9(75)	1–11
Glina et al. [11]	47	Crural edge ligation	23(49)	18.9
Lue [18]	64	DDV + CV resection ligation	36(56)	2–26
Gilbert and Stief [10]	5	Spongiolysis	0(0)	6–8

DDV, Deep dorsal veins; *CV*, cavernous veins

induced rigid erections for satisfactory intercourse, while before surgery, these patients had presented only a partial tumescence. In these patients, psychological factors could explain why they did not recover normal erection, and they were referred for psychologic treatment.

Complications

Few problems have been observed after this kind of surgery. Blood loss is rarely a problem. Edema appears in the immediate follow-up but resolves spontaneously very quickly. This slight complication is mainly present with infrapubic incision due to ligature of the lymphatics and is rarely observed with circumcision or lateral incision. Penile shortening, sensory loss due to extensive surgery, or excessive scarring at the base of the penis can be observed. Priapism can be observed, but this severe problem is very rare and is due to excessive venous resection.

Discussion

Venous surgery for impotence has recently gained in importance. The absence of venous blood trapping in the penis during the erect state produces soft erections inducing sexual dysfunction. The physiopathological mechanism responsible for this failure has not yet been clearly identified, but this phenomenon may be due to incompetence of dilated sinusoïd spaces or to the loss of elasticity of the tunica albuginea that becomes unable to compress the subalbugineal venous plexus and the emissary veins during tumescence. It does not seem to be due to alteration of the adrenoceptors of the veins [8, 14]. The different surgical procedures described here do not invade the corpora cavernosa and are limited to the veins. For that reason, the immediate results are certainly not completely satisfactory and relapses can be observed a few months after surgery. Patient selection is also very important. Patients with arterial disease must be rejected: if the arterial inflow is reduced, ligation of the veins does not lead to sufficient penile tumescence to induce an erection. These patients might benefit from deep dorsal vein arterialization if they are less than 55 years of age [4, 27]. However, the results are not encouraging in patients with severe arterial lesions [2, 38].

An alternative type of anastomosis – sature of the epigastric artery on to the deep dorsal vein and the dorsal artery – has been proposed [13]. This surgery seems to give good results in patients that respond to intracavernous papaverine injection [13]. However, we do not believe that such patients are candidates for vascular surgery since they develop normal pharmacological erections.

In older patients with arterial and venous insufficiencies, intracavernous injections of vasoactive drugs produce pharmacologically induced erections which was not possible before correction of the venous leak. Reduction of venous outflow decreases the amount of drug necessary and avoids secondary effects due to immediate liberation of the drug into the systemic circulation [36]. Patients with neurological alterations are certainly not candidates. However appropriate methods for investigating penile innervation must be found. The measurement of the bulbocavernous reflex latency time is an indirect method, but measurement of the electrical activity in the corpus cavernosum should allow the study of the autonomic motor system function that normally regulates penile function [30].

Vascular surgery should be reserved for patients in whom complete restoration of erectile function is probable. Major resection of the venous return should give the best immediate and also long-term results. Venous surgery should not be limited to the veins opacified at cavernosography but it must be extended, in our opinion, to the two main drainage veins of the corpora cavernosa: the deep dorsal and cavernous veins. The complexity of the penile venous system is so variable that the choice of incision is very important. The lateral or the circumferential and penoscrotal incisions make all the different veins accessible.

Perioperative measurement of the erectile flow rates is mandatory and allows the operation to be monitored. If no reduction in flow rate is seen after resection of several veins, there is leakage through other veins, which must also be ligated.

Patients with suspected veno-occlusive dysfunction should be carefully examined using a multidisciplinary approach. Cavernovenous leakage is demonstrated by cavernosometry and cavernosography, erectile flow rates being the most important criteria. The use of pharmacocavernosometry should reduce the false positive results because papaverine provokes distension of the sinusoïds and seems to reproduce the normal physiological environment. The cavernovenous leakage syndrome certainly requires further investigation. Resection of the deep venous network can restore erection even though the physiopathological mechanism is not yet clear. This surgery increases erectile function in patients without arterial disease and does not exclude penile prosthesis implantation if it fails. A better understanding of erectile physiology will improve our diagnostic and surgical approach to impotent patients.

References

1. Austoni E, Bellorofonte C, Mantovani F (1987) Improved results with intracavernous vasoactive drug infusion following new surgical techniques for vasculogenic impotence. World J Urol 5:182–189
2. Balko A, Malhotra CM, Wincze JP et al. (1986) Deep penile vein arterialization for arterial and venous impotence. Arch Surg 121:774–777
3. Bar-Moshe O, Vandendris M (1988) Treatment of impotence due to perineal venous leakage by ligation of crura penis. J Urol 139:1217–1219
4. Bennet AH, Rivard DJ, Blanc RP, Moran M (1986) Reconstructive surgery for vasculogenic impotence. J Urol 136:599
5. Buvat J, Lemaire A, Buvat-Herbaut M, Dehaene JL, Marcolin G, Desmons F (1980) Impuissances avec fuite veineuse. Ann Urol (Paris) 20 (5):323–330
6. Casey WC, Woods RWW (1982) Anatomy and histology of penile deep dorsal vein: venous cushion and proximal "sphincter". Urology 19:482–485
7. Ebbehoj J, Uhrenholdt A, Wagner G (1980) Infusion cavernography in the human unstimulated and stimulated situations and its diagnostic value. In: Zorgniotti AW, Ross (eds) Vasculogenic impotence. Proc 1st Int Conf on Corpus Cavernosum Revascularization, Thomas, Springfield, pp 191–196

8. Fontaine J, Schulman CC, Wespes E (1987) Postjunctional alpha-1-and alpha-2-like activity in human isolated deep dorsal vein of the penis. Br J Pharmacol 89:493

9. Fournier GR, Juenemann KP, Lue TF, Tanagho EA (1986) Mechanism of venous occlusion during canine penile erection: an anatomic demonstration. J Urol 137:163

10. Gilbert P, Stief C (1987) Spongiosolysis: A new surgical treatment of impotence caused by distal venous leakage. J Urol 138:784–786

11. Glina S, Reichelt AC, Leâo PP, Siqueira Marcondes Dos Reis JM (1988) Impact of cigarette smoking on papaverine-induced erection. J Urol 140:523–527

12. Glina S, Puech-Leâo P, Marcondes Dos Reis JM, Reichelt AC, Chao S (to be published) Surgical exclusion of the crural ending of the corpora cavernosa: late results. Eur Urol

13. Hauri D (1986) A new operative technique in vasculogenic impotence. World J Urol 4:237–249

14. Kirkeby HJ, ForDan A, Sorensen S, Andersson KE (1989) Alpha-adrenoceptor function in isolated penile circumflex veins from potent and impotent men. J Urol 142:1369–1371

15. Krane RJ, Goldstein I, Saenz de Tejada I (1989) Impotence. N E J 1648–1656

16. Lewis RW (1988) Venous surgery for impotence. Urol Clin North Am 15 (1):115–121

17. Lewis RW, Puyau FA, Bell DP (1987) Another surgical approach for vasculogenic impotence. J Urol 136:1210–1212

18. Lue TF (1989) Penile venous surgery. Urol Clin North Am 16:607–611

19. Lunglmayr G, Nachtigall M, Gindl K (1988) Long-term results of deep dorsal penile vein transsection in venous impotence. Eur Urol 15:209–212

20. Newman HF, Northrup JD, Devlin J (1964) Mechanism of human penile erection. Invest Urol 1:350

21. Parrott LH, Sholes AH, Rice JC Lewis RW, Kerstein MD (1989) Penile vein dissection: a study of its long-term efficacy in impotence. World J Urol 7:169–172

22. Puech-Leâo P, Reis JMSM, Glina S, Reichelt AC (1987) Leakage through the crural edge of corpus cavernosum. Eur Urol 13:163–165

23. Puyau FA, Lewis RW (1983) Corpus cavernosography: pressure, flow and radiography. Invest Radiol 18:517

24. Stief C, Wetteraurer U (1983) Quantitative and qualitative analysis of dynamic cavernographies in erectile dysfunction due to venous leakage. Urology 34:252–257

25. Treiber U, Gilbert P (1989) Venous surgery in erectile dysfunction: a critical report on 116 patients. Urology 34:22–27

26. Tudoriu T, Bourmer H (1983) The hemodynamics of erection at the level of the penis and its local deterioration. J Urol 129:741–748

27. Virag R, Zwang G, Dermange H, Legman M (1981) Vasculogenic impotence: a review of 92 cases with 54 surgical operations. Vasc Surg 15:9–17

28. Virag R, Frydman D, Legman M, Virag H (1984) Intracavernous injection of papaverine as a diagnostic and therapeutic method in erectile failure. Angiologie 35:79

29. Wagner G, Uhrenholdt A (1989) Blood flow by clearance in the human corpus cavernosum in the flaccid and erect state. In: Zorgniotti AW, Ross (eds) Vasculogenic impotence. Proc 1st Conf on Corpus Cavernosum Revascularization, Thomas, Springfield, pp 44–46

30. Wagner G, Gerstenberg T, Levin RJ (1989) Electrical activity of corpus cavernosum during flaccidity and erection of the human penis: a new diagnostic method? J Urol 142:723–725

31. Wespes E, Schulman CC (1984) Parameters of erection. Br J Urol 56:416–417

32. Wespes E, Schulman CC (1985) Venous leakage: surgical treatment of a curable cause of impotence. J Urol 133:796–798

33. Wespes E, Schulman CC (1987) Vascular impotence. World J Urol 5:144–149

34. Wespes E, Schulman CC (1988) Systemic complication of intracavernous papaverine injection in patients with venous leakage. Urology 21 (2):114–115

35. Wespes E, Schulman CC (1990) Study of the penile venous system and hypothesis on its behavior during erection. Urology 36 (1):68–72

290 E. Wespes: Diagnostic and Surgical Approach

36. Wespes E, Delcour C, Struyven J, Schulman CC (1984) Cavernometry-cavernography: its role in impotence. Eur Urol 10:229–232
37. Wespes E, Delcour C, Struyven J, Schulman CC (1986) Pharmacocavernometry-cavernography in impotence. Br J Urol 58:429–433
38. Wespes E, Corbusier A, Delcour C, Vandenbosch G, Struyven J, Schulman CC (1989) Deep dorsal vein arterialisation in vascular impotence. Br J Urol 64:535–540
39. Wespes C, Rondeux C, Schulman CC (1989) Effect of phentolamine of venous return in human erection. Br J Urol 63:95–97
40. Williams G, Mulcahy MJ, Hartnell G, Kiely E (1988) Diagnosis and treatment of venous leakage: a curable cause of impotence. Br J Urol 61:151–155

Alloplastics in the Treatment of Erectile Dysfunction

U. Jonas

In contrast to other mammal species such as the whale, dog, bear, gibbon, or otter, the human male does not have a penile bone inside his penis to enforce erection. Despite earlier surgical efforts to treat erectile impotence by the resection of the dorsal vein of the penis it seemed logical that Bogoras in 1936 used a part of rib cartilage in order to reinforce rigidity in the penis. However, the rib cartilage and bone implants were reabsorbed after several months and therefore the effect abolished [7, 22, 24].

The first alloplastic implants were described in 1952 – according to unpublished data by Scardino – using acrylic prostheses. These devices were originally positioned between the corpora cavernosa; however, they were less successful than polyethylene prostheses which were implanted inside the tunica albuginea. Loeffler et al. stated that "It might seem like meddlesome surgery to insert a foreign body of considerable size into the adult male penis, but to the patient with an organic impotence, otherwise in good health and with normal desires, this is a real problem that is worth trying for correction." In 1966, Beheri already reported on 700 penile implants. He used two polyethylene rods and placed each one inside the corpora cavernosa [6, 22, 25, 39, 42, 51].

After having finally found the appropriate material (silicone rubber) and the exact implantation site (inside the tunica albuginea), prosthetic surgery for the treatment of erectile impotence became more and more popular, despite the fact that by creating space inside the corporal body, corporal tissue with eventual residual function had to be destroyed. In 1973, Scott and coworkers described a completely new concept using inflatable silicone cylinders which could be filled voluntarily via a pump which became implanted in the scrotum, transporting fluid to the cylinders from a reservoir which was positioned behind the rectus muscle (Fig. 1). In 1976, Small-Carrion designed a prosthesis which was much easier to implant and had less complications, but which had the disadvantage of a more-or-less permanent erection due to the rigid rods which were positioned inside the corpora cavernosa (Fig. 2) [52, 55].

Comparing the rods designed by Small and Carrion with the inflatable penile implants described by Scott and coworkers, the individual features could be summarized as follows: the *rods* consisted of a simple design, the device itself was of low cost, the surgical procedure was simple and could be

U. Jonas et al. (Eds.) Erectile Dysfunction
© Springer-Verlag Berlin Heidelberg 1991

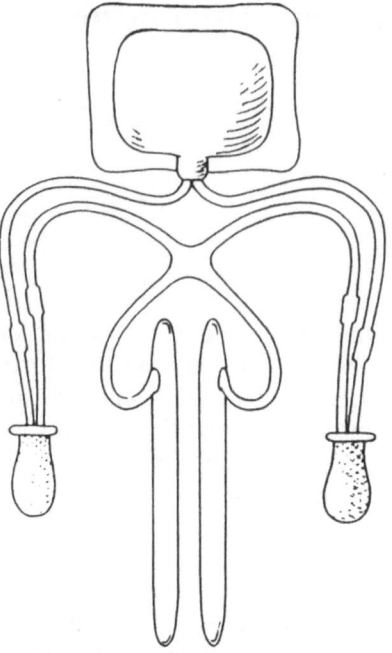

Fig. 1. The original inflatable penile prosthesis [13]

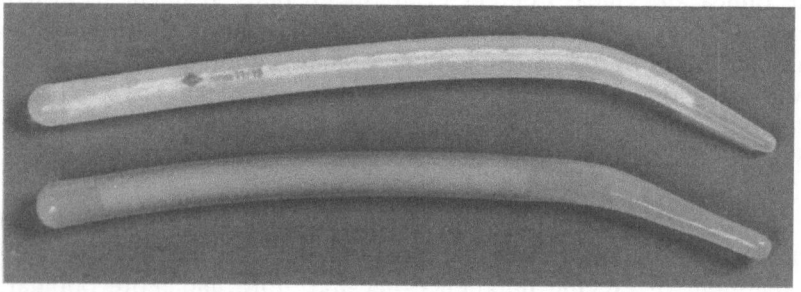

Fig. 2. Semirigid, malleable devices. Small-Carrion (*bottom*) and Jonas (*top*) penile implants

performed by each trained surgeon. Its disadvantages, however, were the permanently erected penis, possible impaired micturition, and a cosmetic appearance which diminished acceptance of this type. The inflatable device had the advantage of being the only device which produced a more-or-less "physiologic" erection and voluntarily controlled "erected" and "flaccid" position of the penis. Its disadvantages were mechanical and hydraulic problems with a possible need for reoperation and exchange of parts in more than 30%, the need for pumping prior to intercourse, possible unequal filling of the cylinders with the consequence of the penis becoming conic in shape, especially in its distal part. However, these two devices started the develop-

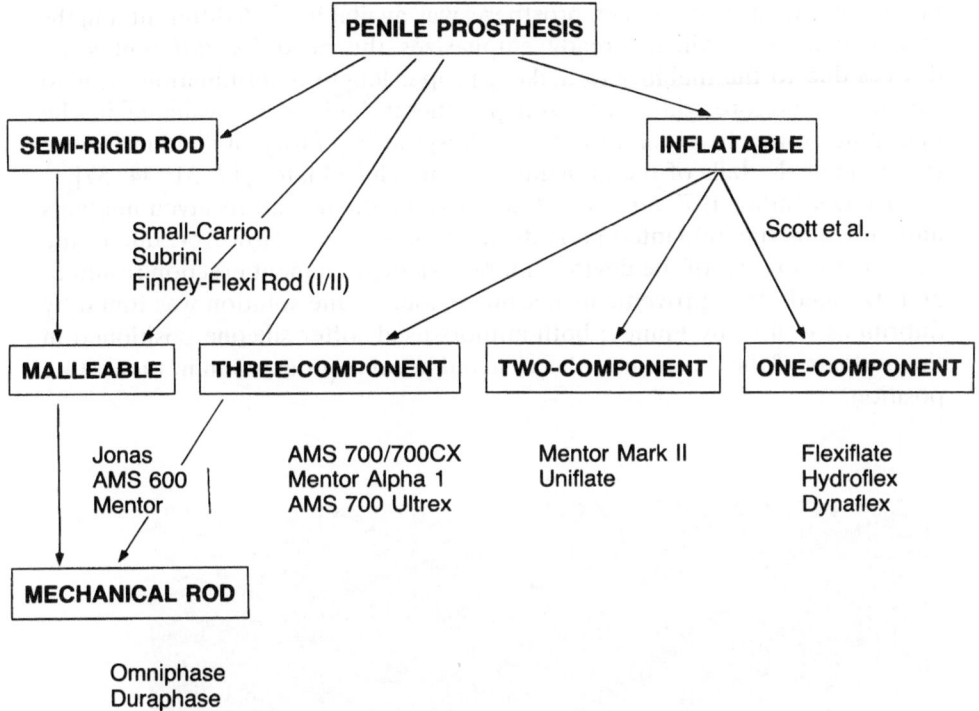

Fig. 3. Alloplastics in erectile dysfunction

ment and design of numerous new prostheses throughout the last 17 years such as the penile implants described by Subrini, Finney, Jonas, and Mentor [15, 17, 20, 21, 30–32, 59].

In order to sort out the different prostheses available in 1990, a brief description of the available possibilities is shown in Fig. 3. The rod prostheses are more or less outdated and were replaced by the malleable devices (if a noninflatable prosthesis was used).

Thus, today's distinction is between the malleable devices versus the one-, two-, or three-component inflatable devices. In the following some features of the individual penile prostheses are reviewed, and special attention is given to the specific characteristics which make these devices different from the others.

Malleable Devices

In 1975 Small and Carrion described their device; it consisted of a pair of silicone rod prostheses (see Fig. 2, bottom) which were implanted through a midline perineal incision. The prosthesis was available in 16 different lengths and 3 diameters, which already emphasizes the need for different sized devices due to the inability to make a proper length determination prior to surgery. Therefore, different sized prostheses had to be available in the operating room. In order to decrease hospital inventory, individual device trimming at the tails of the implants was introduced later [17, 31, 44, 57].

By December 1977 already a total of 260 patients had received implants and only 3 of 106 implanted patients had a poor result. However, due to the rigid characteristics of the device a more-or-less permanent erection resulted, and the need for improvements became evident. One solution was found by Subrini as well as by Finney; both authors used softer silicone positioned in the midpart of the device in order to avoid permanent erection in the resting position.

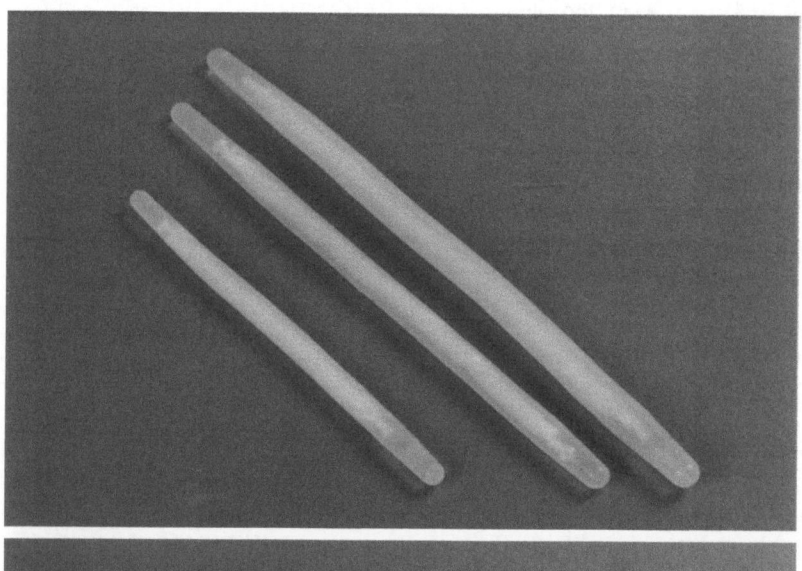

a

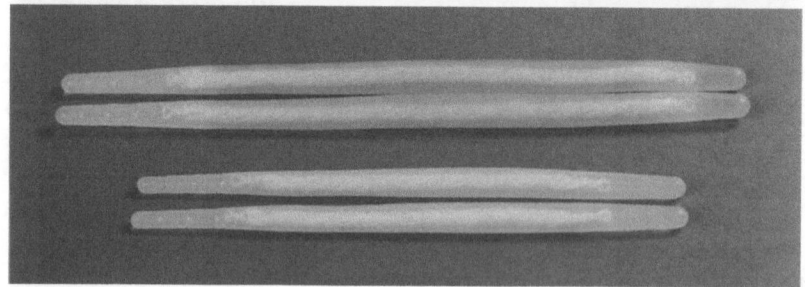

b

Fig. 4a,b. Jonas silicone-silver penile prosthesis. **a** Standard version. A total of 22 pairs of different sized prostheses (in three different diameters) are available for individual fit. **b** Trimming tip version. Proximally, the device may be trimmed up to 3 cm, only four pairs in two different diameters are necessary to fulfill all length requirements

Subrini described his preliminary experience in 1974. Between 1970 and 1982 he operated on a total of 283 impotent patients with an overall failure rate of only 1.7%. Success ranked as high as 95% after primary surgery and 98.3% if surgery had to be performed a second time.

Finney's device, the "flexirod hinged silicone penile implant," was described in 1977. Due to the hinge (in the midpart of the device, as described) in the "resting position," the penis was allowed to hang down rather "normally"; for intercourse it was brought up manually with satisfying rigidity. In 1980 he published the experience with implants in 253 patients. Complications occurred in 5% and only two devices extruded through the urethra. His data showed an overall success rate of around 95%. The feature of this device was that the proximal end could be trimmed intraoperatively. Therefore after a preoperative length estimation (pubis to midglans) from 27 different sized prostheses a correct and custom fit could be made for each patient [17, 19, 30, 56, 59, 60].

A different way of combining the features of malleability with simple design was done by Jonas when in 1978 he published a report on silicone silver penile prosthesis (see Figs. 2, top, 4a,b). This device was characterized by silver wires embedded inside the silicone rubber to stabilize the penis in different positions: downwards or against the body during the resting position or in an erection for intercourse. Despite the fact that the silver strands could break after numerous bendings (following approximately 5000 double bendings on a stimulator at one specific point) the silver never protruded the silicone rubber nor was the function inhibited by fractures of the silver wires (stability). In order, however, to avoid future discussions of whether or not broken silver strands could lead to negative results, since approximately 1984, the individual silver strands were embedded in thermoplastic Teflon, making further breakages impossible (Fig. 5a,b).

The original device (standard version) was manufactured in three different diameters (9.5 mm, 11 mm, and 13 mm in lengths between 17 and 24 cm). A total of 22 different prostheses were available (Fig. 4a).

In order to diminish costs the trimming-tip version was introduced, a device which could be shortened at its proximal end making only two pairs of different lengths necessary in two different diameters (Fig. 4b). In a multicenter trial performed in the early 1980s based on 1834 patients with implants an overall success rate of close to 95% was achieved. Early complications were seen in 5.1%, later in 2.8%; only 19 of the 1834 implants had to be removed (1.04%).

The concept of a metal strand inside the malleable silicone prostheses for reliable and flexible stability was copied later in the AMS Malleable 600 prosthesis in which instead of Teflon-coated silver strands a steel-capped, fabric-wrapped stainless steel core was used. Further features were the removable silicone jacket and the rear-tip extenders.

The MENTOR malleable penile prosthesis also contains a silver strand; however, this strand is coiled in a spiral, giving a corkscrew appearance. The

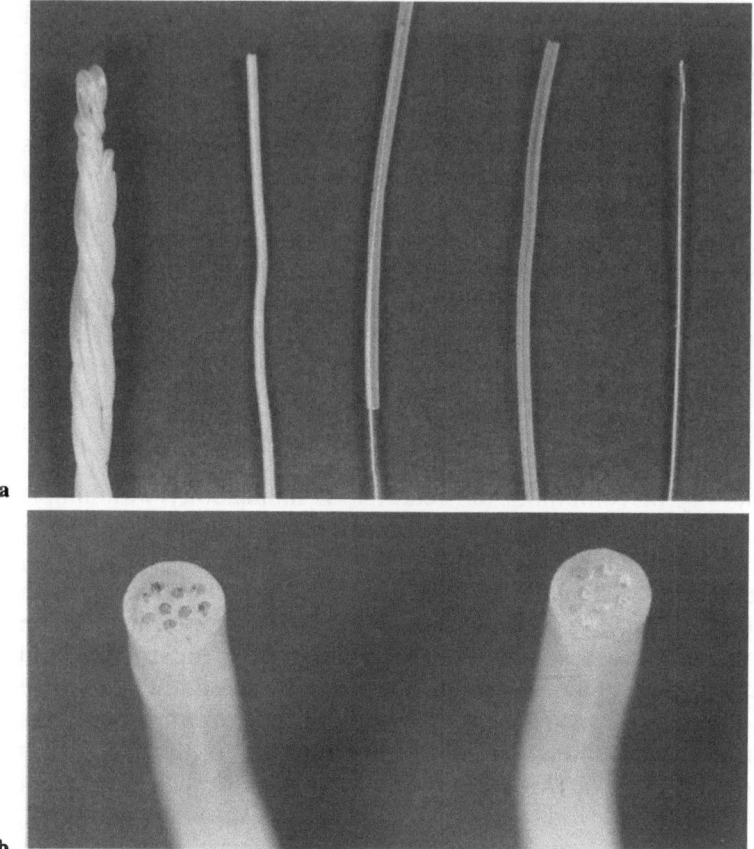

Fig. 5a,b. Jonas silicone-silver penile prosthesis. **a** Special design covering the individual silver strands by thermoplastic Teflon (**b**). The result is the separation of the silver strands avoiding breakage after continuous bending

silver strand is only positioned in the midportion of the device, therefore the proximal end can be trimmed to the exact length required [2, 26, 28, 30, 31, 38, 63, 65].

Rather new developments were the Omniphase and Duraphase. In both devices, rigidity and flaccidity is controlled using articulating segments, a stainless steel cable, and a spring on each end of the central part.

The Omniphase is a self-contained rod-type cylinder with a mechanical activator to transform the device from a natural-like flexed appearance to good rigidity. There is only one pair of devices necessary; however, there is a set of proximal and distal tip extenders which have to be screwed on to the central part intraoperatively.

In order to achieve exact positioning of the activator, a "sizing chart" is necessary for individual length determination. The device is deactivated by

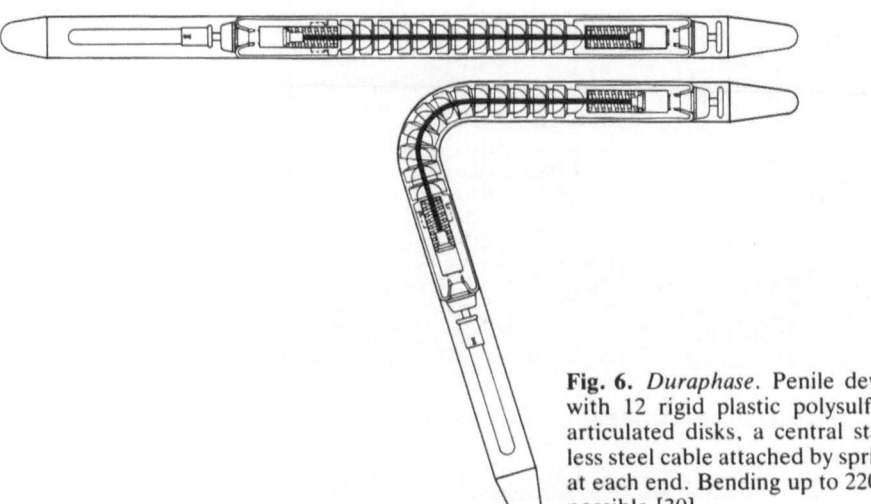

Fig. 6. *Duraphase.* Penile device with 12 rigid plastic polysulfone articulated disks, a central stainless steel cable attached by springs at each end. Bending up to 220° is possible [30]

bending it down, thus unlocking the articulating segments inside the device; it is activated simply by moving the device in the erectile position, thus locking the segments inside the device.

The Duraphase penile prosthesis was a further development of the Omniphase. It consists of 12 rigid polysulfone articulated disks with a centrally placed stainless steel cable and 2 spring mechanisms. The allowed angle of all 13 disk interspaces is 220° (Fig. 6).

According to the results of a multicenter trial consisting of 63 patients published in 1990, mechanical complications included cable breakage in four instances, and 55 out of 57 patients were satisfied with the results. The authors were encouraged by this preliminary experience, which showed fewer complications than the inflatable devices had and especially stressed the features of excellent bendability, superior concealability, and perfect rigidity. Longer follow-up, however, and a larger patient population will be necessary for final judgement of the quality of this specific device [29, 50].

Inflatable Devices

After the rather unsuccessful attempts before the 1970s (Lash, Loeffler [39, 42]), the tremendous breakthrough in alloplastic surgery for the impotent men came in February 1973 when the first inflatable penile prosthesis was implanted by Scott and coworkers (see Fig. 1). Already by 1979, 21 physicians had already performed penile implantation in a total of 1243 patients at different centers. The success rate was 91.5%; however, as stated by practically all authors in this period of time, there was a repair rate of around 30%.

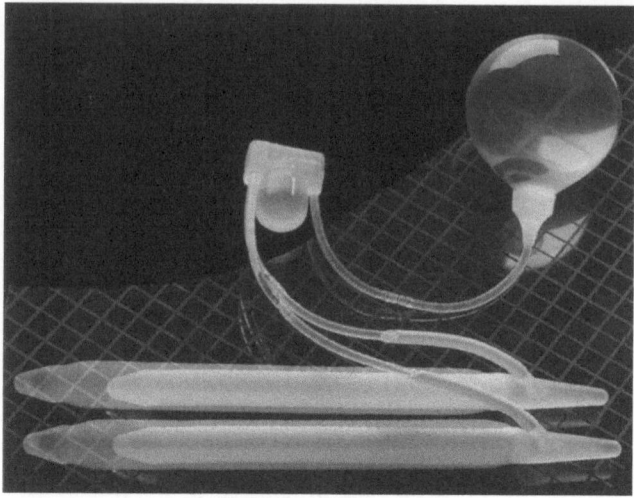

Fig. 7. *AMS-700*. Example of a three-component inflatable device. Available as: (1) 700 CX with cylinder diameter of 12 mm; (2) 700 CXM with cylinder diameter of 9.5 mm; (3) 700 Ultrex with cylinder diameter of 12 mm; expansion during inflation both in length and in width. For further explanation see text [36]

Three-Component Prostheses

From 1973 up to 1990 numerous alterations and improvements were applied. Today's device, the AMS 700 CX has apparently mastered the majority of problems such as kinking of the tubings, cylinder wall aneuryms, and unequal filling of the device. The AMS 700 CX now has a 3-ply cylinder wall minimizing the risk of cylinder bulging; the diameter of each cylinder can expand from 12 up to 18 mm, improving prosthetic erection in circumference; and tubing connectors allow easy handling and safe connection of the tubes to and from the cylinder [1, 14, 15, 20, 21].

The AMS 700 CX was developed from the original inflatable Scott device (see Fig. 1) and consists of *three components*: the *cylinder*, the *pump* and the *reservoir* (Fig. 7). This concept also became adapted in the Mentor inflatable penile prosthesis, described for the first time in 1983 [57].

The essential difference between the very similar looking devices, however, is the material: the Mentor device is manufactured from Bioflex polyurethrane, which was quoted to be more durable and less elastic than silicone. Such material should last longer and prevent cylinder aneuryms. In 1987 the results on 202 implantations were reported: Reoperation was necessary in 8%, of these approximately 50% were due to technical problems, and the rate of complications dropped down to 3.5%. Again, using this device good results were obtained in far more than 90% [44]. The latest Mentor development is the Alpha 1 inflatable penile prosthesis, which features cylinders and pump that are firmly connected, leaving only *one* connector between the pump and reservoir. This diminishes mechanical problems [13, 46].

The latest improvement in the *three-component* inflatable device is the AMS 700 Ultrex penile prosthesis which expands in circumference and extends in length within the corpora cavernosa up to 18 mm. This should give the patient a more natural prosthetic erection than before. The cylinders consist of an inner and outer silicone layer and a woven Lycra and Dacron middle layer. The two-way stretch of this middle layer permits girth expansion and length extension (see Fig. 7).

Preliminary clinical experience in 51 patients with a follow-up from 7 to 11 months showed the mechanical and functional success. No mechanical revisions were necessary [3].

Two-Component Prostheses

In order to reduce the possibility of mechanical failure many attempts have been made to reduce components, connectors, tubes in the concept of inflatable devices. Another consideration was ease of surgical implantation, to offer a penile implant as "pre-prepared" as possible so as to reduce fitting, trimming, and fillings to an acceptable minimum.

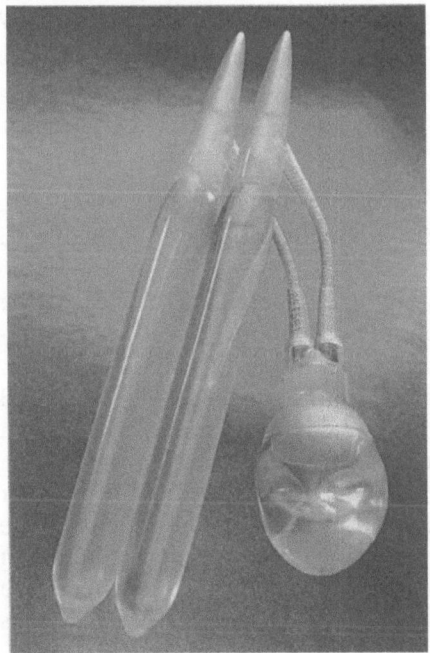

Fig. 8. Mentor-Mark II. Example of a two-component penile implant. Depending on the surgical approach two versions are available. "S" – scrotal, "I" – infrapubic. For further explanation see text [37]

The Mentor Mark II prosthesis is an inflatable penile prosthesis which is preassembled and has no connectors, making any trimming and connecting procedures unnecessary (Fig. 8). The device, however, has to be filled interoperatively by the surgeon. Due to the connectorless one-piece device, depending on the surgical approach, scrotal and infrapubic types are available. In this two-component device, pump and reservoir are combined as "resipump." Twelve differently shaped devices are offered for individual length fitting. In a Mayo Clinic study of 84 patients followed up to 13 months, especially the 13-mm prosthesis was seen to be nearly equal to the three-component devices. Surgical implantation time was reduced to on average 30 min; complications were similar to other devices, such as infection (3.6%), removal due to fluid loss (1.2%), and cylinder erosion (1.2%). The overall success rate was 95.2%.

The second two-component inflatable penile implant is the Uniflate 1000. It features (similar to the Mentor Mark II) a combination of a one-piece device (consisting of pump, reservoir, and cylinders) and a trimmable proximal tail extender as in the Flexirod (see above). In two different diameters (11 and 13 mm) a total of 16 devices varying in length are available. The implantation approach suggested is from a peno-scrotal incision. Included in the kit (as in the Jonas device) is a sizer for determining the exact length. The proximal trimmable tail may be cut down to individual size to allow an exact length adjustment during surgery. Care should be taken that the tubing exit is properly placed at the corporotomy incision without coming into contact with the penile cylinders in order to avoid kinking and tubing abrasion. In this device, also, the fluid content can be adjusted individually [5, 45, 62].

One-Component Prostheses

There are three different types of one-component prostheses available to date.

The Flexiflate II combines the inflatable (self-containing) device with a proximal trimming tail for individual length adaptation (Fig. 9). This one-component device contains pump and reservoir inside the penile cylinder, avoiding any tubings or connectors. An erection is created when the fluid inside the device is transported from an expandable outer cylinder through a special valve to an nonexpandable inner cylinder thus producing rigidity.

An erection is produced easily by squeezing the distal end of the cylinder prior to intercourse. The prosthesis is deflated by bending and squeezing the penile shaft to force the fluid to flow back into the outer cylinder, resulting in flaccidity. Initial experiences by Sagalowski in 25 cases with a postoperative follow-up showed that the device functioned well, however, five revisions were reported.

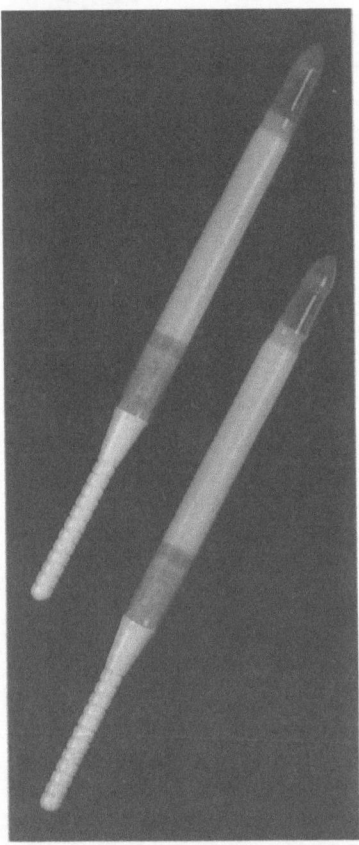

Fig. 9. Flexi-Flate II penile one-component. Pump and reservoir are integrated inside the cylinder; the proximal tip can be trimmed for exact fitting [40]

The AMS Hydroflex self-contained penile prosthesis functions in a very similar way (Fig. 10). It consists of two prefilled cylinders. Again, in each cylinder there is a reservoir at the rear end, an inflation pump and deflation valve, and finally an inflation chamber. Again through repeated pumping close to the glans the fluid moves from the rear reservoir into the inflation chamber and the penis becomes erect. When continuous pressure is applied to the deflation valve which is just behind the inflation pump, the fluid returns in the rear reservoir, and the penis becomes flaccid. The device comes in two different cylinder diameters, 11 and 13 mm, and four different lengths, and all typical surgical approaches may be used for implantation. Preliminary clinical implantation results in 140 patients showed uncomplicated surgery with satisfactory results. A penoscrotal approach mainly used, in 64%.

The last modification of the Hydroflex is the AMS Dynaflex. Here, however, further clinical experience has to provide proof of satisfactory function [8, 53, 61].

Today, the principle types of penile implants are the malleable, semi-rigid and (one- to three-component) inflatable devices. The still existing requests

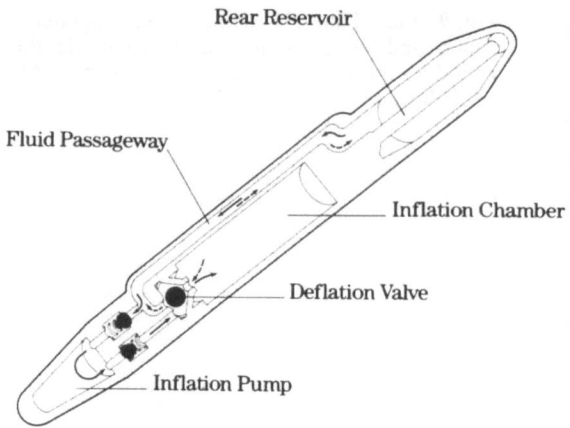

Rear Reservoir

Fluid Passageway

Inflation Chamber

Deflation Valve

Inflation Pump

Fig. 10. AMS-Hydroflex one-component, self-contained penile prosthesis. The cross section shows the mechanics inside the device [42]

for further improvements are based on the patient's wish for a more and more normal and "physiological" sex life. However, in the assessment of success, next to the overall rate from well above 90% "excellent results" in all types used, the postoperative complication rates as well as the chance for necessary repeated surgery plays an important role.

Looking back to the beginning of penile implants in the late 1960s and early 1970s it is evident that an effective treatment choice was already available without knowing too much (or anything at all) about the mechanisms of erections and the underlying pathophysiology. Only in the last 5–8 years has more and more knowledge been gathered to diagnose impotence and to distinguish the different causes of erectile failure with the possibility of applying a cause-related therapy such as intracorporal injections, reconstructive surgery or venous ligation, shifting the role of penile implants towards the end of all therapeutic efforts. It is fair to say today that alloplastics should only be discussed after all other therapeutic modalities have failed or if the patient refuses one of the less invasive or reconstructive treatment modalities. The "mechanical success" rate following penile implant at around 95% is excellent, and more and more data indicating that patients and partners are handling their sex lives very well are available, even in impotence following spinal cord injury. Still, more efforts should be devoted to the psychological impact for patient and partner, and sophisticated pre-, peri- and postoperative guidance for both partners is mandatory [9, 16, 37, 41, 58].

Surgical Techniques

Different "classical" surgical approaches are known which are more-or-less compatible and may be used for the majority of the devices. The choice of approach is finally based on the surgeon's own experience; no general rule can be established advocating one or the other specific access. The surgical approaches are:

- Perineal
- Midshaft
- Penoscrotal
- Infrapubical
- Subcoronal

Small and Carrion initially suggested the perineal approach. This, however, became more and more abandoned due to the fact that perineally, the aseptic conditions are not the best and postoperative wound care is more difficult. On the other hand, the most critical area of implantation is the distal end of the corpora cavernosa underneath the glans. Starting perineally, the corporal dilatation has to be carried out a rather long way to the distal end, and control of dilatation and prosthesis insertion may be more difficult. If an inflatable device is used, the infrapubic approach seems to be appropriate, since all components may be positioned from one incision. This is also true for the penoscrotal incision; however, in this case a catheter should be placed during surgery to avoid injury to the urethra. Criticism has been made concerning the *subcoronal* approach, generally a hemicircular incision in the sulcus coronarius. It has been suggested that this approach may lead to injury of nerve supply with subsequent loss of sensitivity. This does not hold since all interventions along the corporus cavernosum are carried out in a longitudinal fashion, thus avoiding trauma to the nerves and vessels by pushing them away. The approach used by the author is the subcoronal approach, which has been applied in more than 300 cases. It is seen as the method of first choice since no catheter is necessary during implantation, and there is practically no visible scar left behind after surgery (Fig. 11). The implantation of a penile implant (first surgery) in a non-postpriapism patient does normally not cause any problems and may even be performed under local anesthesia. However, it may be difficult following previous surgery, after priapism or in trauma patients when the corpora are fully or partially no longer exist. In these patients the fibrotic corpora may need to be cored or lyodura or vascular prostheses used to cover the penile implant and prevent proximal and distal migration. As a specific aid a specially designed proximal tip extender may be used which can be screwed to the ischiopubic rami in order to fix the device in its proximal end (Fig. 12). It also may be difficult to dilate the corpora, or it may even be almost impossible after repeated surgery and/or infection or after priapism. In these cases a small blade knife or the Qtis urethrotom may be used to core the corpus prior to dilatation. For these maneuvers it is wise to scalp the whole penis down to the base, or if necessary through a second infrapubic incision, in order to have good control during corporal dilatation (Fig. 13). In case of the "Concorde" deformity surgical reposition of the glans may be necessary.

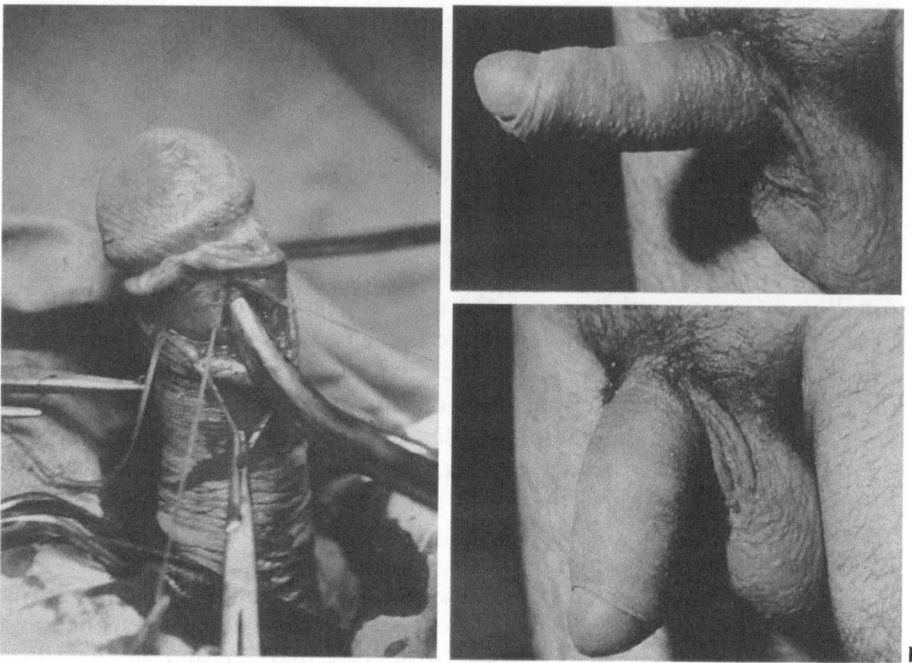

a   b

Fig. 11a,b. Implantation of a penile prosthesis using the subcoronal approach. **a** Following a hemicircular incision. Identification of the corpora covernosa, dilatation proximally (crura) and distally (glans), and subsequent insertion of the appropriate sized device. **b** Situation following implantation. Note the good cosmetic result in the "resting" position (*below*) using a malleable device (Jonas) with practically invisible scar

The etiology of patients receiving penile implants (based on 2641 cases) is shown in Fig. 14. In patients with Peyronie's disease the malleable devices seem to be superior to the inflatable ones in straightening the deformity. Excising the plaques is generally no longer necessary. Another very specific indication may be the paraplegic patient who may need a malleable device in order to give a better support for the condom urinal [4, 12, 18, 27, 30, 33, 35, 36, 40, 49, 55].

Fig. 12a–d. Penile prosthesis implantation. Technique to prevent proximal migration. ▶ **a** Special tip extender (ESKA) to screw the device to to the bone. **b** Parascrotal incision to expose the ischiopubic rami. The tip extender is slipped over the prosthesis. **c** Rear-tip extender fixation with a osteosynthetic screw. **d** X-ray control following implantation

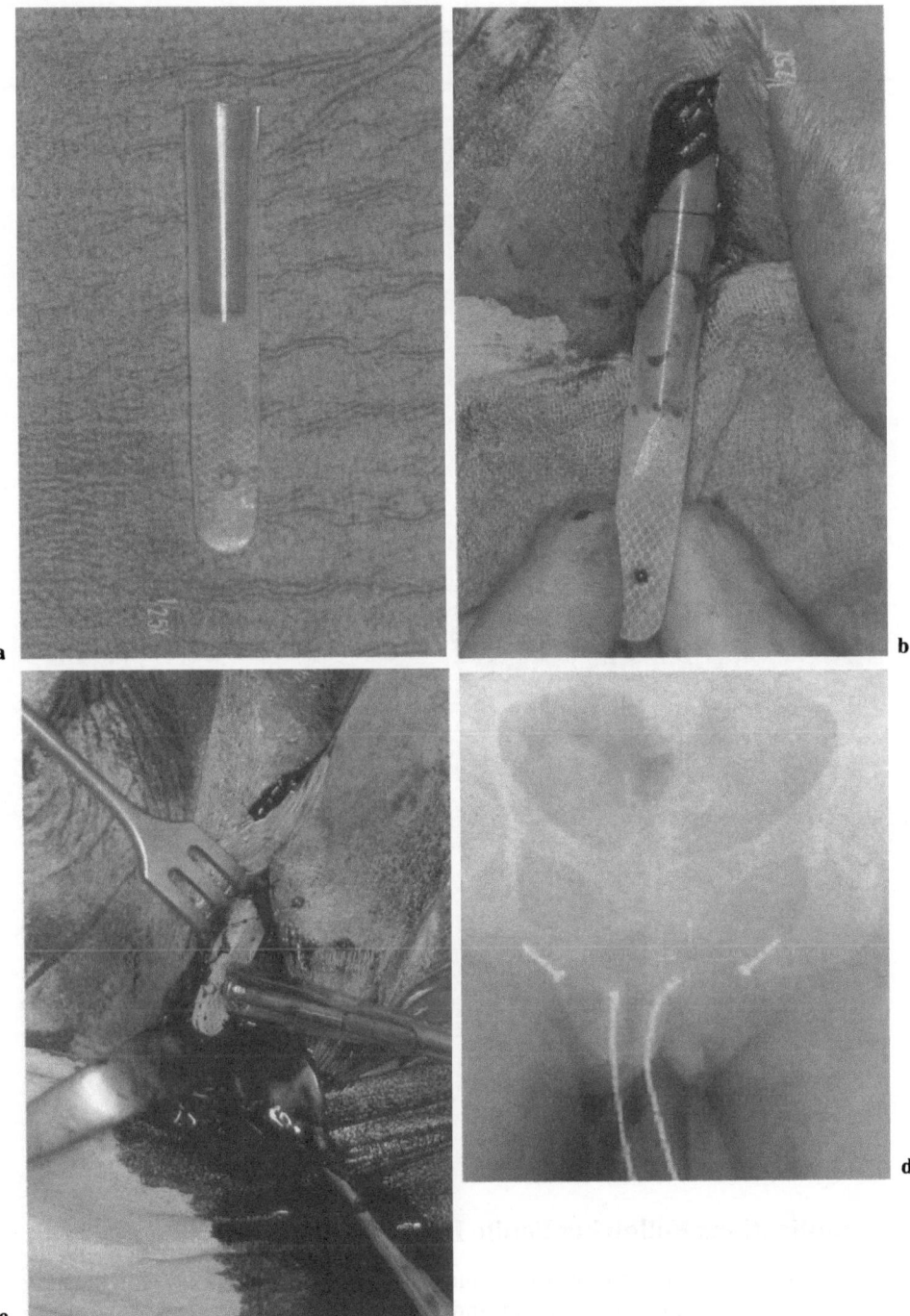

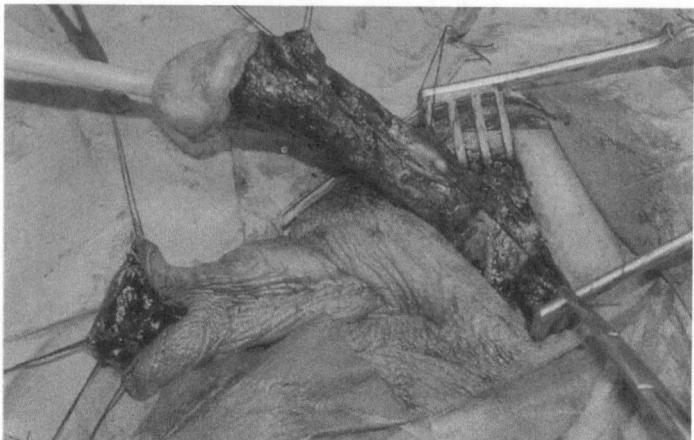

a

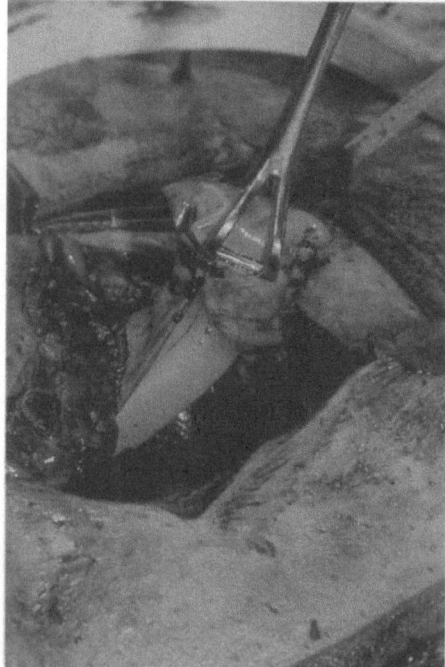

b

Fig. 13a,b. Fourth attempt at penile implantation in completely destroyed corpora cavernosa. **a** For better identification during preparation and dilatation of the corpora, the penis is developed through a second infrapublic incision. **b** Lyo-dura is used to avoid proximal migration: Windsack technique

Complications Following Penile Implantation

Prosthetic infection is the most problematic complication following surgery since the combination of infection and foreign body requires removal of the prosthesis; after 3 months of good healing, however, a reimplantation may be done. The patients most affected with infection problems are the diabetics

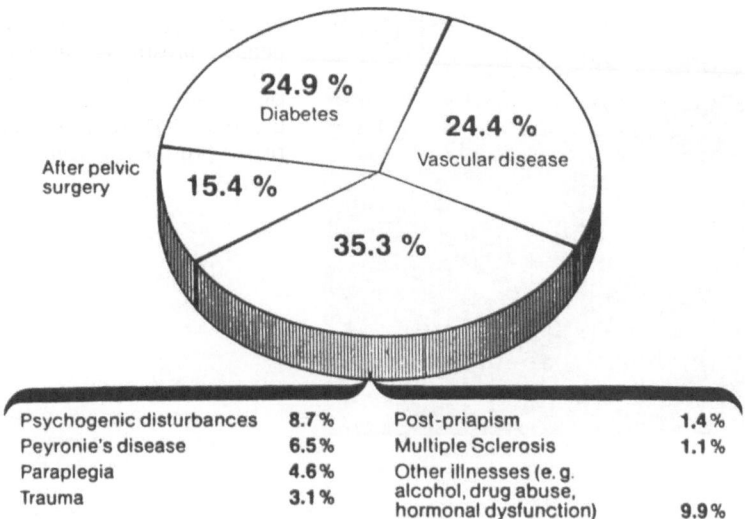

Psychogenic disturbances	8.7%	Post-priapism	1.4%
Peyronie's disease	6.5%	Multiple Sclerosis	1.1%
Paraplegia	4.6%	Other illnesses (e. g.	
Trauma	3.1%	alcohol, drug abuse, hormonal dysfunction)	9.9%

Fig. 14. Causes which led to the implantation of a penile prosthesis (based on etiology of 2641 patients)

where special care must be taken to avoid wound healing problems. The author's own experience has shown that local or systemic antibiotic treatment is completely unsuccessful if the device is infected. Therefore, especially when the device communicates through the open wound, removal is the only possible treatment in order to avoid septic exacerbation. In these cases placement of suction drains may be useful. If, especially in case of the diabetic patient, the infection is not controlled efficiently after removal of the device, necrosis of the corpora may develop. This fact further backs the absolute need for removal of an infected device as soon as possible. The postoperative complication rates due to infection described in the literature are seen to be as high as 8.3%. Therefore specific attention has to be given to preoperative preparation, intraoperative handling and postoperative care [10, 43, 47, 54, 64, 66].

Postoperative Management

Once the devices have healed nicely, there are no further problems to be expected besides infection (see above) and erosion. An infection certainly will provoke an erosion. The most crucial point for an implant perforation is the distal end of the device. The patient has to be informed to use the device in a "physiological" manner, he has to be aware that the friction during intercourse is an important factor to provoke perforation of the prosthesis. If

308   U. Jonas

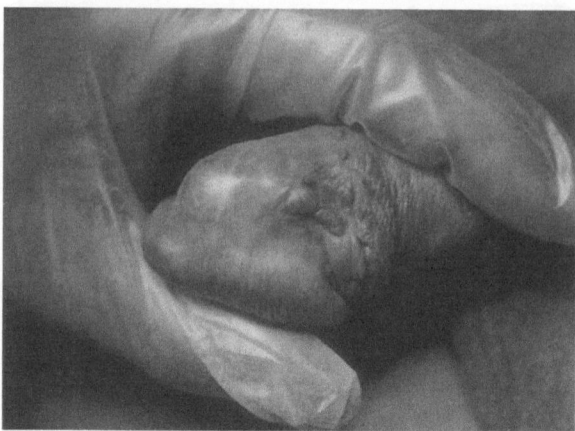

Fig. 15. Status following penile prosthesis implantation. The device is too short, leading to the "SST" deformity. There is a high risk of prosthesis perforation

the partner has no vaginal secretion during sexual stimulation, a lubricant may be advisable.

Exact intra-operative length measurement is mandatory: if the device is too long, post-operative pain and finally prosthesis erosion may result. However in too short a device, the "Concorde" deformity with kinking of the glans during intercourse may occur and perforation laterally through the corpus cavernosum may be possible (Fig. 15).

Endoscopy is possible after implantation, especially if an inflatable device has been implanted. With a malleable prosthesis, the length of the penis may be the limiting factor of endoscopy. Special long instruments are commercially available (Storz); however, the penis may also be twisted around up to 270° for endoscopic work-up. This shortens the penis and enables the examination, still it may become problematic if, for example, a bladder tumor at the dome has to be resected.

Prosthesis reimplantation may be necessary for different problems. The data from the literature show that reimplantation may also lead to satisfying results. However, due to scarring and fibrosis, the penis can shorten, and the first surgical attempt still offers the most promising results [11, 23, 34, 48].

Due to more and more sophisticated diagnostic techniques, the specific causes of impotence can be identified and a cause-related therapy will follow. Due to the fact that treatment modalities which are not or minimally invasive or surgically reconstructive are available, these modalities should be used *prior* to the implantation of a penile prosthesis. Nevertheless penile implants still offer the best rate of success, over 95%, independent of the type of prosthesis is used. The inflatable devices are the most elegant and the ones which best imitate physiological behavior; however, they are still limited by a significant mechanical failure rate. Therefore the different types of devices must be presented to the patient prior to surgery, and he should decide what type of prosthesis he would like to have implanted, after being fully informed of the advantages and disadvantages of the individual types. In case of complications or after removal of the device, reimplantation is possible. This, however, requires a more difficult surgical procedure with a decreased chance of success. Proper indication, careful patient selection, and sophisticated postoperative control not only of the mechanical aspects but also of the psychogenic impact is mandatory to fulfill the patient's and his partner's need of sexual satisfaction. However, the expectations of both the patient and his partner are often too high and both must learn to cope with the new situation.

References

1. American Medical Systems Inc. (1979) A summary of clinical experience to date with the AMS inflatable penile prosthesis. AMS-special report. AUA-annual meeting, New York
2. American Medical System Inc. (1983) AMS malleable 600. AMS product information
3. American Medical System Inc. (1990) A report of the clinical evaluation of the 700 Ultrex™ penile prosthesis. AMS publication 00926
4. Ball TP (1982) Surgical repair of penile "SST" deformity. Urology/Urotech 12
5. Barrett DM (1989) Uniflate 1000 experience with 84 patients. In: Surgitek (ed) Uniflate[R] – 1000 clinical market study. 1989 update. Surgitek information
6. Beheri GE (1966) Surgical treatment of impotence. Plast Reconstr Surg 38:92
7. Bogoras NA (1936) Über die volle plastische Wiederherstellung eines zum Koitus fähigen Penis (Penisplastica totalis). Zentralbl Chir 63:1271
8. Boyd S, Bruskewitz R, Fishman I, Furlow WL, Montague DK, Mulcahy JJ, Scott FB (1985) A report of the clinical trials for the AMS Hydroflex™ self-contained penile prosthesis. AMS publication 50512-E
9. Carrion HM Chaikin LB (1983) Subjective analysis of penile implant. World J Urol 1:260
10. Carson CC, Robertson CN (1988) Late hematogenous infection of penile prostheses. J Urol 139:50
11. Datta NS (1981) Cystoscoping patients with semirigid penile prosthesis. Urology 18/4:403
12. Denil F, Schreiter F (1990) Prothesenchirurgie in vorgeschädigten Schwellkörpern – erste Erfahrungen mit der Windsack-Technik. Urologie Poster 2:55
13. Engel RME, Smolev JK, Hackler R (1987) Mentor inflatable penile prosthesis. Urology 29/5:498
14. Fein RL (1988) Cylinder problems with AMS 700 inflatable penile prosthesis. Urology 31/4:305
15. Fein RL, Winton L, Needell MH (1983) Revision of high-riding kinking Scott penile prosthesis pump. Urology 22/4:416
16. Finkle AL, Finkle CE (1984) Sexual impotency. Counselling of 388 private patients by Urologist from 1954–1982. Urology 23:25
17. Finney RP (1977) New hinged silicone penile implant. J Urol 118:585
18. Finney RP (1984) Coring fibrotic corpora for penile implants. Urology 24:73
19. Finney RP, Sharpe JR, Sadlowski RW (1980) Finney hinged penile implant: experience with 100 cases. J Urol 124:205
20. Fishman IS, Scott FB, Leight JK (1984) Experience with inflatable penile prosthesis. Urology (Special Issue) 23/5:86
21. Furlow WL (1978) Current status of the inflatable penile prosthesis in the management of impotence. Mayo Clin updated. J Urol 119:363

22. Furlow WL (1981) Sex prosthetics. In: Wagenknecht LV, Furlow WL, Auvert J (eds) Genitourinary reconstruction with prostheses. Thieme, Stuttgart New York
23. Gasser TC, Larsen EH, Bruskewitz RG (1987) Penile prosthesis reimplantation. J Urol 137:46
24. Gee WF (1975) A history of surgical treatment of impotence. Urology 5:40
25. Goodwin, WE, Scott WW (1952) Phalloplasty. J Urol 68:903
26. Grein U, Noll F, Schreiter F (1989) Die Behandlung der erektilen Dysfunktion mit Penisprothesen. Urologe [A] 28:266
27. Herschorn S, Barkin M, Comisarolo R (1986) New technique for difficult penile implants. Urology 27:463
28. Houseplan DM, Amis ES jr (1989) Penile prosthetic implants: a radiographic atlas. Radio Graphics 9/4:707
29. Hrebinko R, Bahnson RR, Schwentker FN, O'Donnell WF (1990) Early experience with the Duraphase penile prosthesis. J Urol 143:60
30. Jonas U (1978) Silikon-Silber-Penisprothese. Aktuel Urol 9:179
31. Jonas U (1983) 5-years' experience with the silicone-silver penile prosthesis: improvements and new developments. World J Urol 1:251
32. Jonas U, Jacobi GH (1980) Silicone-silver penile prosthesis: description. Operative approach and results. J Urol 123:865
33. Kaufman JJ (1982) Penile prosthetic surgery under local anaesthesia. J Urol 128:1190
34. Kaufman JJ, Lindner A, Raz S (1982) Complications of penile prosthesis surgery for impotence. J Urol 128:1192
35. Kelámi A (1976) Infrapubic approach for Small-Carrion prosthesis in erectile impotence. Urology 8:164
36. Kelámi A (1980) Peyronie disease and surgical treatment – a new concept. Urology 15:559
37. Kockott G (1986) Impotenz. Urologe [A] 25:90
38. Krane RJ, Freedberg PS, Siroky MS (1981) Jonas silicone-silver penile prosthesis: initial experience in America. J Urol 126:475
39. Lash H (1968) Silicone implant for impotence. J Urol 100:709
40. Leach GE (1986) Transscrotal approach for insertion of inflatable penile prosthesis. Urology 27:465
41. Light JK, Scott FB (1981) Management of neurogenic impotence with inflatable penile prosthesis. Urology 17/4:341
42. Loeffler RA, Samegh ES, Lash H (1964) The artificial os penis. Plast Reconstr Surg 34:71
43. Maatman TJ, Montague DK (1982) Intracorporeal drainage after removal of infected penile prosthesis. Urology/Urotech 42
44. Malloy TR, Wein AJ, Carpeniello VL (1982) Improved mechanical survival with revised inflatable penile prosthesis using rear-tip extenders. J Urol 128:489
45. Mentor Corp (1989) Mark II inflatable prosthesis. Surgical protocol. Mentor Corp information
46. Merrill DC (1983) Mentor inflatable penile prosthesis. Urology 22/5:504
47. Montague DK (1987) Periprosthetic infections. J Urol 138:68
48. Morgenstern JH, Stein BS, Kendall AR (1982) Complications in patient with triple penile prostheses. Urology 20/5:530
49. Mulcahy JJ (1987) A technique of maintaining penile prosthesis position to prevent proximal migration. J Urol 137:294
50. Mulcahy JJ, Krane RJ, Lloyd LK, Edson M, Siroky MB (1990) Duraphase penile prosthesis – results of clinical trials in 63 patients. J Urol 143:518
51. Pearman RO (1972) Insertion of a silastic penile prosthesis for the treatment of organic sexual impotence. J Urol 107:802
52. Scott EB, Bradley WD, Timm GW (1973) Management of erectile impotence. Urology 2:80
53. Segalowski RL (1986) In: Surgitek (ed) Flexi-Flate: clinical experiences. Surgitek information

54. Shelling RH, Maxted WC (1980) Major complications of silicone penile prosthesis. Urology 15:131
55. Small MP (1976) Small-Carrion penile prosthesis: a new implant for management of impotence. Mayo Clin Proc 51:3
56. Small MP (1978) Small-Carrion penile prosthesis: a report on 160 cases and review of the literature. J Urol 119:365
57. Small MP, Carrion HA, Gordon JA (1975) Small-Carrion penile prosthesis. Urology 5:479
58. Stewart TD, Gerson SN (1976) Penile prosthesis: psychological factors. Urology 7:400
59. Subrini L (1982) Subrini penile implants. Surgical, sexual and psychological results. Eur Urol 8:222
60. Subrini L, Couvelaire R (1974) Le traitement chirurgical de l'impuissance virile par intubation prothétique intravacerneuse. J Urol Nephrol 80:269
61. Surgitek (1987) Surgitek^R Flexi-Flate II: intracorporeal inflatable penile implant. Surgical procedural guide.
62. Surgitek (1989) Surgitek^R Uniflate 1000^R inflatable penile implant. Surgical procedural guide. Surgitek information
63. Tawil E, Hawatmeh IS, Apte S, Gregory JG (1984) Multiple fractures of the silver wire strands as a complication of the silicone-silver wire prosthesis. J Urol 132:762
64. Thomalla JV, Thompson ST, Rowland RG, Mulcahy JJ (1987) Infectious complications of penile prosthetic implants. J Urol 138:65
65. Timm GW (1981) A summary and discussion of life testing – conditions, results and conclusions – engineering test report. Dacomed information
66. Walther PJ, Andriani RT, Maggic MI, Carson CC III (1987) Fournier's gangrene: a complication of penile prosthetic implantation in a renal transplant patient. J Urol 137:299

Special Aspects

Erectile Impotence Due to Spinal Cord Injury

W.F. Thon

Introduction

Each year approximately 10 000 new causes of spinal cord injury occur in the USA, the majority in patients who are 25 years old or younger. In West Germany, 9399 new cases were registered between 1978 and 1987 (cited by [30]); 70% were men.

Sexuality in spinal cord injured patients is an important issue. Sexual activity persists and is enjoyed by a large group of spinal cord injured men [15]. Oral-genital sexual activity is practiced by 70% of all paraplegic and quadriplegic men [7]. In most cases, spinal cord injured men consider resuming sexual activity [9] because they are not fully incapacitated.

Penile erection involves psychological, hormonal, vascular, and neurological factors. The essential event instituting an erection is regulated by the autonomic nervous system. In 1863, Eckhardt first reported that electrical stimulation of the pelvis nerves produced a penile erection in the dog. In 1938, Semans and Langworthy [24] showed that hypogastric nerve stimulation during an erection caused a sudden detumescence. In 1947, Root and Bard [25] demonstrated that a full erection was still possible in the male cat even after removal of the sacral cord when a female cat in estrus was present. In cases of transection above the level of sympathetic outflow, this erectile ability disappeared.

In patients with spinal cord injury the level of transection will determine the preservation or loss of erectile potency. Chapelle et al. [6] described three types of erection in spinal cord injured men.

1. Reflexogenic erections following complete spinal transection cranial to T10/T12 vertebrae, occurring from direct genital stimulation via the afferent limb in the pudendal nerves and efferent limb through the pelvic parasympathetic nerves.
2. Psychogenic erections from tactile, auditory, olfactory, or visual stimuli to the cerebral cortex mediated through the sympathetic (thoracolumbar) pathways in cases of cord injury caudal to T12.
3. Mixed reflexogenic-psychogenic erections occurring when the cord injury is caudal to T10/T12 vertebrae and cranial to S2.

U. Jonas et al. (Eds.) Erectile Dysfunction
© Springer-Verlag Berlin Heidelberg 1991

Reflex erections occur as long as the conus medullaris is intact. In spinal cord injured patients, reflex erections are about four times more common than psychogenic erections [4]. Reflexogenic erections occur in almost 100% of patients with transection of the cervical cord, while most patients with sacral lesions are impotent. Only in a small number of cases is potency preserved due to thoracolumbar outflow (psychogenic erections).

In a large series outlining the sexual function of 529 spinal cord injured patients, Bors and Comarr [4] reported that erections were most frequent in patients with incomplete upper neuromotor lesions. Erections were more frequent in patients with complete upper motor neuron lesions than in those with complete lower motor neuron lesions.

Tsuji and associates [32] confirmed these results in their study of 638 spinal cord injured patients. Those having incomplete lesions showed an erectile capability of 67% versus 50% in those with complete lesions. While erectile potency is maintained on average in 70% of spinal cord injured patients, ejaculation is preserved in only 7% [1].

Neurogenic impotence occurs if the release of neurotransmitter substances of the autonomic penile nervous system is impaired. The parasympathetic system responds to local and psychogenic stimuli, the sympathetic system to psychological stimuli only. Several neurotransmitter substances are released during pelvic cavernous nerve stimulation in order to initiate hemodynamic changes that occur during penile erections. Integrity of the somatic nervous system (pudendal nerve, dorsal penile nerve) is necessary to sustain rigidity. The spinal nuclei for control of erection are located in the intermediolateral gray matter at the S2–S4 and T10–L2 Levels. Together with the axons of the nuclei for the bladder and rectum, the sacral nuclei axons form the sacral visceral efferent fibers. Most fibers join the sympathetic fibers to form the pelvic plexus [19].

Diagnostic Evaluation

In cases of spinal cord injured men with erectile dysfunction, etiology seems obvious. However, in some patients, impotence is caused not only by transection, but also by psychological and/or vascular disorders. Therefore it is necessary to carefully evaluate vascular, hormonal, psychological, and neurogenic involvement. As in every patient with erectile impotence, work-up consists of a complete history with a sexual psychological interview, physical examination, laboratory blood test (including testosterone and prolactin), Doppler sonography of the penile arteries [11], intracavernous pharmaco-testing with real-time monitoring by RigiScan during visual erotic stimulation [13], and a sophisticated neurophysiological evaluation. When indicated by pharmacotesting, pharmacocavernosography and pharmacocavernosomertry are performed to evaluate the veno-occlusive mechanism (Bookstein et al. 1987) [3].

Neurophysiological Testing

Previous methods evaluating men with erectile dysfunction and spinal cord injury relied on testing S2–S4 function by anal sphincter tone, perianal sensation, and subjective testing of the bulbocavernous reflex (BCR). Nowadays, the integrity of the nervous afferent and efferent pathway and sacral spinal cord is evaluated using biothesiometry, somatosensory evoked potentials (SSEP), BCR latency time, corpus cavernosum electromyography, and genital skin potentials.

Biothesiometry

Peripheral and central dorsal nerve afferent pathways can be evaluated using a biothesiometer. The biothesiometer determines the penile vibration threshold [24]. This electromagnetic device provides a vibration stimulus at a fixed frequency, but with variable amplitude.

SSEP Testing

Peripheral afferent function can be assessed by measuring the conduction velocity in the dorsal nerve of the penis [5, 12]. The central afferent pathway can be investigated by recording the cortical pudendal evoked response [16, 23]. The cortical pudendal response is recorded using surface electrodes placed at specific sites corresponding to projections from the central nervous system. The time from initiation of the stimulus to the peak of spinal response indicates the peripheral conduction time, the time to the cerebral response provides the total conduction time. The difference between the two latency' times represents the central conduction time. SSEP testing is used to evaluate the peripheral and central afferent pathways of penile sensation. Impaired dorsal nerve activity does not enable the patient to sustain an erection and is known as dorsal nerve impotence [14].

BCR Latency Time

BCR latency measurement is a standardized method used to diagnose injury to somatic penile innervation [26, 31]. The test examines the integrity of normal afferent and efferent fibers of S2–S4. The motor responses to stimulating electrodes on the shaft of the penis are recorded by placing concentric needle electrodes in the bulbocavernosus muscles. Maximum latency, temporal dispersion, and minimum and maximum side differences are recorded. Patients with complete sacral spinal cord lesions show an abscence of the reflex. In incomplete sacral cord lesions, lateralized latency differences can be documented. The difficulty in interpretating the results is due to the unknown contribution of the motor efferent pathway.

Electrical Activity of the Corpus Cavernosum (EACC):
Single Potential Analysis of Cavernous Electric Activity (SPACE)

Wagner et al. [34] first described a test to define the integrity of the autonomic penile nervous system. Up to this time, autonomic penile neuropathy could only be evaluated by corpus cavernosum biopsy, electron microscopy, and neurotransmitter immunohistology. Wagner et al. [34] recorded continuous electromyographic activity in the corpus cavernosum using a coaxial needle electrode inserted into one of the cavernous bodies. Autonomic neuropathy could be demonstrated by severe "dyscoordination" of the smooth muscles in cases of denervation. Stief et al. [29] recorded salves of 28–41s, positive and negative whips, spikes, and bursts in patients with spinal cord injury.

Genital Skin, Potential Recording

Recording sensory potentials from the genital skin area seems to be useful for evaluating sympathetic functions involving the genital region. Since the sympathetic fibers mediating sudomotor activity and those subserving erection are bound closely together, any pathological process affects both functions [10]. Therefore, this test indirectly allows evaluation of the sympathetic pathway in patients with erectile dysfunction.

An ever-increasing sophistication in technology is presently available to assess the integrity of nervous penile innervation. Further experience with these new methods will help us to make a more accurate diagnosis concerning nervous impairment in patients with erectile dysfunction.

Treatment

The standard treatment for patients with spinal cord injury and erectile impotence has been *the penile prosthesis*. A higher incidence of erosion, extrusion and infection is reported in patients with neurogenic impotence [8, 21]. Causes of noninfected erosions are usually pressure necrosis of the corpora cavernosa and penile skin due to a combination of decreased blood flow and decreased penile skin sensation. Because of this sensory deficit, hydraulic prostheses should be preferred to semirigid prostheses in order to prevent erosion. The number of penile prosthesis implantations is decreasing because other therapy alternatives such as *penile intracorporal injection therapy* with vasoactive drugs [2, 28] and *constriction suction devices* have been successfully used [22, 36]. Vasoactive drugs used for intracavernous pharmacotherapy are papaverine [33], papaverine and phentolamine [37], and prostaglandin E1 [35]. Intracavernous injection therapy with these vasoactive substances mimics endogenous neurotransmitter activity and causes similar physiological responses to those observed during pelvic nerve stimulation. Potential dangers of the autoinjection therapy, especially in spinal cord injured men, are sustained erections, fully developed priapism, and intracorporal fibrosis. To avoid prolonged erections, which can also occur after the injection of a low dose due to denervation hypersensitivity, it is advisable to monitor drug dose testing using real-time RigiScan during visual sexual or genital stimulation. Patients and their partners are instructed in the proper injection technique and are provided with an injection pen (Andropen).

Vacuum constriction devices may assist in achieving and maintaining an erection sufficient for vaginal intercourse. In men with neurogenic and venogenic etiologies, intracavernous injection therapy can be combined with the use of a vacuum constriction device or implemented after penile venous surgery [17]. Preliminary results with electrode implantation indicate that an erection pacemaker seems feasible in humans [18, 20]. Because most spinal cord injured patients have intact cavernous nerves and neurovascular bundles the implantation of electrodes around the cavernous nerves appears to be a possible therapy alternative.

The majority of spinal cord injured men can receive successful treatment with regard to their spontaneous erectile capacity. The described treatment modalities can lead to a significant improvement in their quality of life.

References

1. Bennet CJ, Seager SW, Vasher EA, McGuire E (1988) Sexual dysfunction and electroejaculation in men with spinal cord injury: Review. J Urol 139:453–457
2. Bodner DR, Lindan R, Leffler E, Kursh ED, Resnick MI (1987) The application of intracavernous injection of vasoactive medications for erection in men with spinal cord injury. J Urol 138:310–311
3. Bookstein JJ, Valiji K, Parsons L, Kessler W (1987) Penile pharmacocavernosography and cavernosometry in the evaluation of impotence. J Urol 137:772–776
4 Bors E, Comarr AE (1960) Neurological disturbances of sexual function with special reference to 529 patients with spinal cord injury. Urol Surv 10:191–222
5. Bradley WE, Lin JTY, Johnson B (1984) Measurement of the conduction velocity of the dorsal nerve of the penis. J Urol 131:1127–1129
6. Chapelle PA, Durand J, Lacert P (1980) Penile erection following complete spinal cord injury in men. Br J Urol 52:216–219
7. Cole TM, Chilgren R, Rosenberg P (1973) A new programme of sex education and counselling for spinal cord injured adults and health care professionals. Paraplegia 11:111–124
8. Collins KP, Hackler RH (1988) Complications of penile prostheses in the spinal cord injury population. J Urol 140:984–985
9. Comarr AE (1970) Sexual function among patients with spinal cord injury. Urol Int 25:134–138
10. Ertekin C, Ertekin N, Mutlu S, Almis S, Akcam A (1987) Skin potentials (SP) recorded from the extremities and genital regions in normal and impotent subjects. Acta Neurol Scand 76:28–36
11. Gall H, Bähren W, Scherb W, Stief C, Thon WF (1988) Diagnostic accuracy of Doppler ultrasound technique of the penile arteries in correlation to selective arteriography. Cardiovasc Intervent Radiol 11:225–231

12. Gerstenberg TC, Bradley WE (1983) Nerve conduction velocity measurement of dorsal nerve of penis in normal and impotent males. Urology 21:90–92
13. Giesbers AAGM, Bruins JL, Kramer AEJL, Jonas U (1987) New methods in the diagnosis of impotence: RigiScan penile tumescence and rigidity monitoring and diagnostic papaverine hydrochloride injection. World J Urol 5:173–176
14. Goldstein J (1988) Evaluation of penile nerves. In: Tanagho EA, Lue TF, McClure RD (eds) Contemporary management of impotence and infertility: Williams & Wilkins, Baltimore HongKong London Sidney, pp 70–83
15. Higgins GE Jr (1979) Sexual response in spinal cord injured adults: a review of the literature. Arch Sex Behav 8:173–196
16. Kaneko S, Bradley WE (1987) Penile electrodiagnosis: Penile peripheral innervation. Urology 30(3):210–212
17. Lue TF (1989) Penile venous surgery. Urol Clin North Am 16(3):607–611
18. Lue TF, Tanagho EA (1988) Erection pacemaker. In: Tanagho EA, Lue TF, McClure RD (eds) Contemporary management of impotence and infertility. Williams & Wilkins, Baltimore HongKong London Sidney, pp 157–159
19. Lue TF, Zeineh, SJ, Schmidt RA, Tanagho EA (1984) Neuroanatomy of penile erection: Its relevance to iatrogenic impotence. J Urol 131:273–280
20. Lue TF, Schmidt RA, Tanagho EA (1985) Electrostimulation and penile erection. Urol Int 40:60–64
21. Montague DK (1987) Periprosthetic infections. J Urol 138:68–69
22. Nadig PW, Ware JC, Blumoff R (1986) Noninvasive device to produce and maintain an erection-like state. Urology 27:126–31
23. Opsomer RJ, Guerit JM, Wese FX et al (1986) Pudendal cortical somatosensory evoked potentials. J Urol 135:1216–1218
24. Padma-Nathan H, Levine F (1987) Vibratory testing of the penis. J Urol 137:210 A
25. Root WS, Bard P (1947) The mediation of feline erection through sympathetic pathways with some remarks on sexual behavior after differentiation of the genitalia. Am J Physiol 150:80–85
26. Scherb WH, Bähren W, Gall H, Thon WF (1988) Neurophysiologic parameters in evaluation of erectile dysfunction. Acta Urol Belg 56:154–161
27. Semans J, Langworthy OR (1938) Observations of the neurophysiology of sexual function in the male cat. J Urol 40:836–846
28. Sidi AA, Cameron JS, Dykstra DD, Reinberg Y, Lange PH (1987) Vasoactive intravavernous pharmacotherapy for the treatment of erectile impotence in men with spinal cord injury. J Urol 138:539–542
29. Stief CG, Djamilian M, Schaebsdau F, Truss MC, Schlick W, Abicht JH, Allhoff EP, Jonas U (1990) Single potential analysis of cavernous electric activity – a possible diagnosis of autonomic impotence? World J Urol 8:75–79
30. Stöhrer M (1989) Alterations in the urinary tract after spinal cord injury – diagnosis, prevention and therapy of late sequelae. Word J Urol 7:1–7
31. Tackman W, Porst H, van Ahlen H (1988) Bulbocaverosus reflex latencies and somatosensory evoked potentials after pudendal nerve stimulation in the diagnosis of impotence. J Neurol 235:219–225
32. Tsuji I, Nakajma F, Morimoto J, Nounaka Y (1961) The sexual function in patients with spinal cord injury. Urol Int 12:270–280
33. Virag R (1982) Intracavernous injection of papaverine for erectile failure. Lancet 2:938
34. Wagner G, Gerstenberg T, Levin RJ (1989) Electrical activity of corpus cavernosum during flaccidity and erection of the human penis: a new diagnostic method? J Urol 142:723–725
35. Waldhauser M, Schramek, P (1988) Efficiency and side effects of prostaglandin E1 in treatment of erectile dysfunction. J Urol 140:525–527
36. Witherington R (1989) Vacuum constriction device for management of erectile impotence. J Urol 141:320–322
37. Zorgniotti AW, Lefleur RS (1985) Autoinjection of the corpus cavernosum with a vasoactive drug combination for vasculogenic impotence. J Urol 133:39–41

Subject Index

accessory internal pudendal artery 141
acetylcholine (Ach) 22, 50, 63
activities
– electrical 61
– rhythmic 61
adrenoceptor
– α_1- 61
– α_2- 61
alloplastic(s) 291
– implants 218
– inflatable penile prosthesis 298
α_1 adrenoceptor 61
α_2 adrenoceptor 61
AMS
– 700 CX 298
– 700 ultrex 299
– dynaflex 301
– hydroflex self-contained penile prosthesis 301
– malleable-600 295
anastomosis, arterioarterial 266
anatomy 3
androgen receptors 52
anxiety, performance 97
arterial
– disease, occlusive 147
– impotence, idiopathic 271
– inflow 126
– malformation, penile 151
– revascularization 262
arterioarterial anastomosis 266
arteriography 127
– pharmacoarteriography 137, 243
arterioles 47
arteriosclerosis 34
arteriosclerotic
– alterations 148
– lesions 139
artery/arteries
– cavernosal 116, 145, 240
– deep or profunda 6
– dorsal 6, 115, 145
– epigastric, inferior 246

– hypogastric 6, 141
– internal pudendal 6, 139, 163
– – accessory 141
atherosclerotic disease 241
ATP 22
autoinjections, intracavernosal 218
autonomic
– innervation, cavernous 194
– nervous system 9, 69
– neuropathy 187
AV shunt, venous leakage 266
avoidance behavior 97

BCR (bulbocavernous reflex) 178, 194
behaviour, avoidance 97
Buck's fascia 5
bulbocavernous muscle 181

calcium 58
– channel blockers 65
cAMP (cyclic adenosine monophospate) 51
cardiovascular (CV)
– complications 111
– responses 187
catheterization, superselective 139
cavernitis 111
cavernosal (see cavernous/cavernosal)
cavernosography 163, 165
cavernosometry 163
cavernous/cavernosal
– artery 116, 145, 240
– autonomic innervation 194
– electrical activity 197
– – single potential analysis of (SPACE) 164,194
– nerves 27
– vein 45
– – ligature 253, 285
cavernovenous leakage 282–284
CGRP (calcitonin gene-related peptide) 22, 51, 105

U. **Jonas,** Medizinische Hochschule Hannover,
FRG; **N. F. Dabhoiwala,** University of
Amsterdam, **F. M. J. Debruyne,** University of
Nijmegen, The Netherlands (Eds.)

Endourology

New and Approved Techniques

1988. XI, 162 pp. 99 figs. 22 tabs.
Hardcover DM 118,– ISBN 3-540-18415-5

Endourology provides a summary of the different
endourological modalitites, especially the more
advanced and controversial techniques, such as
the antegrade resection of urethral valves, the
transperineal I 125 seed implantations, the spoon-
loop resectoscope, flexible endoscopy, teflon
injection to correct vesicoureteral reflux, stone
manipulation in calyceal
diverticula, as well as the
extraperitoneal pelvios-
copy. These techniques
are supported by
descriptions of the
standard endourological
procedures.

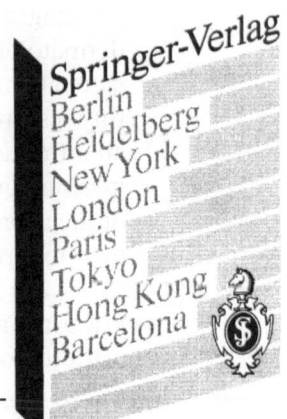

Springer-Verlag
Berlin
Heidelberg
New York
London
Paris
Tokyo
Hong Kong
Barcelona

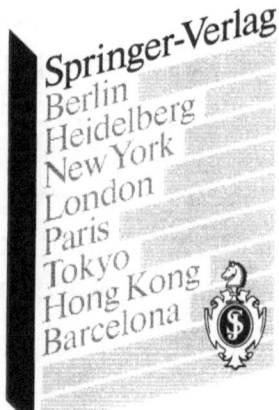